ELECTRODIAGNOSIS OF NEUROMUSCULAR DISEASES THIRD EDITION

ELECTRODIAGNOSIS OF NEUROMUSCULAR DISEASES THIRD EDITION

JOSEPH GOODGOLD, M.D.
Director, Electrodiagnostic Service,
Institute of Rehabilitation Medicine and University Hospital,
New York University Medical Center

And the Howard A. Rusk Professor, and Chairman,
Department of Rehabilitation Medicine,
New York University School of Medicine

ARTHUR EBERSTEIN, Ph.D.
Professor, Department of Rehabilitation Medicine,
New York University School of Medicine

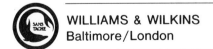

WILLIAMS & WILKINS
Baltimore/London

Made in the United States of America

First Edition, 1972
Reprinted 1973
Reprinted 1975
Reprinted 1976
Second Edition, 1978
Reprinted 1979
Reprinted 1980

Library of Congress Cataloging in Publication Data

Goodgold, Joseph.
Electrodiagnosis of neuromuscular diseases.

Includes bibliographical references and index.
1. Neuromuscular diseases—Diagnosis. 2. Electrodiagnosis. 3. Electromyography. I. Eberstein, Arthur. II. Title. [DNLM: 1. Electrodiagnosis. 2. Electromyography. 3. Neuromuscular diseases—Diagnosis. WE 550 G651e]
RC925.7.G66 1983 616.7′4′07547 82-17622
ISBN 0-683-03686-6

Composed and printed at the
Waverly Press, Inc.
Mt. Royal and Guilford Aves.
Baltimore, MD 21202, U.S.A.

This book is dedicated to

Mildred S. Goodgold

and

Marion Eberstein

for their continued understanding, devotion, and encouragement.

Preface to the Third Edition

The publication of the third edition of *Electrodiagnosis of Neuromuscular Diseases* has provided an opportunity to update the contents and to add new material that notably serves to reflect the dynamic nature of clinical electrodiagnosis.

The basic purpose of this book has not changed. This edition presents a comprehensive and critical introduction to the practice of electromyography, nerve conduction studies, reflexology, and evoked cerebral potentials at a level suitable for the serious student as well as the more advanced practitioner. Current knowledge regarding basic concepts and a rigorous review of modern techniques were intentionally integrated in one text. This approach enhances the acumen of the practitioner as well as demonstrates the logical reasoning and ultimate interpretation of the findings for the other interested physicians.

The performance of these electrophysiological studies do not fall into the category of "laboratory" tests, carried out by technicians. Rather they are physician oriented and truly represent an extension of the history and physical examination used in clinical assessment of diseases of the neuromuscular system.

If meaningful interpretation of the electrodiagnostic observations is to prevail, a solid knowledge of medicine, especially in the neurological realm, must be engrafted on an equally concrete informational base of anatomy, pathology, physiology, and fundamental electronics. These subjects do not uniquely fall within the absolute domain of any single medical specialty, such as neurology, neurosurgery, rehabilitation medicine, or orthopaedics. Successful completion of training is keyed to a period of full time training in an established (and busy!) department which has been organized to accomplish this educational mission. With due regard to a candidate's background, at least 12 to 18 months of what really amounts to preceptorship seem to be a minimal, and essential, postresidency interval.

This book has been conceived to meet the need for a comprehensive, critical, and modern introduction to basic concepts and to provide current information regarding neurophysiological evaluation of disorders of skeletal muscles and peripheral nerves. Discussion of some of the older methods of examination (chronaxie, etc.) have been intentionally minimized or omitted.

The principles underlying electromyography and nerve stimulation studies are presented in a form suitable for the physician planning to specialize as well as for the main group of physicians who rely on the results to augment clinical dignosis—the neurosurgeon, neurologist, orthopaedist, physiatrist, and others. In this sense, the text furnishes a rigorous introduction which is neither elementary nor specialized. No prior training in electrodiagnostic technique is assumed. However, this is not a simple manual delineating methods of procedure. Instead, the subject is carefully developed from a fundamental level so that the reader may fully understand the logical reasoning and acumen behind the procedures carried out and arrive at an ultimate interpretation which has clinical significance.

A fundamental approach to the formulation of the concepts which are presented has been adopted throughout this book. The basis of the electrical activity recorded from muscles or nerves and a complete discussion of volume conduction are introduced in the first section, followed by a review of the instrumentation system necessary to perform the electrodiagnostic studies. This area is covered in a simple, descriptive manner and provides the reader with an understanding sufficient to select, utilize, and realize the limitations of the apparatus. After these instructional chapters, the technique and concepts of electromyographic examination and nerve conduction studies are developed. The order for presentations we have found best over the years of teaching these subjects proceeds from a discussion of normal to the findings in myopathy and neuropathy. Examples of cases which are unusually instructive have been included. Pitfalls and errors of procedure and interpretation have been presented and discussed for various abnormalities.

Important facts of neuroanatomy, pathology, neurology, or internal medicine are briefly reviewed whenever necessary to present a clear picture of the abnormal state and to define the purpose of the various testing procedures. The section on root compression lesions demonstrates how helpful this type of review may be to the clinician. If the electromyographer, for example, is not aware of the implications of lateral vs. medial herniation of an intervertebral disc, his value as an essential member of the diagnostic team is considerably weakened.

In regard to content, we are deeply indebted to Bhagwan T. Shahani, M.D., and Robert R. Young, M.D., from the Department of Neurology, Harvard Medical School, Boston, Massachusetts, for the excellent discussion on Reflexology; to Goodwin M. Breinin, M.D., Chairman and Professor of the Department of Ophthalmology, New York University Medical Center, for his contribution on Ocular Electromyography; and to Drs. Joan B. Cracco, Associate Professor, and Roger Q. Cracco, Professor and Chairman, Department of Neurology, State University of New York, Downstate Medical Center, Brooklyn, New York, for their comprehensive section on Somatosensory Evoked Potentials.

We are likewise indebted to the American Association of Electromyography and Electrodiagnosis for permission to reproduce as an appendix their publication "A Glossary of Terms Used in Clinical Electromyography."

Many sections of the previous editions have been altered and include updated comments on the resting potential, spontaneous electrical activity, motor unit recruitment, Guillain-Barré syndrome, H reflex, F wave, etc. There is a new chapter on Somatosensory Potentials, a new section on macro EMG, and an entirely rewritten chapter on Myasthenia Gravis.

Throughout the years many friends and colleagues have helped us by pointing out typographical, grammatical, photographic, and occasional substantive errors that have insidiously crept into the text. We are ever grateful to all, but particularly to David G. Simons, M.D., who meticulously reviewed and positively critiqued each and every chapter.

Joseph Goodgold, M.D.
Arthur Eberstein, Ph.D.

Contents

chapter 1

Anatomy of Nerve and Muscle—A Review

The anatomic system of primary interest in clinical electrodiagnosis consists essentially of the peripheral nerves, the myoneural junctions, and the skeletal muscles. During normal behavior, these three components interact with each other to bring about the contraction and relaxation of a muscle. Electromyography and nerve conduction measurements may be used to determine abnormalities occurring in the three subdivisions; however, the interpretation of the findings depends on a thorough understanding of basic neuromuscular anatomy and physiology.

THE FUNCTIONAL NERVOUS SYSTEM

The motor nerve fibers which innervate striated voluntary muscles except those in the head are axons of cells in the anterior gray matter of the spinal cord (Fig. 1.1). Those fibers which supply the head, such as the muscles of mastication, facial expression, and eye movement, emerge from the brain stem in close association with certain cranial nerves. In either case they are considered peripheral nerves because the peripheral nervous system is defined to include all of the nerves and associated ganglia.

Besides functioning as a receptor for nerve impulses, the muscles (as well as the tendons) contain sensory organs which serve as a *source* of nerve impulses. The Golgi tendon organs are highly specialized sensory receptors in series with the skeletal muscle fibers and detect tension applied to the tendon during muscle contraction or stretch; muscle spindles are sensory receptors which detect change in length of the muscle fibers and the rate of change in length. Signals from these receptors are sent back to the central

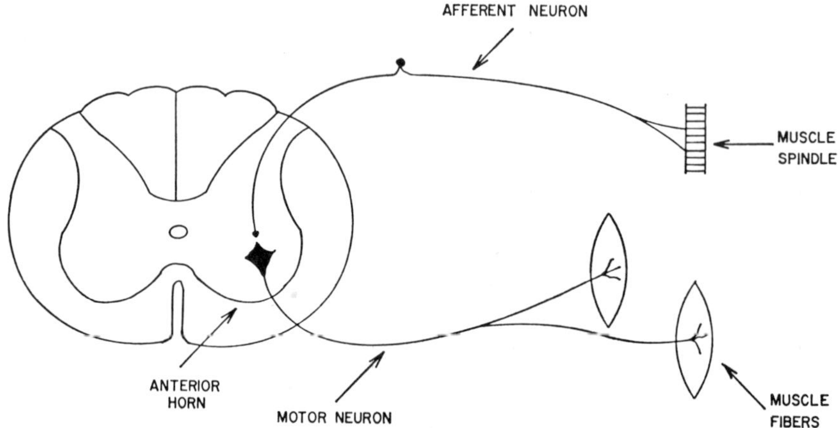

FIG. 1.1. Diagram showing innervation of skeletal muscle fibers by a motor neuron. Impulses are conducted away from the central nervous system in the motor neuron and toward the central nervous system in the afferent neuron.

nervous system via the sensory nerve fibers which are part of the peripheral nervous system.

The junction between the terminal branch of the nerve fiber and the muscle fiber is located at the midpoint of the muscle fiber and is called the motor end-plate (Fig. 1.2). Each terminal axon generally contributes to the formation of a single end-plate innervating one muscle fiber.

However, Coers (1, 2) showed 2.3% of the limb muscle fibers have double end-plates, and that these end-plates always come from the same nerve fiber. Coers and Woolf (3), in their extensive investigation of biopsy specimens from normal muscles, state that they never observed in human limb muscles the innervation of a single muscle fiber by two different axons. The only muscle fibers in man found to have multiple end-plates (i.e., more than two) are located in the extraocular muscles (4, 5).

Cholinesterase staining demonstrates the presence of two kinds of nerve endings: (a) large, heavily staining compact discs which innervate the twitch fibers and are called *en plaque* endings; (b) smaller, lighter staining droplets arranged in clusters or chains along the single muscle fiber, which are classified as *en grappe* endings and innervate the tonic fibers (5). It has not been established as yet whether the multiple junctions on one muscle fiber are derived from one neuron or from several neurons.

Myoneural junctions are not spread all over the muscle, but are usually concentrated in confined zones. In the majority of muscles there is only one zone of innervation, the shape of which depends on the form and pattern of insertion of the muscle fibers on the tendon. For example, in muscles in which the fibers lie parallel to each other from one end to the other, as in the soleus or peroneus brevis, the innervation zone runs in a line across the

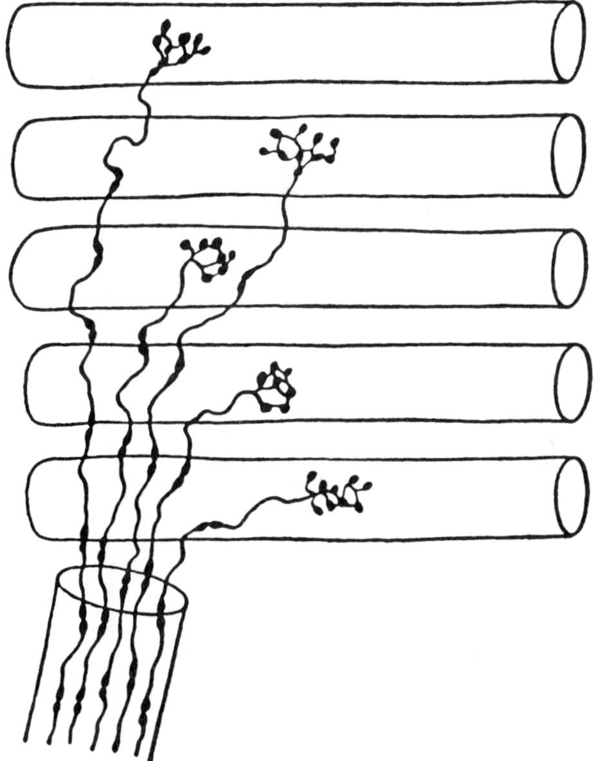

FIG. 1.2 Diagram of normal terminal innervation pattern of skeletal muscle fibers. (From C. Coers and A. L. Woolf: In *The Innervation of Muscle*. Blackwell Scientific Publications, Ltd., Oxford, England, 1959.)

center and perpendicular to the muscle fibers (Fig. 1.3). In the pennate muscles, like the flexor carpi radialis or palmaris longus, the line of innervation is curved as it passes through the midportion of the muscle fibers (Fig. 1.3). In the sartorius and gracilis muscles, instead of one zone of innervation there appear to be numerous scattered bands (3). This does not necessarily indicate multiple innervation of individual fibers, because it has been shown that the fibers do not run the entire length of the muscle (6, 7). The scattered zones probably represent simple innervation of short fibers linked in series. Knowledge of the extent of the zone of innervation is important in the evaluation of certain normal spontaneous electrical activity.

The zone of innervation usually lies near the *motor point*, which is the point where the motor nerve enters the muscle. The motor point may be identified clinically as the site where a twitch may be evoked in response to minimal electrical stimulation. Localization of the motor point permits the innervation zone to be exposed and biopsy specimens to be accurately

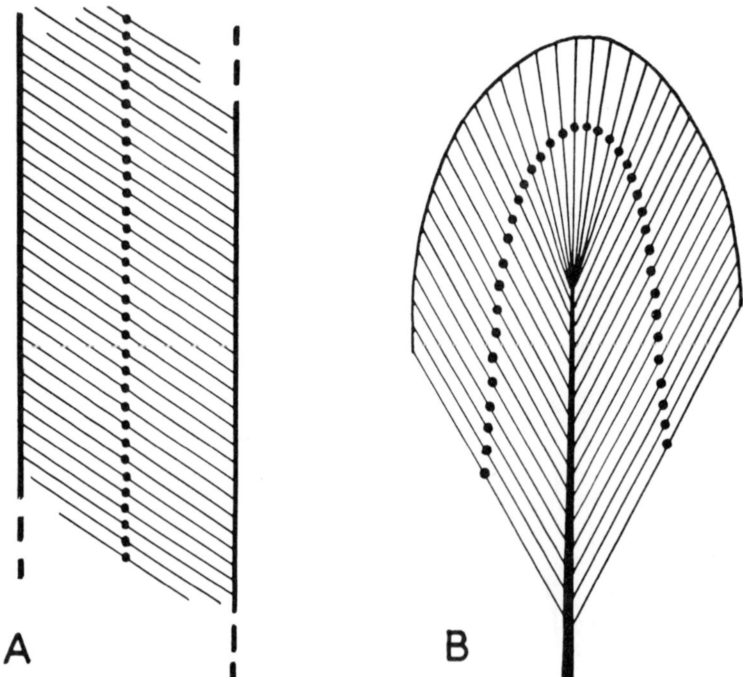

FIG. 1.3. Diagram of terminal innervation band distribution. *A*, muscle in which fibers run in a parallel manner; *B*, circumpennate muscle. (From Coers and A. L. Woolf: In *The Innervation of Muscle*. Blackwell Scientific Publications, Ltd., Oxford, England, 1959.)

obtained in certain muscles with little difficulty. Coers (8), who developed a biopsy technique which depended on first finding the motor point by electrical stimulation, believes that in some muscles the motor point does not represent the entrance of the nerve into the muscle. It is the terminal branches of the nerve nearer the skin surface which are accessible for stimulation and correspond to the motor point. Whether the motor point represents the nerve entrance or the terminal branches, it is important to remember that the motor point is a fixed anatomic site.

SKELETAL MUSCLE

Each muscle is bound by a connective tissue sheath called the *epimysium* (Fig. 1.4). At various intervals the connective tissue passes from the surface into the muscle to form coarse sleeves, the *perimysium*. Smaller and smaller groups of muscle fibers are surrounded until ultimately the subdivisions of the perimysium result in the bundling together of about 12 or more muscle fibers into a discrete group, the muscle *fascicle*. The muscle fascicle is the smallest unit of the muscle that can be seen by the naked eye. The final

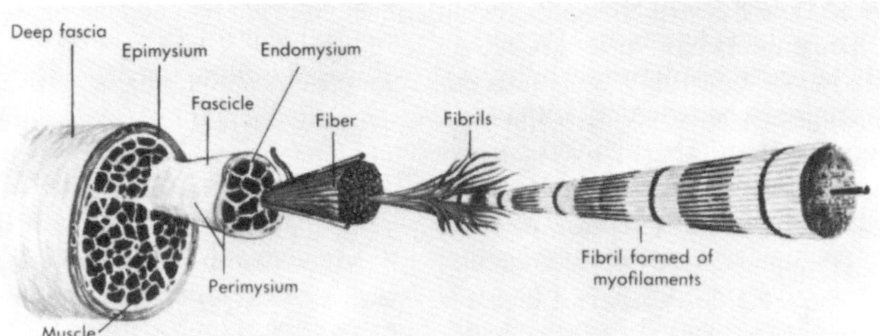

FIG. 1.4. Cross-section of skeletal muscle showing relationship of various anatomic structures. (From W. D. Gardner and W. A. Osburn: In *Structure of the Human Body*. W. B. Saunders Co., Philadelphia, 1967.)

distribution from the perimysium consists of a delicate network of fine connective tissue fibers which branches to surround each muscle fiber to form the *endomysium*, which serves to hold the capillaries and nerve fibers in place and secure the muscle fibers to each other.

Individual muscle fibers range from 0.01 to 0.1 mm in diameter and from 2 to 12 cm in length. The average fiber diameter increases from 0.01 mm in the newborn to about 0.05 mm in the adult (9). For short muscles, the muscle fibers extend the entire length of the muscle. For long muscles, however, a single fiber may extend only through a short distance of the total length. Within a fascicle, one end of the fibers terminates at a tendon and the other terminates in long tapering points which are overlapped by other muscle fibers and securely bound together by the reticular endomysium between them. Several muscle fibers may be attached end to end in this manner with the final fiber in the fascicle extending to the tendon at the other pole of the muscle. These fibers, tied together in series, act exactly as a single fiber of the same total length; it shortens by approximately one-half its length during contraction.

Histochemical studies have shown that human skeletal muscles do not consist of a grouping of homogeneous fibers but instead are composed of at least three types, each differing in enzymatic activity. Histochemically, the different fibers have been designated as Type I, Type II, and "intermediate."

Type I fibers are rich in mitochondrial oxidative enzymes, such as succinic dehydrogenase and cytochrome oxidase, but poor in phosphorylase, glycogen, and myofibrillar adenosine triphosphatase (ATPase). Type II fibers, conversely, are rich in phosphorylase, glycogen, and ATPase but poor in the oxidative enzymes (Table 1.1). Type II fibers also have a high content of mitochondrial α-glycerophosphate dehydrogenase (10, 11). Thus the two types of fibers contrast in energy metabolism; Type I fibers are concerned with aerobic metabolism, whereas Type II fibers are essentially concerned with anaerobic metabolism. Fibers intermediate in enzyme activity between Types I and II have also been recognized.

Type I muscle fibers have long contraction times and are highly resistant to fatigue, whereas Type II fibers have short contraction times and fatigue rapidly. Type I fibers have a low threshold of activation and a firing rate of 8 to 10 per sec; Type II fibers have a higher threshold, are activated with a rapid vigorous contraction, and fire in short, irregular bursts at 16 to 50 per sec. A low level sustained contraction will stimulate the Type I fibers. The axons supplying the Type I motor units have smaller diameters and lower conduction velocities than those connected to Type II motor units.

In man, when the muscles are histochemically stained to exhibit these

TABLE 1.1. Relative Amount of Histochemical Staining within Human Muscle Fibers*

Reaction†	Muscle Fiber Reactivity	
	Type I	Type II
DPNH dehydrogenase	High	Low
TPNH dehydrogenase	High	Low
Succinate dehydrogenase	High	Low
Cytochrome oxidase	High	Low
Dihydroorotic acid dehydrogenase	High	Low
Benzidine peroxidase (probably myoglobin)	High	Low
Menadione-mediated α-glycerophosphate dehydrogenase	Low	High
DPN-linked lactate dehydrogenase (PMS, azide)‡	Low	High
DPN-linked α-glycerophosphate dehydrogenase, (PMS, azide)	Low	High
Phosphorylase	Low	High
Glycogen	Low	High
UDPG-glycogen transferase	High§	Low§
Argyrophil reaction	Medium	Medium
ATPase, myofibrillar	Low	High
ATPase, edetic acid low pH activated	High	Low
ATPase, "wet"	Medium	Medium
Antimyosin fluorescent antibody	Medium	Medium
Tyrosine	Medium	Medium
Esterase	High	Low
Osmium tetroxide	Medium	Medium
Oil red O	High	Low

* The relative amount of staining is consistent but does not necessarily represent the relative enzyme content of the two fiber types if technical factors exert a false localization influence.

† Abbreviations used are: DPNH, reduced diphosphopyridine nucleotide; TPNH, reduced triphosphopyridine nucleotide; DPN, diphosphopyridine nucleotide; PMS, phenazine methosulfate; UDPG, uridine diphosphate glucose; ATPase, adenosine triphosphatase.

‡ Reversed without PMS and azide.

§ Reversed in occasional specimens.

From W. K. Engel: Selective and nonselective susceptibility of muscle fiber types. Arch. Neurol. (Chicago), *22:* 98, 1970.

differential enzymatic characteristics, a cross-section presents a mosaic pattern of lightly and darkly stained fibers (Fig. 1.5); the different fiber types appear to be uniformly distributed through the muscle (12, 13). In any one region of a skeletal muscle, there may be an intermingling of approximately 10 different fiber types. There does not appear to be any muscle composed entirely of one fiber type. In contradistinction, in animal muscles a particular histochemical fiber type may be concentrated in a single area of the whole muscle. For example, in the mouse, Type I and intermediate fibers are situated deeply, near to the bone in the normal triceps, tibialis anterior, and gastrocnemius, whereas Type II fibers are found in the most superficial part of the muscle. In the soleus, the fibers are all of the Type I and intermediate classes (14).

In recent years, investigators (15, 16) have shown that the contractile characteristics of the various histochemical fiber types are also different. Isometric twitch measurements indicate that the contraction times (time from the start of the twitch to its peak tension) vary, with some fibers contracting much faster than others, so that a classification into slow twitch and fast twitch fibers is feasible. An example of twitch tensions recorded from a normal human rectus abdominis muscle biopsy showing both types of responses is given in Figure 1.6. There is also some evidence (15, 17) that the conduction velocities along the muscle fiber may be a function of fiber type.

All human skeletal muscle fibers are considered to be twitch fibers because they produce a mechanical twitch response for a single stimulus and generate a propagated action potential. This feature is quite distinct from the observations in frog muscle, where two major types of fibers are present, the fast or twitch fibers and the slow or tonic fibers. Tonic fibers do not respond to stimuli with twitches but with continuous, graded contractions. The extrinsic eye muscles represent a sole exception in humans, in that fibers with "tonic" characteristics may be present. Electron microscopic and cholinesterase staining studies show that some of these fibers have an afibrillar ultrastructure and multiple nerve endings.

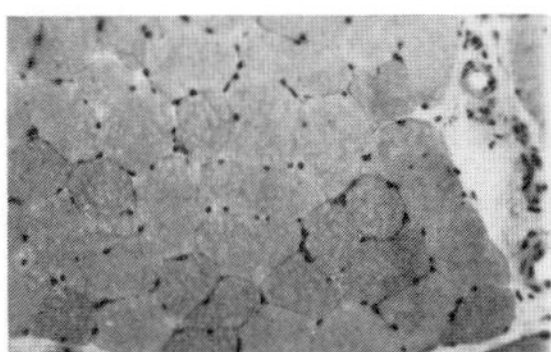
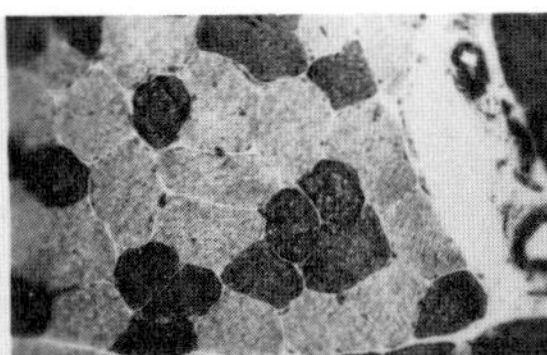
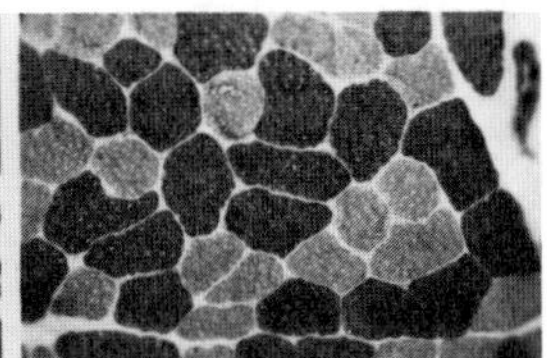

FIG. 1.5. Serial sections of normal pectoralis major muscle. *Left*, hematoxylin and eosin stain; *center*, Type I fibers darker (DPN diaphorase); *right*, Type II fibers darker (adenosine triphosphatase). ×63. (Courtesy of John Pearson, M.D., Department of Pathology, New York, University Medical Center, New York, New York.)

THE MOTOR UNIT

Within a muscle, the axon from a single motor nerve cell arborizes into many terminal branches. Each branch is attached to an individual muscle fiber. The branching of the axon permits a single neuron to stimulate a group of muscle fibers. For example, an electrical impulse traveling along a single axon induces the contraction of approximately 2000 fibers in the gastrocnemius. The functional unit of the neuromuscular system thus differs from the structural units of the nerve and muscle systems which are, respectively, the neuron and the muscle fiber. The functional unit of the neuromuscular system is the *motor unit; it consists of the anterior horn cell, its axon, and all of the muscle fibers innervated by that axon* (Fig. 1.7). Modern study of the motor unit began when Liddell and Sherrington first

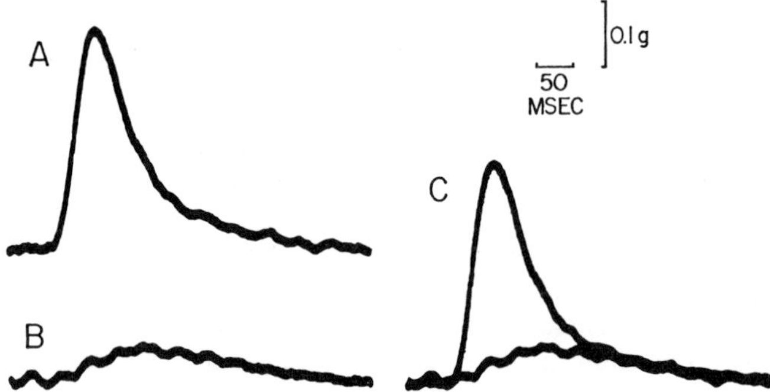

FIG. 1.6. Twitch tensions of a rectus abdominis muscle biopsy showing fast twitch response (*A*) and slow twitch response (*B*). Responses *A* and *B* are superimposed in *C*. (From A. Eberstein and J. Goodgold: Slow and fast twitch fibers in human skeletal muscle. Am. J. Physiol., *215:* 539, 1968.)

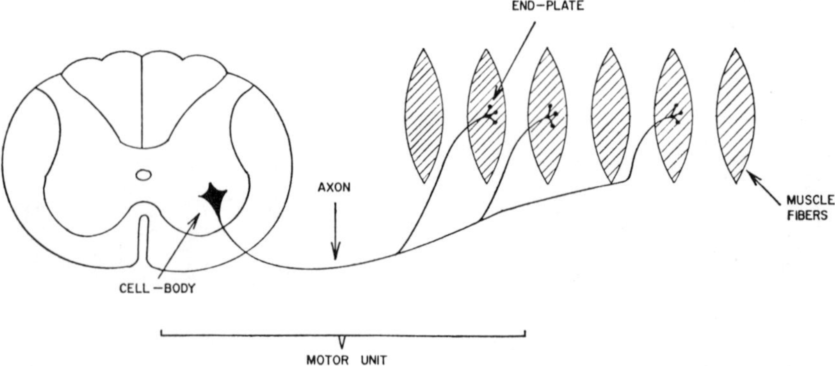

FIG. 1.7. Diagram indicating the single motor unit: the anterior horn cell, axon, and all of the muscle fibers innervated by the axon.

used the term in 1925 (18). The concept was developed as a result of studies on the reflex activity of the spinal cord, the motor unit being considered the final common path of the nervous system.

The number of muscle fibers in a single motor unit varies widely for the different skeletal muscles (Table 1.2). A large muscle with many fibers which is involved in relatively gross movements may include hundreds of muscle fibers in a motor unit, whereas a muscle concerned with precise movements may have a small number of muscle fibers per motor unit. This is seen, for example, in the gastrocnemius and laryngeal muscles, which have 1934 and two to three muscle fibers per motor unit, respectively.

The number of muscle fibers per motor nerve fiber is expressed as the *innervation ratio*. This is usually computed by dividing the total number of muscle fibers in a muscle by the total number of motor nerve fibers. It is difficult to determine the exact number of motor nerve fibers in the nerve trunk because muscle afferent (sensory) and small motor nerve fibers supplying the intrafusal muscle fibers are also present. If only the large nerve fibers are considered (including both motor and sensory components), the calculated innervation ratio will be substantially lower than the correct value. Some investigators have attempted to increase the accuracy by assuming that 40% of the large-sized nerve fibers are afferent. One investigator (19) was able to determine the innervation ratio in the laryngeal muscles by actually observing the different twigs of the same branch of the nerve innervating the various muscle fibers.

It is generally agreed that the individual fibers of a motor unit are not all grouped together but rather involve more than single fasciculi. There is considerable intermingling of fibers derived from different motor neurons. Although direct evidence that this is true in human muscle is difficult to obtain and as yet not available, recent histochemical studies (22, 23) have clearly shown the diffuse anatomic distribution of the motor units in rat muscle. In these studies, single ventral root nerve fibers innervating the

TABLE 1.2. Number of Muscle Fibers per Motor Unit in Various Human Muscles

Muscle	No. of Large Nerve Fibers	No. of Muscle Fibers	Calculated No. of Motor Units	Mean No. of Fibers per Motor Unit	Reference
Platysma	1826	27,100	1096	25	20
First dorsal interosseous	199	40,500	119	340	20
Lumbricalis I	155	10,038	93	108	20
Anterior tibialis	742	250,200	445	562	20
Gastrocnemius, medial	965	1,120,000	579	1934	20
Laryngeal muscles				2–3	19
External rectus				9	20
Temporalis				936	21
Masseter				640	21

anterior tibialis muscle were isolated and electrically stimulated repetitively. Immediately after the cessation of stimulation, the muscle was excised and frozen, and cross-sections were stained for glycogen. It was assumed that tetany exhausted the muscle cell glycogen so that the unstained muscle fibers represented those fibers innervated by the single stimulated nerve fiber. The results showed extensive overlapping of the motor units. The majority of fibers of a single motor unit were not in contact with other fibers of the same unit; only two or three fibers of the same unit were occasionally adjacent to each other. Further observations indicated that the fibers which belong to a given motor unit are homogeneous histochemically (22, 23). Although there may be considerable intermingling of fibers of different units, it appears that there is no overlapping of fiber types within the single motor unit; Type I muscle fibers are innervated by Type I motor neurons.

TYPES OF NERVE FIBERS

The peripheral nerve trunk contains sensory and motor fibers of various diameters, conduction speeds, action potential configurations, and refractory periods. Examination of the action potentials of various nerves reveals that the fibers can be classified into different types known as A, B, and C* fibers. The A fibers are large myelinated fibers which innervate skeletal muscle and also conduct afferent impulses from the proprioceptive receptors in skeletal muscles as well as receptors in the skin. The B group consists of small myelinated, efferent, preganglionic fibers found only in autonomic nerves. The C fibers are unmyelinated pre- and postganglionic sympathetic fibers, also found as afferents mediating various modalities of sensation (deep pain).

A typical peripheral nerve such as the sciatic nerve contains both A and C fibers. The individual fibers are not of equal size but, in fact, cover a wide range of diameters. The A fibers, especially, constitute a group of which the most prominent variable is the diameter. In mammalian nerve fibers, the diameter of A fibers can vary from 1 to 22 μ. For example, the diameter spectrum of afferent nerve fibers innervating the soleus muscle is shown in Figure 1.8. It is obvious in this as well as other muscle nerves that the fibers fall into two distinct groups. One group, constituting the large diameter fibers, represents the motor fibers connected to the extrafusal muscle fibers, and the other group of smaller diameter fibers innervates the intrafusal fibers of the muscle spindles.

The nerve fibers can be subdivided in terms of their conduction velocity as well as their diameters. Because the internal longitudinal resistance is

* C Fibers are differentiated into s. C and d.r. C fibers. The s. C group represents the efferent postganglionic sympathetic axons having pronounced negative and positive afterpotentials. The d.r. C Group is the small afferent axons found in peripheral nerves and dorsal roots having no negative afterpotential but a large positive afterpotential which can be converted into a negative deflection with repetitive activity.

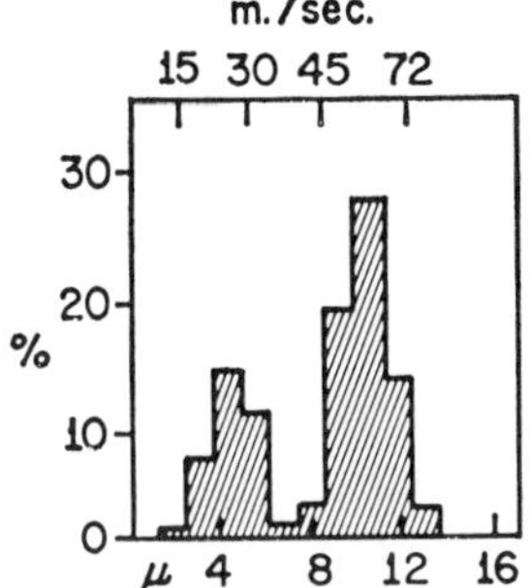

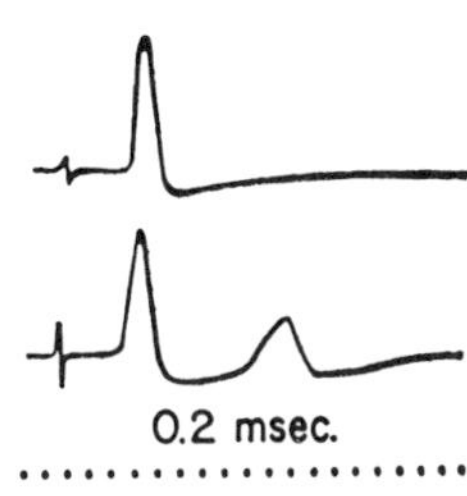

FIG. 1.8. Diameter spectrum and compound action potential of motor fibers supplying soleus. *Left*, distribution of fiber diameters and velocity spectrum; *right*, *upper trace*, compound action potential elicited by maximal stimulus for large diameter fibers; *right*, *lower trace*, stronger stimulus elicited second deflection attributable to small diameter fibers. (From T. C. Ruch and H. D. Patton; *Physiology and Biophysics*, ed. 19. W. B. Saunders Co., Philadelphia, 1965. *Left*, originally from J. C. Eccles and C. S. Sherrington: Proc. R. Soc. Lond. [Biol]. *106:* 326–357, 1930; *right*, originally from S. W. Kuffler, C. C. Hunt, and J. P. Quillain; J. Neurophysiol., *14:* 28–54, 1951.)

inversely proportional to the diameter, the large diameter fibers should conduct at a greater velocity than the smaller diameter fibers. This appears to be the case and can be demonstrated by recording the action potentials of a nerve at some distance from the site of stimulation. When the stimulus is gradually increased in strength, the action potential amplitude increases until it reaches a maximum. Further increase in stimulus does not increase the amplitude any more but causes a change in shape of the action potential. The response at the higher stimulating intensity is called the *compound action potential* and represents the subgroups of the A fibers successively adding their responses to the total (Fig. 1.8). For the A fibers, the conduction velocities have been found to be linearly related to the fiber diameters (Fig. 1.9).

If the intensity of stimulation is increased further, another peak in the response is observed at a later time. This represents the activity of the nonmyelinated C fibers. Myelinated B fibers are found only in autonomic nerves. A drawing of the action potential of the saphenous nerve of the cat illustrating the amplitude and time relationship between the various fiber groups is given in Figure 1.10.

It is conventional to designate the successive peaks of the compound action potential of the A fibers in a nerve by the Greek letters α, β, γ, δ. Because the peaks result from activity in fibers conducting at different velocities, the Greek letters designate the different rates of conduction; that is, α represents the first peak or highest conducting fibers, β the next peak with a lower conduction velocity, and, similarly, γ and δ the third and fourth peaks. Correspondingly, the same Greek letters may be used to categorize

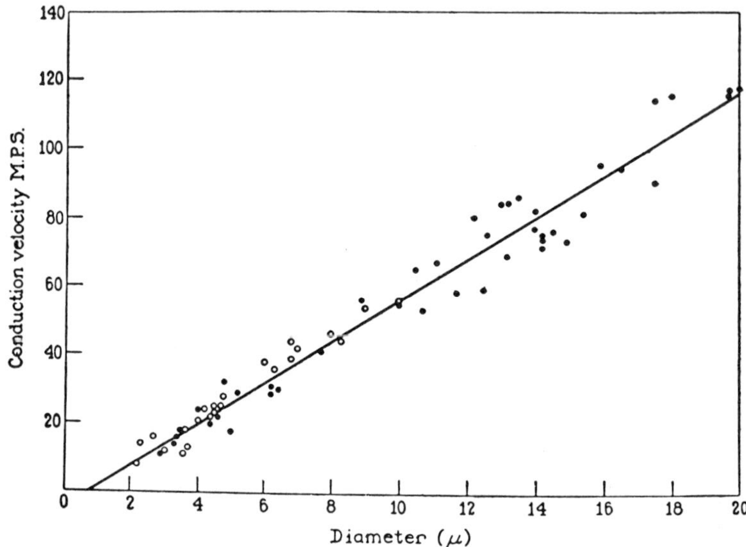

FIG. 1.9. Curve showing linear relation between conduction rate and diameter of mammalian myelinated nerve fibers. (From T. C. Ruch and H. D. Patton: In *Physiology and Biophysics*, ed. 19. W. B. Saunders Co., Philadelphia, 1965. Originally from H. S. Gasser, Ohio J. Sci., *41:* 145–159, 1941.)

the different groups according to fiber diameter; e.g., α represents the large diameter A fibers and δ the smallest diameter A fibers.

Besides the variation in fiber diameter and conduction velocity, another demonstrable difference between the nerve fibers is the threshold of electrical stimuli applied externally. As the stimulus intensity is increased, the various components of the response appear in succession, that is, first the activity from the Aα fibers, then those from the Aβ, Aγ, and Aδ, and finally the potentials from the C fibers. In other words, fibers with a low rate of conduction have a relatively higher threshold of stimulation. This relationship is important to the clinical electrophysiologist. By selecting the intensity of stimulation, the fastest conducting fibers may be activated to the exclusion of the slowly conducting ones. The response to this particular stimuli may then be recorded.

Lloyd's Roman numeral classification (24) is frequently used, instead of the Greek letters, to designate the different *sensory* fibers in a nerve. In this classification the fibers are grouped according to diameter: Group I, 12 to 20 μ; Group II, 6 to 12 μ; Group III, 1 to 6 μ. Group IV consists of the C fibers. It is current practice to use both types of classification interchangeably. The fiber diameter classification may be roughly equated to the "compound action potential" classification in the following manner: Aα corresponds to Groups I and II, Aδ corresponds to Group III.

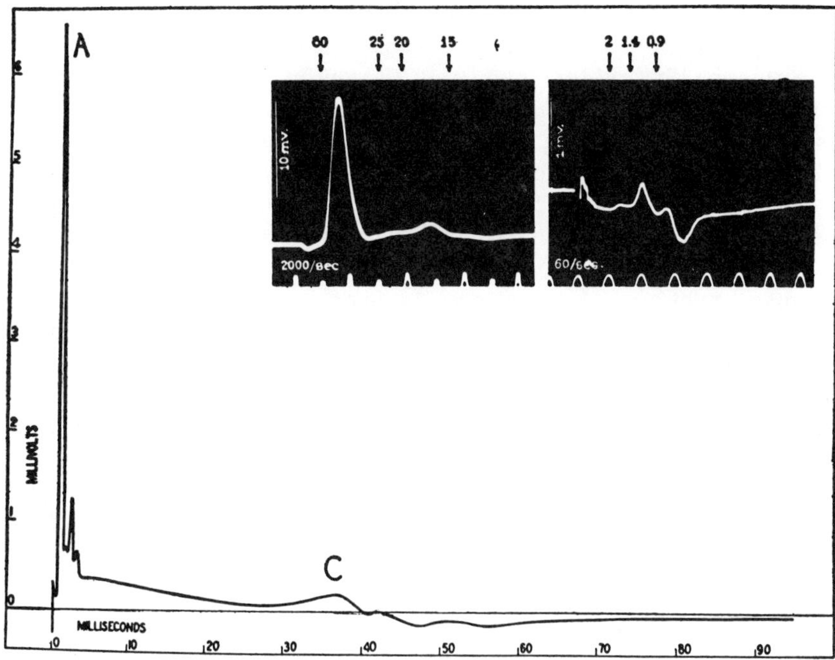

FIG. 1.10. Scale drawing of complete compound action potential of mammalian saphenous nerve. *Inset, left*, A fiber components; *insert, right*, C fiber components. *Numbers above arrows* give maximal conduction rates (meters per second) of each component. (From T. C. Ruch and H. D. Patton: In *Physiology and Biophysics*, ed. 19. W. B. Saunders Co., Philadelphia, 1965. Originally from H. S. Glasser; J. Appl Physiol., *9:* 88–96, 1938, and Ohio J. Sci., *41:* 145–159, 1941.)

It is important to remember, especially when performing nerve conduction studies, that the usual peripheral nerve is not a bundle of homogeneous fibers but, instead, is composed of both motor and sensory fibers. The fibers show considerable variation in diameter, conduction velocities, and threshold to stimulation.

STRUCTURE OF THE MUSCLE FIBER

Nerve and muscle fibers have many features in common. Both are long cylindrical structures enclosed by thin functional membranes capable of excitation and propagation of impulses. Despite these similarities, nerve and muscle fibers differ considerably in their function and internal structure. The function of muscle is to contract by means of a complex process occurring within the fiber. Understanding the contractile process requires a knowledge of the fiber's internal structure. The following brief description is limited to that of skeletal muscle, although many of the same features are found in cardiac muscle.

The individual muscle fiber is a self-contained system with multiple nuclei distributed just underneath its *sarcolemma*. The sarcolemma is a thin sheath enclosing the fiber. Within the fiber is the semifluid cell plasma or intracellular fluid called the *sarcoplasm*. Packed closely together in the sarcoplasm are a large number of long, thin, thread-like structures called the *myofibrils*. The myofibrils, like the fiber itself, are cross-striated, and the striations of the various myofibrils are properly aligned so that the light and dark bands run across the whole fiber. The myofibril is the functional unit of the muscle contraction. The contraction of a muscle fiber is produced by shortening of the many myofibrils which compose the fiber.

Electron microscope studies reveal that the myofibrils in turn arc made up of still smaller filaments. These myofilaments are of two types, thick and thin. The thick and thin filaments are the sarcoplasmic proteins, myosin and actin, respectively. These myofilaments are closely packed and longitudinally aligned parallel to each other. They are oriented so that similar myofilaments lie side by side with some overlap at the ends of the actin and myosin (Fig. 1.11). This arrangement explains the characteristic cross-striations of the muscle fibers as observed with the light microscope and of the myofibrils as

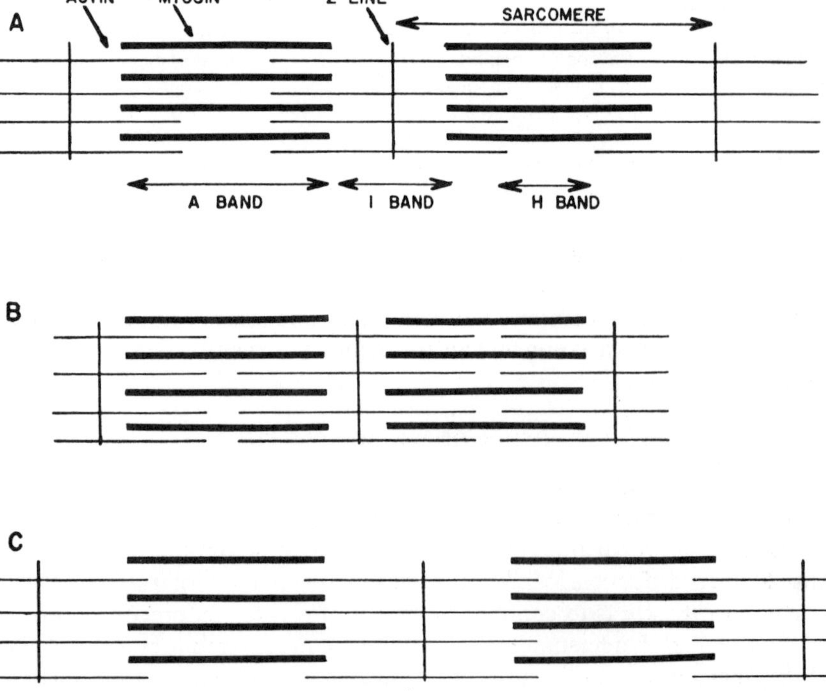

FIG. 1.11. Drawing illustrating arrangement of filaments at rest (*A*), during contraction (*B*), and stretched (*C*).

seen with the electron microscope. The dark band, called the A (anisotropic) band, is divided in the center by a lighter region called the H band; the light I (isotropic) band is divided in its center by a dark stripe called the Z line. The region between two adjacent Z lines is called a *sarcomere* and represents a repetitive unit of the muscle fiber. The I band is composed of actin filaments; the H band contains myosin filaments; and the A band consists of myosin and the overlapping actin filaments. Myosin is the more abundant protein in muscle. Two other major proteins are incorporated into the thin filaments: tropomyosin and troponin.

Electron microscope and X-ray diffraction studies indicate that the actin and myosin filaments are connected by "bridges" or "cross-links." In the region of overlap between thick and thin filaments, electron micrographs show that the bridges occur at regular intervals. The bridges represent a mechanical linkage between filaments and are responsible for the structural continuity along the length of the muscle fiber. They are considered to be the structural basis for the development of tension and shortening of the muscle.

According to the sliding filament hypothesis developed by H. E. Huxley and J. Hanson, the active shortening of muscle fibers is caused by the thick and thin filaments sliding into one another. That is, the myofilaments themselves do not change in length during a contraction but slide past one another; the actin filaments move farther into the A bands and thereby increase the amount of overlap. Conversely, stretching the muscle fiber pulls the thin filaments out of the A bands and decreases the overlap. The force necessary to pull the thin filaments into the A band as the muscle contracts is believed to be generated by interaction between the filaments and the bridges.

In the narrow spaces between the myofibrils, an extensive network of tubules and vesicles has been observed with the electron microscope. This highly organized, membrane-limited system has been named the *sarcoplasmic reticulum*. The tubules run parallel to each myofibril, and at certain fixed positions in the sarcomere some of the tubules combine to form a vesicle that surrounds a myofibril (Fig. 1.12). Longitudinal sections of a muscle fiber show at these fixed positions three elements, or a triad structure. Two of the elements belong to the vesicles of the sarcoplasmic reticulum. The third, located in the middle of the triad, runs transversely through the fiber. This latter network of tubules, called the T-system (or transverse system), has no visible connection with the tubules of the sarcoplasmic reticulum but is in close contact with them. Thus, the T-system is a separate network which extends to the membrane surface and is opened to the extracellular space.

There is strong evidence which suggests that the sarcoplasmic reticulum and the T-system are involved with uptake and release of calcium ions in

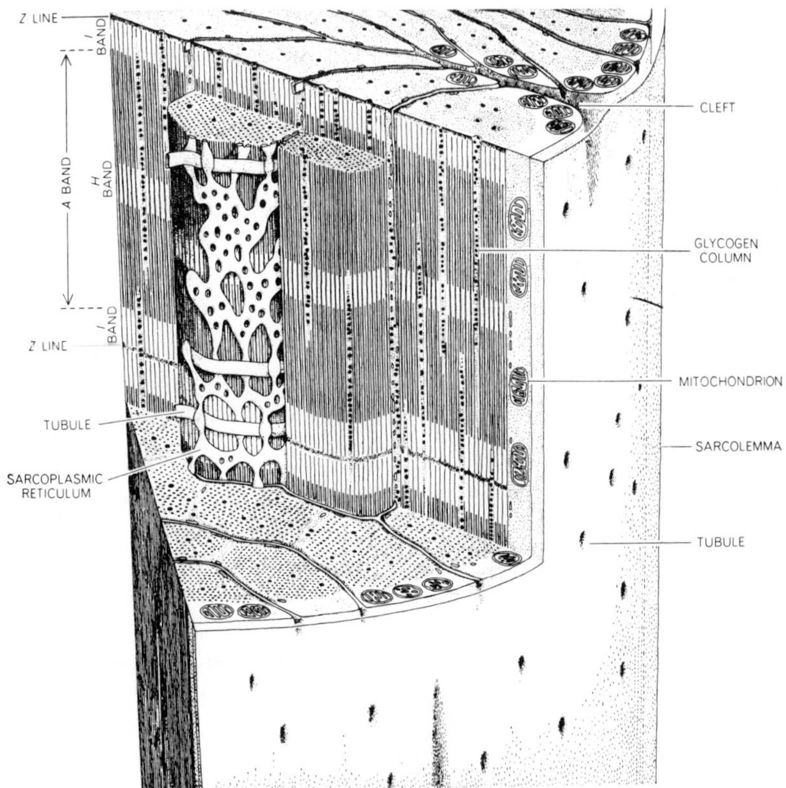

FIG. 1.12. Drawing of a giant barnacle illustrating structure of a single muscle fiber. (From G. Hoyle: How is muscle turned on and off? Sci. Am., *222:* 87, April 1979.)

triggering the contraction of the myofibrils as well as in controlling their relaxation. The well ordered arrangements of tubules throughout the muscle fiber may explain how all of the myofibrils are stimulated to contract simultaneously as well as provide a path for the inward flow of energy-supplying substances and an outward flow of metabolic waste products.

In addition to actin and myosin, two other major proteins involved in muscle contraction are to be found in the fiber and are incorporated in the thin filaments: tropomyosin and troponin. Tropomyosins are long, thin molecules that form a continuous strand on the surface of the actin molecules. Troponins are globular in shape and are affixed near one end of each tropomyosin. The troponin-tropomyosin complex, bound uniformly along the whole length of the actin filaments, is required for calcium to participate in the regulation of the contraction-relaxation cycle (Fig. 1.13). To understand the cooperative interaction of the different proteins, it is first necessary to realize that myosin molecules are long, thin rods with two globular heads at one end (Fig. 1.14). The heads have sites where the chemical activity involved in the contraction process takes place. To form the thick filaments, myosin molecules are assembled with the parallel thin rods forming the backbone and the heads projecting from the surface over most of the filament length except for a bare region in the center. The projections, which are the cross-bridges observed in the electron microscope, are always oriented in one direction on one side of the middle and in the opposite direction on the other side.

The four proteins, as well as adenosine triphosphate (ATP) and calcium, must be present for muscle to contract. The series of events which takes place in the muscle cell and results in contraction and relaxation of the muscle cell can be described as follows:

1) The nerve signal arrives at the muscle cell, causing depolarization of the surface membrane. The propagated action potential spreads into the interior of the cell along the transverse tubules.

2) The potential changes in the tubules stimulate the adjacent, but unconnected, terminal cisternae of the sarcoplasmic reticulum to release calcium from membrane-bound storage sites into the fluid surrounding the filaments (Fig. 1.15). The mechanism by which the transverse tubules stimulate the sarcoplasmic reticulum is unknown, but it has been suggested that the depolarization of the membrane of the T-system may result in the depolarization of the membrane of the terminal cisternae and induce calcium release.

3) The free calcium binds to troponin, which then modifies the position of

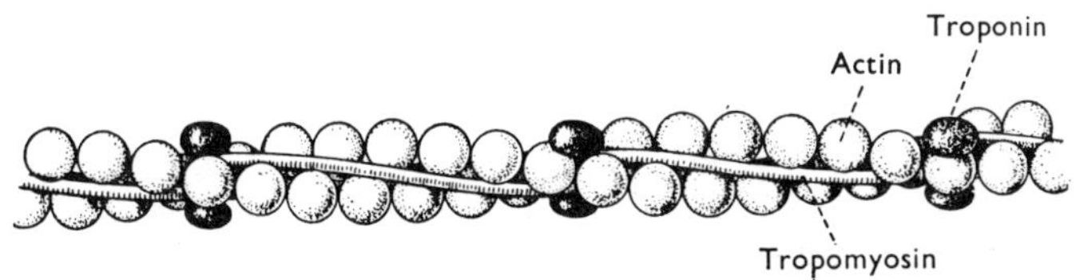

FIG. 1.13. A model for the fine structure of the thin filament showing the ordered arrangement of the troponin and tropomyosin molecules along the actin molecule. (From S. Ebashi, M. Endo, and I. Ohtsuki: Control of muscle contraction. Q. Rev. Biophys., *2:* 364, 1969.)

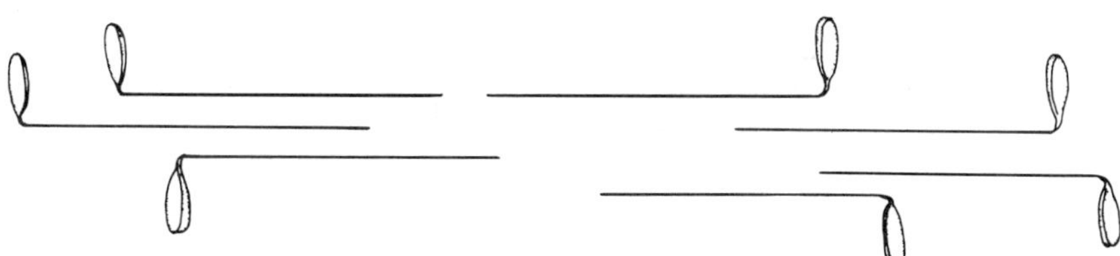

FIG. 1.14. Drawing of myosin molecules showing the two globular heads at one end of the long, thin rods.

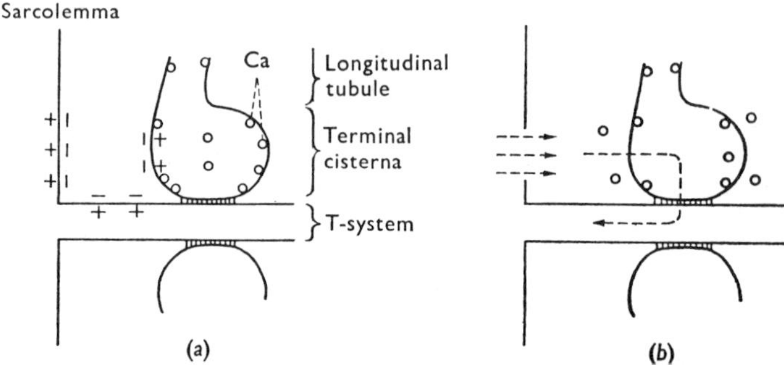

FIG. 1.15. Diagram illustrating the electrical events in the excitation-contraction coupling; (*a*) resting state; (*b*) excited state. The *arrows* show the current flow caused by excitation of the sarcolemma. (From S. Ebashi, M. Endo, and I. Ohtsuki: Control of muscle contraction. Q. Rev. Biophys., 2: 368, 1969.)

tropomyosin in the filament so that an active complex can be formed between myosin and actin. Troponin is the only calcium-receptive protein in the contractile system but is not directly involved in controlling the interaction of actin and myosin. Tropomyosin acts as the mediator of information from the troponin to actin; for example, if troponin is free from calcium, then tropomyosin blocks the attachment of myosin-actin cross-bridges and contraction is inhibited. However, once troponin becomes saturated with calcium, tropomyosin shifts in position relative to actin, which permits the formation of cross-bridges and contraction of the muscle.

4) Shortening and the development of muscle tension ensue from a rotation of the angle, pulling the actin filaments past the myosin filaments.

5) Shortly after its release, calcium is again accumulated by the sarcoplasmic reticulum by actively transporting it from the sarcoplasm. Protein kinase, activated by cyclic AMP (adenosine 3′:5′-cyclic phosphate), may play an important role in the uptake of calcium by the sarcoplasmic reticulum. In cardiac muscle, stimulation of calcium-activated ATPase activity and an increase in the rate of calcium accumulation by the sarcoplasmic reticulum are observed in the presence of protein kinase and cyclic AMP (25). The removal of free calcium prevents the further interaction of myosin and actin, and the muscle relaxes.

Hydrolysis of ATP also provides the energy required for muscle contraction. A specific site on a myosin head combines with a molecule of ATP and, if the sarcoplasmic calcium concentration is sufficiently elevated, forms a cross-bridge with an actin molecule. The ATP subsequently splits into adenosine diphosphate (ADP) and inorganic phosphate and liberates energy which is used to pull actin past the myosin filament for the development of tension. Binding of an ATP molecule to the myosin head dissociates the myosin from the actin; the process is then complete and ready to start a new cycle (26, 27).

REFERENCES

1. Coers, C.: L'exploration fonctionelle et l'étude histologique quantitative des muscles atropies. Acta Clin. Belg., *10:* 244–265, 1955.
2. Coers, C.: Les variations structurelles normales et pathologiques de la junction neuromusculaire. Acta Neurol. Psychiatr. Belg., *55:* 741–866, 1955.
3. Coers, C., and Woolf, A. L.: *The Innervation of Muscle: A Biopsy Study.* Blackwell Scientific Publications, Oxford, 1959.
4. Dietert, S. E.: The demonstration of different types of muscle fibers in human extraocular muscle by electron microscopy and cholinesterase staining. Invest. Ophthalmol., *4:* 51–63, 1965.
5. Zenker, W., and Gruber, H.: Überform, Anordnung, Zahl und Grösse der myoneuralen Synapsen multipel innervierter Skelettmuskelfascern. Z. Mikrosk. Anat. Forsch., *76:* 361–377, 1967.
6. Schwarzacher, H. G.: Zur Lage de motorischer Endplatten un den Skeletmuskeln. Acta Anat. (Basel), *30:* 758–774, 1957.
7. Christensen, E.: Topography of terminal motor innervation in striated muscles from stillborn infants. Am. J. Phys. Med., *38:* 17–30, 1959.
8. Coers, C.: Note sur une technique de prelevement des biopsies neuro-musculaires. Acta Neurol. Psychiatr. Belg., *53:* 759–765, 1953.
9. Buchthal, F., Guld, C., and Rosenfalk, P.: Propagation velocity in electrically activated muscle fibers in man. Acta Physiol. Scand., *34:* 75–89, 1955.
10. Engel, W. K.: The multiplicity of pathologic reactions of human skeletal muscle. In *Proceedings of the Fifth International Congress of Neuropathy,* edited by F. Luthy and A. Bischoff, pp. 613–624. Excerpta Medica Foundation, Amsterdam, 1966.
11. Dubowitz, V.: Enzyme histochemistry of skeletal muscle. Part 2. Developing human muscle. J. Neurol. Neurosurg. Psychiatry, *28:* 519, 1965.
12. Susheela, A. K., and Walton, J. N.: Distribution of histochemical fibre types in normal human muscles. J. Neurol. Sci., *8:* 201–207, 1969.
13. Engel, W. K.: Histochemistry of neuromuscular disease: Significance of muscle fiber types. In *Neuromuscular Diseases, Proceedings of the 8th International Congress, Vienna,* pp. 67–101. Excerpta Medica Foundation, Amsterdam, 1965.
14. Susheela, A. K., and Walton, J. N.: Murine muscular dystrophy: Some histochemical and biochemical observations. J. Neurol. Sci., *7:* 437–463, 1968.
15. Eberstein, A., and Goodgold, J.: Slow and fast twitch fibers in human skeletal muscle. Am. J. Physiol., *215:* 535–541, 1968.
16. Buchthal, F., and Schmalbruch, H.: Contraction times and fiber types in intact human muscle. Acta Physiol. Scand., *79:* 435–452, 1970.
17. Shinozaki, R.: Electrophysiological and histological studies on the human skeletal muscle. J. Okayama Med. Assoc., *74:* 477–507, 1962.
18. Liddell, E. G. T., and Sherrington, C. S.: Recruitment and some other features of reflex inhibition. Proc. R. Soc. Lond. [Biol.], *97:* 488–518, 1925.
19. Ruedi, L.: Some observations on the histology and function of the larynx. J. Laryngol., *73:* 1–20, 1959.
20. Feinstein, B., Lindegard, B., Nyman, E., and Wohlfart, G.: Morphologic studies of motor units in normal human muscles. Acta Anat. (Basel), *23:* 127–142, 1955.
21. Carlsöö, S.: Motor units and action potentials in masticatory muscles. Acta. Morphol. Neerl. Scand., *2:* 13–19, 1958.
22. Edstrom, L., and Kugelberg, E.: Histochemical composition, distribution of fibers and fatiguability of single motor units. J. Neurol. Neurosurg. Psychiatry, *31:* 424–433, 1968.
23. Brandstater, M. E., and Lambert, E. H.: A histological study of the spatial arrangement of muscle fibers in single motor units within rat tibialis anterior muscle. Bull. Am. Assoc. EMG Electrodiagn. *15-16:* 82, 1969.

24. Lloyd, D. P. C.: Neuron patterns controlling transmission of ipsilateral hind limb reflexes in cat. J. Neurophysiol., *6:* 293–326, 1943.
25. Tada, M., Kirchberger, M. A., Repke, D. I., and Katz, A. M.: The stimulation of calcium transport in cardiac sarcoplasmic reticulum by adenosine 3:5 monophosphate-dependent protein kinase. J. Biol. Chem., *249:* 6174–6180, 1974.
26. Weber, A., and Murray, J. M.: Molecular control mechanisms in muscle contraction. Physiol. Rev., *53:* 612–673, 1973.
27. Ebashi, S., Endo, M., and Ohtsuki, I.: Control of muscle contraction. Q. Rev. Biophys., *2:* 351–384, 1969.

chapter 2

A Review of Nerve and Muscle Physiology

Electromyography is the detection and recording of electrical activity from a portion of a muscle. The source of this activity is related to the structure and function of the muscle fiber membrane: specifically, its capability for storing electrical charge and releasing bursts of electrical energy when properly stimulated. To understand the process by which electrical activity is generated, it is necessary to consider the difference in electric potential between the inside of the cell and the interstitial fluid. In this chapter fundamental properties of the transmembrane potential, excitation and impulse propagation, are reviewed, and in a later chapter these are related to the electromyogram.

THE RESTING POTENTIAL

The role of the membrane, either nerve or muscle, is to regulate the interchange of substances between the cell interior and its environment. The nature of the membrane is such that it imposes a restriction on the movement of some ions; that is, certain ions pass freely through the membrane whereas the diffusion of others is severely limited. The result of this selective permeability is an unequal distribution of charged ions across the membrane which, in turn, contributes to the creation of a potential difference. This potential difference is commonly referred to as the resting potential because it represents a steady state condition maintained by utilization of metabolic energy supplied by the cell.

Before discussing the origin of the membrane potential, several basic properties of the living cell membrane must be cited and emphasized:

1) The membrane is about 50 times more permeable to K^+ than it is to Na^+.

2) The membrane has a mechanism to actively transport Na^+ from the inside to outside the cell and K^+ in the opposite direction (the sodium-potassium pump).

3) The membrane is impermeable to the organic anions within the cell.

In the living cell, the intracellular fluid contains organic anions (proteins and phosphates), a high concentration of K^+, and low concentration of Na^+ and Cl^-; whereas in the extracellular space, there are a low concentration of K^+ and high concentrations of Na^+ and Cl^- (Fig. 2.1). *Anions* are negatively charged atoms or molecules which migrate toward the anode in a solution; *cations* are positively charged ones which migrate toward the cathode.

The membrane is pictured as having channels, called membrane *pores*, which permit water and many of the dissolved ions to pass through. The pores for potassium ion diffusion are different from those for sodium ion diffusion.

An exact description of the pores is not yet available, but they are believed to be long protein molecules aligned perpendicular to the surface of the membrane which serve as channels through the membrane for the ions. The pores act as if a "gate" (possibly an electrical charge) controlled the opening, either stopping or allowing ion flow. Since, in the resting state, the membrane is 50 times more permeable to potassium than to sodium ions, it would appear that the potassium pore "gates" are almost all open, whereas the sodium ones are almost all closed. The configuration of the gates (open or closed) is dependent on voltage and time.

Because potassium ions can easily penetrate the membrane and because of their higher concentration within the cell, these cations will diffuse more frequently *out* of the cell than into it. The result is a net efflux of potassium ions. This would tend to make the outside of the membrane more positive

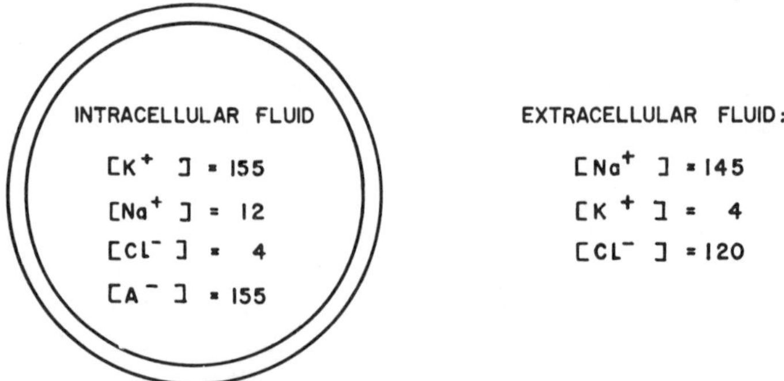

FIG. 2.1. Approximate electrolyte concentrations (μmoles per ml) within mammalian muscle cell and in extracellular fluid.

than the inside (Fig. 2.2). However, in the resting state, the membrane is also permeable to sodium ions, although to a lesser extent than to potassium ions. The sodium ions, by following its concentration gradient, will diffuse slowly *into* the cell and thereby make the inside more positive.

The potential that will develop across the membrane, V_m, as a consequence of ion diffusion due to concentration differences is expressed in the equation first derived by Goldman in 1943 (1) and called the Goldman equation:

$$V_m = \frac{RT}{F} \ln \frac{P_K [K^+]_o + P_{Na} [Na^+]_o}{P_K [K^+]_i + P_{Na} [Na^+]_i}$$

where R = gas constant (8.31 Joules per mole degree absolute); T = absolute temperature; F = Faraday (96,500 coulombs per mole); P_K and P_{Na} = permeability of potassium and sodium, respectively; $[K^+]_o$ and $[K^+]_i$ = concentration of potassium outside and inside the cell; and $[Na^+]_o$ and $[Na^+]_i$ = concentration of sodium outside and inside the cell.

If the permeability of sodium (P_{Na}) is much lower than the permeability of potassium (P_K) than the above equation reduces to the Nernst equation for potassium ions:

$$V_m = \frac{RT}{F} \ln \frac{[K^+]_o}{[K^+]_i}$$

This equation can be simplified for body temperature:

$$V_m \text{ (in mV)} = 61 \log_{10} \frac{[K^+]_o}{[K^+]_i}$$

Taking $[K^+]_o$ equal to 4 μmoles per ml and $[K^+]_i$ to be 155 μmoles per ml, the calculated resting potential is equal to −97 mV, inside negative with respect to outside. The extracellular potential is taken conventionally to be zero. The measured resting potential averages about −90 mV. The calculated "potassium potential" across the membrane is greater than the measured resting potential because the steady influx of small quantities of sodium ions is neglected.

It is important to note from the Goldman equation that the membrane

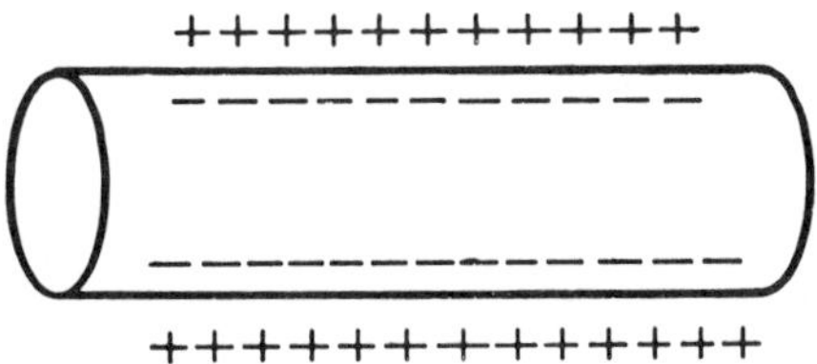

FIG. 2.2. Polarization of charges across membrane: positive charges on outside and negative charges on inside of membrane.

potential can be varied by alteration in ion permeability without any change in the ion concentration gradients.

The continuous influx of sodium ions while the potassium ions are flowing outward would prevent a state of equilibrium to be maintained across the membrane; that is, if only passive ion currents were involved, the intracellular concentrations of sodium would increase and potassium would decrease. Under these conditions, the concentrations of the two ions would eventually be the same on both sides of the membrane and the resting potential would disappear.

This does not occur in the healthy, living cell because there is in the membrane a mechanism for the *active transport* of sodium and potassium ions. This process is called the sodium-potassium pump. Essentially, the "pump" transports sodium from inside the cell to the outside and potassium from outside to the inside. The sodium-potassium pump is usually simply called the sodium pump because the active transport of sodium is more important than that of potassium in the resting state.

Active transport differs considerably from facilitated diffusion in that the latter process requires no energy, whereas in the former, energy must be provided to force ions against concentration and potential gradients. This energy is supplied by the cytoplasm to the membrane in the form of the high energy phosphate compound ATP.

The model that has emerged from various research endeavors to explain the operation of the sodium-potassium pump requires the action of special carrier molecules. These carriers, called sodium-potassium ATPase, are membrane-bound enzymes which can split ATP molecules and utilize the energy released to transport the two cations. Any intracellular sodium ions that come in contact with the inside surface of the membrane will combine with a carrier molecule to form a complex. The carrier-sodium complex diffuses through the membrane to the outer surface where the sodium ions spontaneously split away and pass out of the membrane into the extracellular space.

After the loss of sodium ions, the carrier binds with potassium ions in contact with the outside membrane surface and diffuses back through the membrane to the inner surface. At this point, energy supplied by ATP splitting releases the potassium from the carrier, and the potassium passes into the interior of the cell. The carrier than binds with sodium ions, and the sequence is recycled. In this process, energy is expended only at the inner side of the membrane.

The exact number of K^+ ions coupled to each Na^+ ion translocated is probably not constant. Often three Na^+ ions are transported out for every two K^+ ions transferred into the cell. The linkage may be one for one: one K^+ pumped in for each Na^+ pumped out. The effect of the pump is the same in both cases, a higher concentration of sodium on the outside of the cell.

The action of both active transport and diffusion results in a balance of ion movement in and out of the cell. *Net* ion movement is then zero, and the potential difference across the membrane remains constant or "resting."

Chloride ions are not involved in the active transport process and only play a passive role in establishing ionic equilibrium. The distribution of chloride ions, which are completely permeable through the membrane, is determined by the membrane potential difference. The negatively charged chloride ions flow out of the cell with the positively charged sodium ions, resulting in the high extracellular chloride concentration. This loss of sodium chloride also causes a flow of intracellular water from the cell. In this way, the action of the sodium-potassium pump is important in regulating cell volume.

Summary

The significant factor to be remembered from this discussion is that a potential, called the resting potential, is continuously maintained across the membrane of normal, resting nerve and muscle fibers. The potential arises from the separation of electric charges by the membrane, negative inside and positive outside. With its capacity to store charges, the fiber behaves as a capacitor, i.e., the membrane represents an insulator separating two conductors, the extracellular and intracellular fluids.

RESTING POTENTIAL MEASUREMENT

The potential difference between the inside and outside of the cell can be measured directly either in situ or in vitro. The technique involves placing an electrode inside the cell and another electrode in the extracellular space. The electrode which enters the cell is specially constructed to have a very small tip to minimize damage to the membrane. Conventionally, the electrode is made by drawing out a piece of glass tubing until the tip is less than 1 μ in diameter and filling it with a 3 M solution of KCl. A concentrated KCl solution is used to overcome diffusion potentials between the electrode and the solutes in the adjoining electrolyte and also to minimize the resistance of the electrode. An electrode of this type, employed mainly for intracellular recording, is referred to as a *microelectrode* or a *micropipette electrode.*

The experimental arrangement for recording nerve or muscle fiber resting potentials is illustrated in a schematic drawing (Fig. 2.3*A*). For in vitro measurements the isolated tissue is placed in a chamber containing a physiological salt solution. The two electrodes which are in the bath are connected to a high input impedance voltage amplifier (the impedance of the microelectrode may be around 10 megohms) which, in turn, is connected to a pen recorder or oscilloscope and camera. With both electrodes in the salt solution, the potential difference is zero; as the microelectrode is slowly lowered, a sudden deflection of the oscilloscope beam (or recorder pen) indicates that the membrane has been penetrated and the electrode is in the cytoplasm. The recorded potential indicates −70 to −90 mV, negative inside with respect to the bath, and remains at a constant level until the electrode is removed from the fiber (Fig. 2.3*B*). This potential difference measured between inside and outside the cell is the membrane resting potential.

MEMBRANE EXCITABILITY

We have established that a resting potential is developed and maintained by the cell because of certain unique properties of the membrane. In addition to these properties, the membranes of nerves and muscles possess another

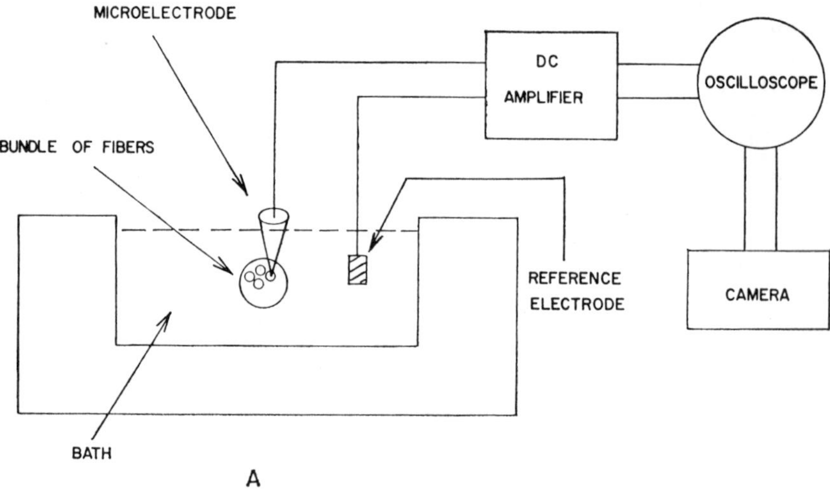

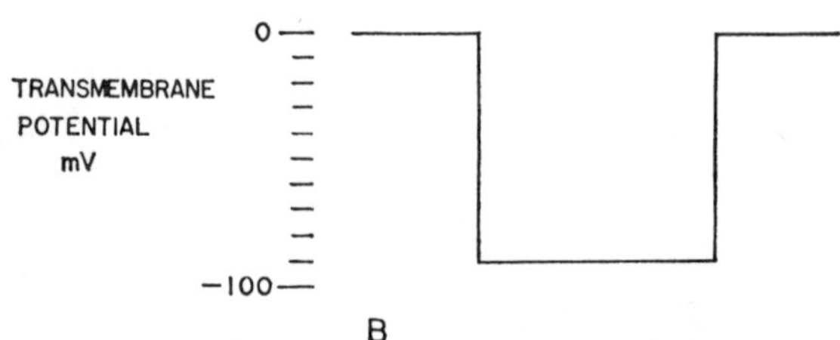

FIG. 2.3. *A*, experimental in vitro measurement of intracellular potentials of single fibers. *B*, resting potential measurement as observed on oscilloscope. Potential between microelectrode and reference electrode drops to −90 mV when microelectrode passes through membrane, and then returns to base line when electrode is removed.

distinctive feature: excitability. When the transmembrane potential is reduced below a threshold level, changes in membrane permeability occur which are unique to excitable cells. The most significant result of these changes is an action potential which propagates along the fiber away from the stimulus site.

Let us first consider what happens to the transmembrane potential when the voltage across the membrane is varied. Experimentally, this can be observed by inserting two microelectrodes into the same fiber (nerve or muscle) within a short distance of each other (Fig. 2.4*A*). One electrode connected to a square wave pulse generator is used to change the membrane potential by passing a current through the membrane; the other electrode is connected to a DC amplifier and records any variations in potential across the membrane. In Figure 2.4*B* the responses of the membrane to three different stimuli are shown. In stimulus *1*, a current passed from outside to inside the cell results in an increase in transmembrane potential. This means that the outside of the membrane is more positive with respect to the inside or, stated another way, that the membrane is *hyperpolarized*. The membrane potential increases from −90 to −120 mV in this example.

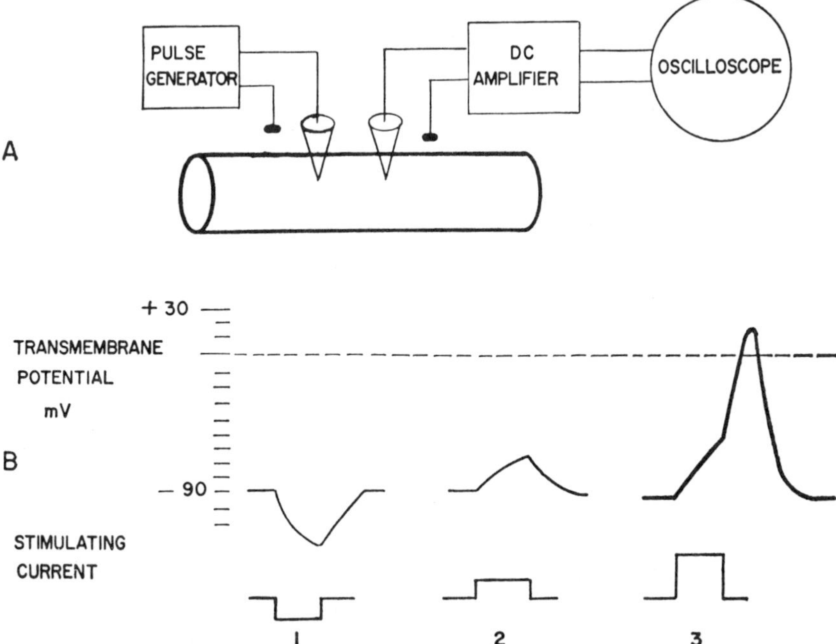

FIG. 2.4. *A*, recording of potential changes produced across membrane by square current pulses. Recording electrode is on the *right* and stimulating electrode on the *left*. *B*, with stimulus *1*, membrane is hyperpolarized; with stimulus *2*, membrane is depolarized from −90 mV to −75 mmV; with stimulus *3*, transmembrane potential reaches threshold and action potential is produced.

If the polarity of the pulse generator is changed so that the current flows outward, the membrane is depolarized (Fig. 2.4*B*, stimulus *2*). In this example of a low current, the potential decreases from −90 to −75 mV. This change is considered to be a *local response* of the membrane because the voltage falls back to the resting level when the stimulus current is turned off, without initiating an action potential. However, an increase in the depolarizing current to a level where the transmembrane potential is at threshold (about −55 mV) may produce either a sudden rise in potential to about +20 mV or just a local response (Fig. 2.4*B*, stimulus *3*).

At threshold potential the membrane is at a state of unstable equilibrium; however, any increase in current beyond threshold always results in the rapid rise and fall of the potential, which is called an action potential. Once the membrane has been depolarized above threshold, the generation of the action potential is automatic and no longer controlled by the stimulus.

The rapid depolarization produced by the stimulus alters the specific permeability of the membrane and increases the permeability to sodium. It has been noted that the resting membrane is much less permeable for Na^+ than K^+ and that the Na^+ is higher in concentration on the outside of the fiber. In response to stimulation beyond threshold, the membrane (either nerve or muscle) becomes highly permeable to Na^+ which, consequently, flows inward. This influx of Na^+ further reduces the internal negativity which, in turn, permits more Na^+ to flow inward. Thus, a self-regenerating chain reaction is established between the depolarization and sodium permeability. This activity results in not only depolarization of the membrane but complete reversal of its polarity, that is, from positive to negative on the outside and negative to positive on the inside (Fig. 2.5).

The influx of Na^+ decreases back to its resting level as abruptly as it began, usually after about 1 msec. This decrease and the accompanying increase in K^+ permeability bring the membrane rapidly back to its original polarized state. Repolarization is complete when the permeability to K^+ decreases to its resting level. The entire sequence of changes at the site of

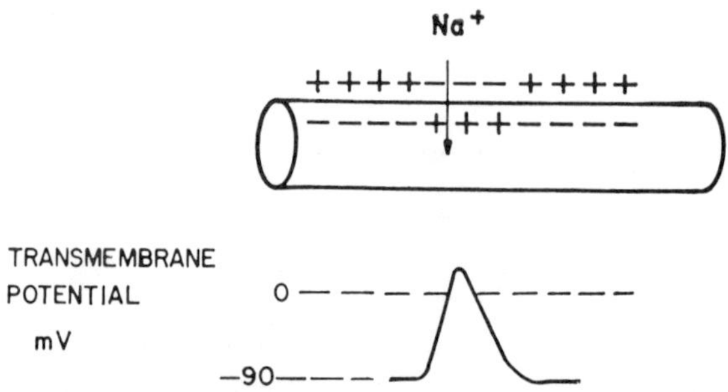

FIG. 2.5. When stimulus exceeds a critical threshold level, sodium flows inward, polarity across membrane reverses, and action potential is obtained.

stimulation, which includes depolarization of the membrane and its spontaneous recovery, occurs within a few milliseconds.

The action potential may be recorded by inserting a microelectrode into the fiber, reference electrode outside, and depolarizing a portion of the membrane with a threshold stimulus. The stimulus may be applied with "surface" or extracellular electrodes instead of intracellular microelectrodes. A typical intracellularly recorded action potential obtained by stimulating with a pair of electrodes placed near the surface of the fiber is illustrated in Figure 2.6. When current flows between the two electrodes, the portion of the membrane underneath the cathode electrode is depolarized, initiating an action potential. The normal action potential is approximately 120 mV in amplitude and 1 to 2 msec in duration.

Summary

An action potential may be initiated in a nerve or muscle fiber by rapidly depolarizing a portion of the membrane to threshold voltage. The depolarization leads to increased sodium permeability and reversal of the resting membrane polarity. Recovery of the membrane back to the resting state

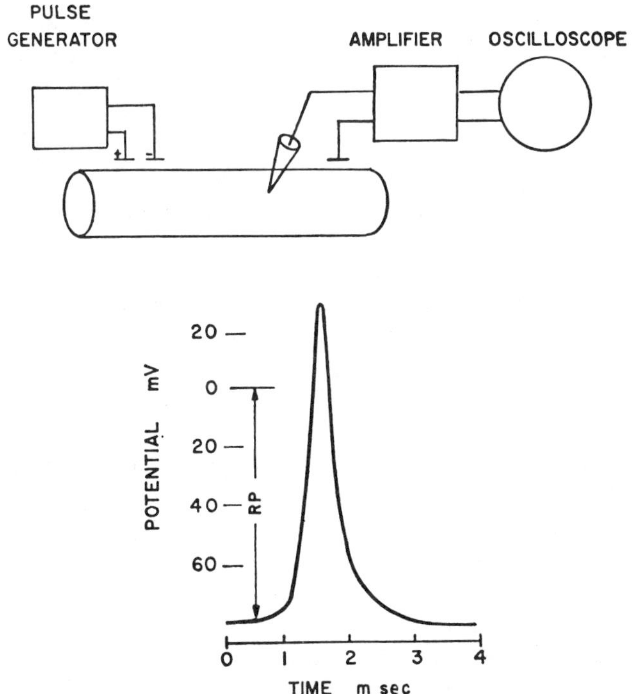

FIG. 2.6. Intracellular recording of action potential initiated with externally applied stimulating electrodes. *Bottom* drawing illustrates typical normal action potential.

follows the spontaneous fall of the sodium permeability and the delayed increase in permeability to potassium.

PROPAGATION OF THE IMPULSE

The action potential, once initiated by a threshold stimulus, propagates along the whole length of a fiber without decreasing in amplitude. This is a basic property of nerve and muscle fibers and is responsible for the transfer of information over relatively long distances from one part of the body to another. Unlike a current of electricity flowing through a wire, the action potential is self-propagating and does not get weaker as it moves away from the site of excitation. This is accomplished by a progressive depolarization of the membrane which is best described by considering the sequences of events occurring after application of a threshold stimulus.

In the resting state, the membrane is charged positive on the outside and negative on the inside, as shown in Figure 2.7*A*. An adequate stimulus will depolarize the membrane in the region of the cathode, resulting in an action potential and, for a few milliseconds, a reversal of the charges on the membrane (Fig. 2.7*B*).

As a consequence of the difference in potential between the depolarized region and the adjacent inactive regions, current flows from the depolarized region through the intracellular fluid to the inactive regions, as shown by the *arrows* in Figure 2.7*C*. The current also flows through the extracellular fluids, through the depolarized membrane, and back to the intracellular space, thus forming a complete local circuit. This local current flowing between the active and adjacent inactive regions acts to depolarize the inactive regions. By reducing the resting membrane voltage, the local current stimulates the neighboring regions to threshold, and action potentials are generated in regions unaffected by the original stimulus (Fig. 2.7*D*). As described in the previous section, the active regions of the membrane recover to the normal resting condition after the period of depolarization. This process is repeated all along the fiber (Fig. 2.7*E*). Thus, from the original site of stimulation, action potentials are propagated in both directions at constant speed.

Because the action potential is self-propagating, energy to maintain the conduction must be supplied by the fiber itself. Local energy resources must be released upon excitation at every point along the fiber. This results in impulses progressing long distances along fibers without any decrement in amplitude.

Up to this point we have discussed propagation along a muscle fiber or an unmyelinated nerve fiber, in which case the membrane is freely exposed to the interstitial fluid. The mechanism of conduction along myelinated nerves is somewhat different. The myelinated fiber has a segmented sleeve or

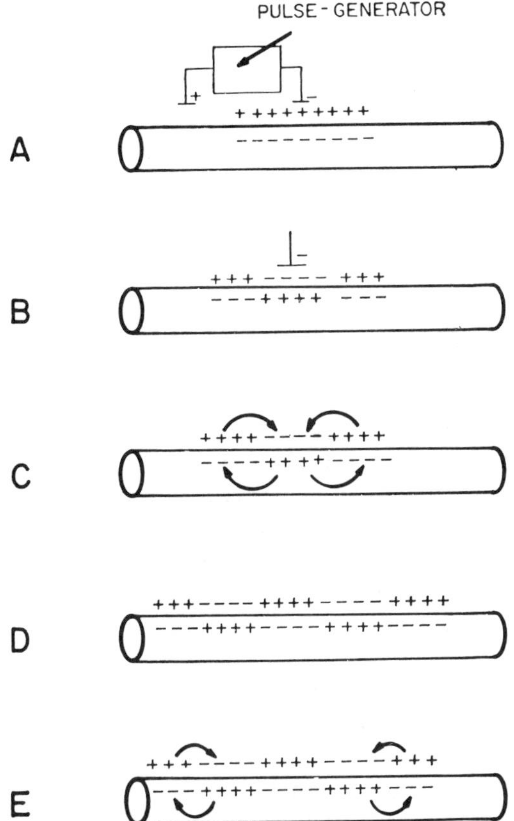

FIG. 2.7. Propagation of impulse. Drawings show sequence of events after depolarization at one point along fiber. (See text for complete description.)

myelin sheath, with areas of the membrane exposed approximately every 2 mm. The interruptions of the myelin sheath are called the nodes of Ranvier (Fig. 2.8). The sheath surrounding the membrane acts as a good insulator, and thus the resting and action potentials appear only at the nodes.

When a myelinated fiber is stimulated, the sites of excitation and the corresponding changes of membrane permeability are only at the nodes. In Figure 2.8, a myelinated fiber is illustrated with one of the nodes depolarized. As with the unmyelinated fiber, a local circuit is established, except that in this case the current flows from one node to another. Current flows from the active node to the adjacent inactive one, depolarizing it and initiating an action potential. In effect, the impulses "jump" from node to node as they progress along the fiber. This type of impulse propagation is called *saltatory conduction*.

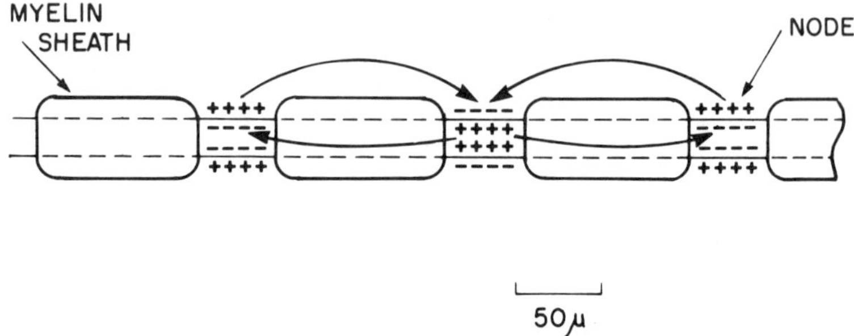

FIG. 2.8. Myelinated nerve fiber illustrating local current flow from node to node resulting in depolarized adjacent nodes.

Summary

Once initiated by a threshold stimulus, impulses propagate along nerve and muscle fibers without decrement. Local current flowing from the depolarized region stimulates the adjacent inactive region and generates action potentials which are conducted away in both directions. In myelinated nerve fibers, the impulses are propagated from node to node along the fiber (saltatory conduction).

STRENGTH-DURATION RELATIONSHIP

In our discussion of the membrane resting potential, it was concluded that the cell acts as a capacitor: an insulating membrane separating two electrolytic solutions. The actual representation of the axon core and membrane in terms of resistors and capacitors is shown in Figure 2.9. It is seen that the equivalent electrical circuit for a segment of the membrane is essentially a resistor and capacitor connected in parallel. These two elements in the membrane affect the time required to change the voltage across the membrane. If a current is suddenly impressed across the membrane, the transmembrane voltage does not change instantly. Because it takes time to alter the charge on the capacitor, the voltage increases slowly. Thus, the effect of the membrane capacitance is to cause the membrane voltage to lag behind the applied current pulse. This implies that the duration of the stimulus pulse must be considered, as well as its strength, when depolarizing the membrane.

To generate an action potential, the membrane must be depolarized to threshold voltage. Two factors are decisive in determining whether the threshold is reached: (a) the strength of the stimulating current and (b) the duration of its flow. If a current pulse applied to a nerve or muscle fiber is allowed to flow sufficiently to charge the membrane capacitance and decrease the membrane potential to threshold, an impulse is initiated. A very weak current requires a long duration pulse, whereas a short duration of current flow is sufficient to excite the fiber with a strong stimulus. This

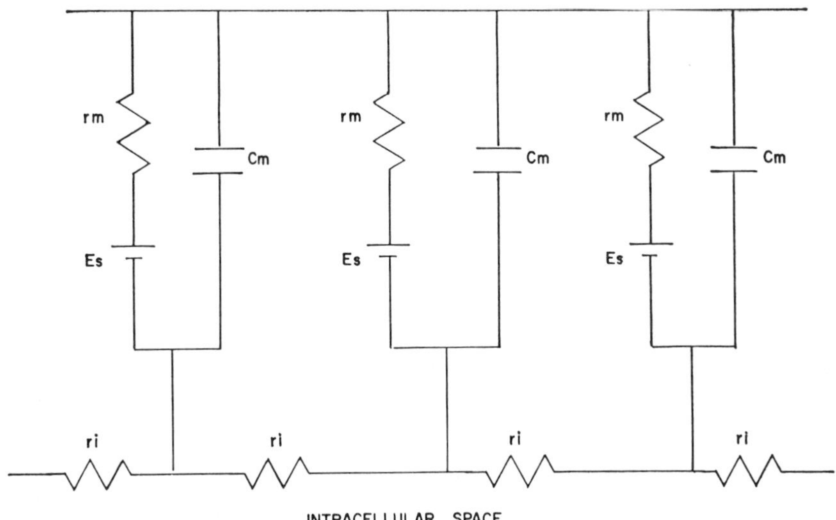

FIG. 2.9. Equivalent electric circuit of nerve or muscle membrane. *Es*, voltage of battery representing a steady potential; *rm*, membrane resistance; *Cm*, membrane capacity; *ri*, longitudinal resistance axoplasm.

relationship between strength and duration of the threshold stimulus is illustrated in Figure 2.10. The general shape of this curve is the same for both nerve and muscle; differences are noted as shifts in the curve along the axes.

The *rheobase* of the strength-duration curve is defined as that current strength which requires a very long current pulse to excite the fiber. Any current below rheobase strength will not excite the fiber for any pulse duration. *Chronaxy* is the length of time a current pulse of *twice the rheobase strength* must flow to depolarize the membrane to threshold. Using the equivalent circuit of the fiber as a starting point, it can be shown that chronaxy is proportional to the membrane time constant. The membrane time constant is membrane resistance multiplied by capacitance ($r_m \times c_m$) and is a measure of the time course of voltage changes for an abruptly applied voltage; that is, the greater the time constant, the longer the time required to reach a certain voltage. Because the membrane capacitance (c_m) for muscle is much higher than that for nerve, the time constant and, likewise, chronaxy are greater in muscle than in nerve.

GRADATION OF MUSCULAR CONTRACTION

Considering that the nerve impulses transmitted to a muscle are all fixed in amplitude and shape, how is it possible for a whole muscle to develop

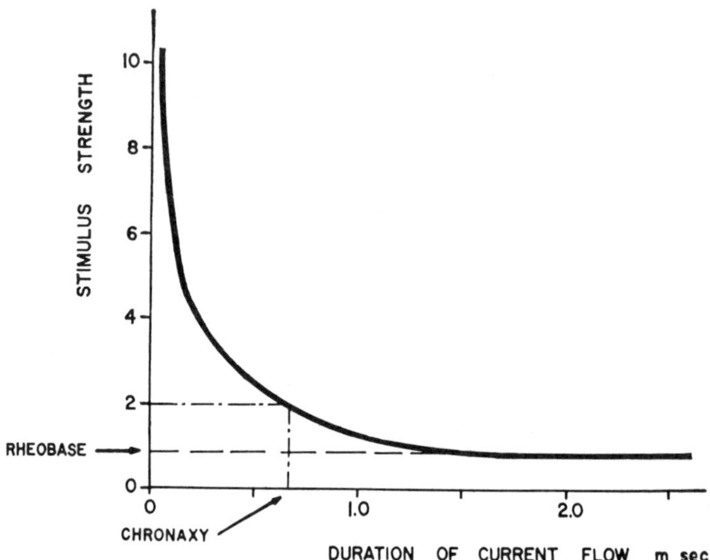

FIG. 2.10. Strength-duration curve showing relation between strength of stimulus current and duration of current flow.

contractions of graded force? The answer to this involves (a) activating new motor units with increasing effort and (b) increasing the frequency of discharge of the individual active motor units.

It will be recalled that the functional unit of the neuromuscular system is the motor unit, which was defined as the anterior horn cell, its axon, and all of the muscle fibers innervated by the axon. The weakest possible tension that can be developed by a muscle is produced by a single action potential propagating along one axon and activating all of these muscle fibers, or, in other words, the tension developed by a motor unit. If increased effort is required, more motor units are activated. This mechanism is called recruitment and is considered to be the most important mechanism for grading tension. The hundreds of motor units in an average muscle allow considerable variation in the mechanical output.

Tension in a muscle can also be graded by varying the discharge frequency of each active motor unit. Within limits, the higher the firing frequency, the greater the developed tension. At the higher frequencies the motor unit twitch tension summates to form a tetanic contraction and an increase in force. Until recently, it was generally accepted that the gradation of tension by variation of the firing rate was effective only for weak efforts, whereas recruitment was the predominant factor at higher tension levels (2–4). Recruitment was considered as the major factor in the grading of the force of a muscular contraction. Milner-Brown et al. (5) after quantifying the forces due to recruitment and the forces due to increased firing rate, claim contrary results. At low force levels where precise control is desired, recruitment proved to be the major mechanism for grading tension, whereas at higher force levels where coarse adjustments are made, increased firing rate was the predominant mechanism. Rate coding appeared to be the chief means of varying tension over most of the physiological range of voluntary contraction, which, Milner-Brown et al. (5) point out, was originally suggested by Adrian and Bronk (6) over 50 years ago. *Spatial* recruitment refers to an increased *number* of motor units being activated; *temporal* recruitment refers to an increased *frequency* of firing of individual motor units.

The total tension generated by a muscle is the sum of the tensions developed by each motor unit. It should be emphasized that motor units are activated at different frequencies and are recruited at different times. Thus, the various units contract asynchronously, and, as a consequence, the summation of the individual tensions produces a fairly smooth and continuous total tension.

REFERENCES

1. Goldman, D. E.: Potential, impedance, and rectification in membranes. J. Gen. Physiol., *27:* 37–60, 1943.
2. Bigland, B., and Lippold, O. C. J.: Motor unit activity in voluntary contraction of human muscle J. Physiol. (Lond), *125:* 322–335, 1954.
3. Das Gupta, A., and Simpson, J. A.: Relation between firing frequency of motor units and muscle tension in the human. Electromyography, *2:* 117–128, 1962.
4. Clamann, H. P.: Activity of single motor units during isometric tension. Neurology (Minneap.), *20:* 254–260, 1970.
5. Milner-Brown, H. S., Stein, R. B., and Yemm, R.: Changes in firing rate of human motor units during linearly changing voluntary contractions. J. Physiol. (Lond.) *230:* 371–390, 1973.
6. Adrian, E. D., and Bronk, D. W.: The discharge of impulses in motor nerve fibres. part II. The frequency of discharge in reflex and voluntary contractions. J. Physiol. (Lond.), *67:* 119–151, 1929.

chapter 3

Volume Conduction and Electromyography

In the preceding chapter action potential initiation and propagation were discussed, and the technique of intracellular recording was carefully described. Although difficult and time consuming, several attempts have been made to record muscle fiber resting and action potentials intracellularly in man in vivo (1–4). Essentially the in vivo technique involved inserting a hypodermic needle through the skin into a muscle belly and then slowly lowering a microelectrode through the cannula into a single fiber. Resting potential data were collected in this manner.

Action potential recording proved to be much more difficult because contraction or slight movement of the fiber resulted in breakage of the microelectrode tip. It is obvious that in spite of the advantage provided by its direct measurement of membrane properties, intracellular recording of muscle potentials has serious shortcomings which preclude routine clinical application. Fortunately, the conductive properties of the whole nerve or muscle permit measurement of electrical activity with *extra*cellular electrodes. As the name implies, these electrodes do not penetrate the cell membrane but detect potential differences external to the fiber and distant from the potential source. The propagated action potential along the fiber and the extracellular potential field are related, and it is this relationship which forms the basis of electromyography.

In this chapter we discuss potentials in a conducting medium and the different shapes of extracellularly recorded action potentials. For an excellent mathematical description of the interrelationships between intracellular and extracellular potentials, the reader is referred to the monograph by Poul Rosenfalck (5).

VOLUME CONDUCTION IN NERVES AND MUSCLES

When the transmembrane potential is decreased to threshold, a rapid reversal of potential occurs which is transient and constitutes the action potential. During this period, local current flow between the active portion of the membrane and the adjacent inactive region acts to depolarize the neighboring region to threshold, initiating a new reversal in polarity and an action potential. This, in turn, provides the conditions for current flow anew and so, as each region progressively depolarizes, the action potential propagates from point to point or node to node. These events describe the activity in and around a typical nerve or muscle fiber. Current flow was considered only near the membrane surface, and conduction into the surrounding medium was not discussed. In the whole muscle or nerve, local current flow is not limited to the membrane surface but spreads throughout the tissue. This follows from the volume-conducting properties of the electrolytic solution surrounding the fibers. A conducting medium through which current will spread from a potential source is called a *volume conductor.*

In Figure 3.1*A* the possible field of current around an impulse is depicted, the current spreading through the extracellular space from the membrane.

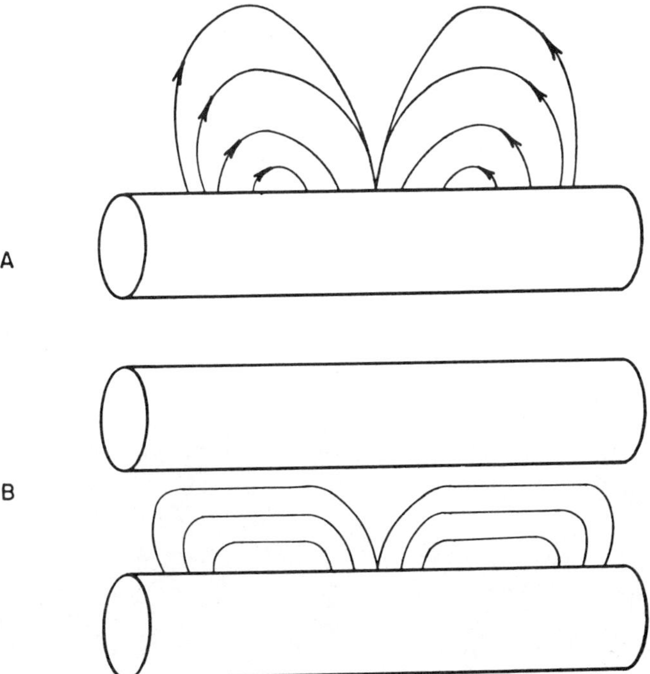

FIG. 3.1. Schematic drawing of volume-conducted current flow. *A*, fiber in isotropic conducting medium; *B*, possible current pattern for active fiber adjacent to inactive fiber.

It should be understood that this drawing represents an idealized condition, that is, one in which the neighboring fibers are not considered and the current spreads uniformly in all directions, as, for example, in an isolated fiber in Ringer's solution. In reality, quiescent fibers surrounding the active one act as good insulators so that the conductivity is not equal in all directions, tending to be resistive when parallel to the fiber and both resistive and capacitive when transverse to it. The result is greater current flow along the fiber than perpendicular to it (Fig. 3.1*B*). Other factors present in muscle, such as fibrous tissue, fat, and blood vessels, can also distort the current flow. It is thus extremely difficult to predict the exact pattern of current flow in the whole muscle.

Associated with the volume-conducted current are, of course, the potential variations. The extracellular action potential represents potential changes outside the fiber caused by electrical activity at the membrane. If no current is flowing in the tissue, then all points in the extracellular space are at equal potential. A potential difference between the active and inactive regions of the membrane becomes a source for current flow and a potential distribution throughout the volume conductor. The potential at a point in the volume conductor can be measured with two electrodes, one in the potential field and the other at some distance from it. The crucial problem is interpreting the recorded response. How is it possible that a monophasic variation in membrane potential can give rise to a di- or triphasic potential as recorded in the extracellular medium? The simultaneous recording of intra- and extracellular potentials from muscle fibers and three different configurations of the externally recorded potential are shown in Figure 3.2. The shape of the extracellular action potential is determined by (a) the distance between the active fiber and the electrode, (b) the properties of the fiber, and (c) the structure and conductivity of the volume conductor surrounding the active fiber.

Attempts have been made to correlate mathematically the extracellular potential with intracellular action potentials. The fundamental study in this

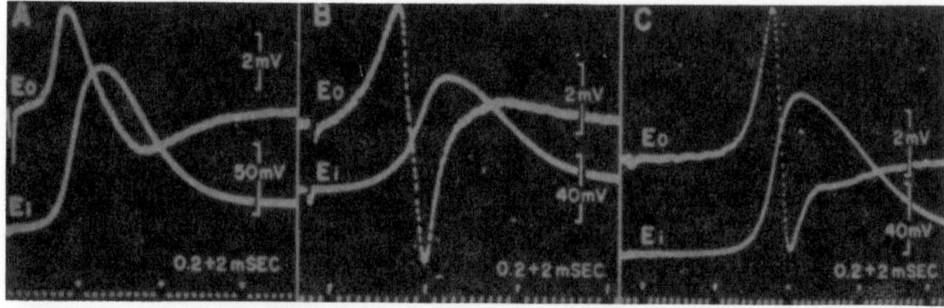

FIG. 3.2. Simultaneous intracellular (E_i) and extracellular (E_o) recordings obtained from fibers of toad sartorius muscle. (From M. Murakami, K. Watanabe, and T. Tomita: Effect of impalement with a micropipette on the local cell membrane. Jap. J. Physiol., *11:* 83, 1961).

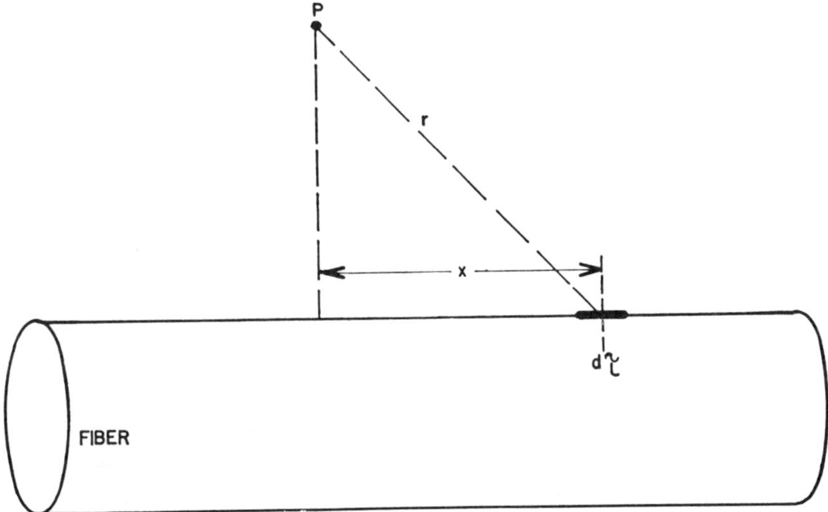

FIG. 3.3. Diagram showing relation between fiber surface and point P used in deriving formula for potential.

field is that by Lorente de Nó (6), whose mathematical analysis of the spread of nerve action currents through a volume conductor was based on classical potential theory. Lorente de Nó found that the field of the nerve action potentials could be considered to arise from a distribution of dipoles* located on the surface of the nerve. He derived an expression for the potential at a point in the field due to impulses propagated along a nerve of unlimited length:

$$\Phi(P) = -\tfrac{1}{4}\pi \int (\partial^2 V_e)/(\delta x^2)\frac{1}{r}d\tau$$

where $\Phi(P)$ is the potential at point P, τ is the volume of the nerve, $d\tau$ is an element of volume, x is measured along the axis of the fiber, r is the distance from the element to point P, and V_e is the monophasic action potential recorded in an oil or air medium (Fig. 3.3).

This equation shows that the amplitude of the volume-conducted action potential declines with distance from the axis of the fiber. Rosenfalck (5), in his own mathematical analysis of intracellular and extracellular potential fields, calculated that the peak-to-peak amplitude decreases 90% within about 0.5 mm from the fiber axis.

This function expresses the relation between the intra- and extracellular potential: the volume potential is proportional to the second derivative

* An electric dipole is a pair of electrically charged particles of equal magnitude and opposite sign which are separated by a very small distance.

($\partial^2 V_e/\partial x^2$) of the monophasic action potential. The second derivative of a typical intracellular action potential is triphasic; the first two phases are about equal in amplitude, with the third, final phase much reduced. The potential, as recorded in the external medium, is greatly reduced in comparison to the potential recorded across the membrane. For an intracellular potential of about 100 mV, the extracellular potential is about 0.33 mV (330 μV) peak to peak. It is pertinent to point out that the sharp positive-to-negative deflection of the extracellular potential corresponds to the rapid rise (depolarization phase) of the transmembrane action potential, and that the third phase occurs during the period of membrane repolarization.

RECORDED EXTRACELLULAR POTENTIALS

Theoretical analyses utilizing classic potential theory indicate that the recorded extracellular potentials are triphasic. Similarly, a nonmathematical approach may be employed to demonstrate the triphasic nature of the potential field (7). This involves examining the effect on a nearby recording electrode of the various ionic currents flowing during conduction of an impulse.

Consider a fiber immersed in a volume conductor and stimulated to threshold at some point, while a short distance away near the fiber surface is located a recording electrode (the second "reference" electrode is at a distant point from the first). Before stimulation there is no external current flow and, therefore, no potential difference between the two electrodes; the base line is at zero (Fig. 3.4*A*). As depolarization at the excited region proceeds, the outward flow of current through adjacent regions of the membrane makes the recording electrode more positive with respect to the reference electrode; that is, the recording is situated over a region which acts as a "source" of current (Fig. 3.4*B*) and thus is at a higher potential relative to the distant electrode. Consequently, the first result of the impulse *approaching* the electrode is a positive or downward deflection.†

A short time later, the region underneath the recording electrode reaches threshold, increases its permeability to Na^+, and reverses its polarity. Current now flows from the adjacent regions into this area. The recording electrode, now situated over a region into which current is flowing, is negative with respect to the reference electrode and an upward deflection is observed (Fig 3.4*C*). This positive-to-negative deflection is steep in slope and corresponds to the sharp rise of the intracellular action potential.

† In the physical sciences, the accepted convention is to display positive potentials "upward" and negative potentials "downward." However, in electrophysiology a reversed convention is in common usage: positive potentials, down; negative potentials, up. Thus in accordance with this convention, also adopted by many electromyographers, our drawings in Figure 3.4 show positive potentials deflected downward and negative potentials upward. Of course, the direction chosen to represent a deflection is completely arbitrary.

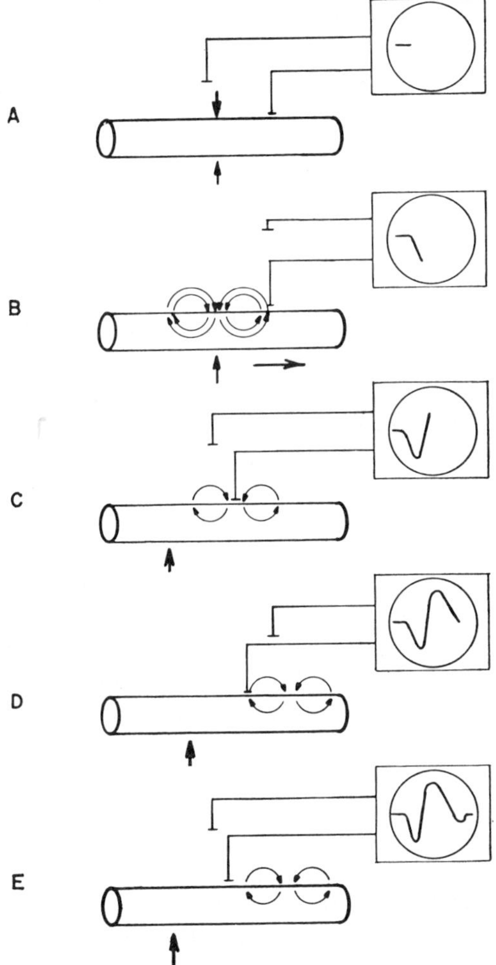

FIG. 3.4. Sequence of events after stimulation of a nerve (at *arrow*) in a conducting medium. Active recording electrode is on surface of nerve and reference electrode is at a distant point. As impulse propagates to right, recorded potential is shown in screen. (See text for complete explanation.) (From M. A. B. Brazier: *The Electrical Activity of the Nervous System*, ed. 3, p. 71. Pitman Medical and Scientific Publishing Co., Ltd., London, 1968.)

As the area under the recording electrode repolarizes, the adjacent region depolarizes. Again the electrode is over a region which acts as a source of current (Fig. 3.4*D*), and its potential is positive relative to the reference electrode. The recorded potential thus progresses downward (negative to positive) from the peak of the negative deflection. As the impulse moves further along the fiber, the recording electrode ceases to be influenced by the current flow, and the observed potential slowly returns to the original base line (Fig. 3.4*E*). The complete potential change produced by an impulse propagated along the fiber is thus triphasic, with a steep linear positive-negative deflection.

In this analysis, the recording electrode was close to the source of the electrical activity or active fiber. The shape of the recorded potential varies considerably with the position of the electrode with respect to the active fibers. Before discussing some examples, it will be helpful to consider first the spatial extent of an impulse; that is, how much of the fiber length is actually involved in the depolarization and repolarization process for an impulse? This may be calculated by multiplying the action potential duration by the conduction speed of an impulse along the fiber. Taking the action potential duration and conduction speed of a human muscle fiber to be approximately 2 msec and 4 m per sec, respectively, the spatial extent of an impulse in human muscle is 8 mm. Thus, activity along 8 mm of fiber length is needed to produce the triphasic response recorded near the fiber.

Extracellular potentials recorded at different points along the nerve and at various distances from it are illustrated in Figure 3.5. One can see immediately that, depending on the location of the recording electrode, potentials of different shape, amplitude, and duration are obtained. In this example, the nerve is arranged such that point $a(x = 0, y = 0)$ represents a point on the nerve where the impulse is initiated, e.g., a cell body. If recording electrodes are placed at different points on the nerve at fixed distances from point $a(x = 0, 7, 15, 26$ mm), we observe potentials *a*, *b*, *c*, and *d*.

At point *a*, the impulse travels only away from the electrode, so that the first change seen by the electrode is depolarization (negative deflection), followed by repolarization (positive deflection). Hence, a diphasic response is recorded. At points further along the nerve (*b* and *c*), triphasic potentials are observed as expected. However, at *d* a diphasic response is seen, a positive-negative deflection. Point *d* is the end of the fiber and represents, in the case of a muscle, recording near the tendon. The third positive deflection is missing because there is no current flow from the region beyond the electrode.

If we now place electrodes at different distances from the fiber, we obtain a new set of curves. For example, by placing electrodes at *c*, *g*, and *k* (all 15 mm from the nerve end) which are 0, 3, and 10 mm from the fiber, we obtain potentials *c*, *g*, and *k*. The electrode *c*, near the membrane surface, records a typical triphasic waveform with a steep positive-negative deflection. Increasing the distance from the fiber (point *g*), the potential is still triphasic but lower in amplitude and slower in the positive-negative rise time. With further movement away from the fiber (point *k*), the amplitude decreases appreciably and the slope becomes considerably slower. It should be clear

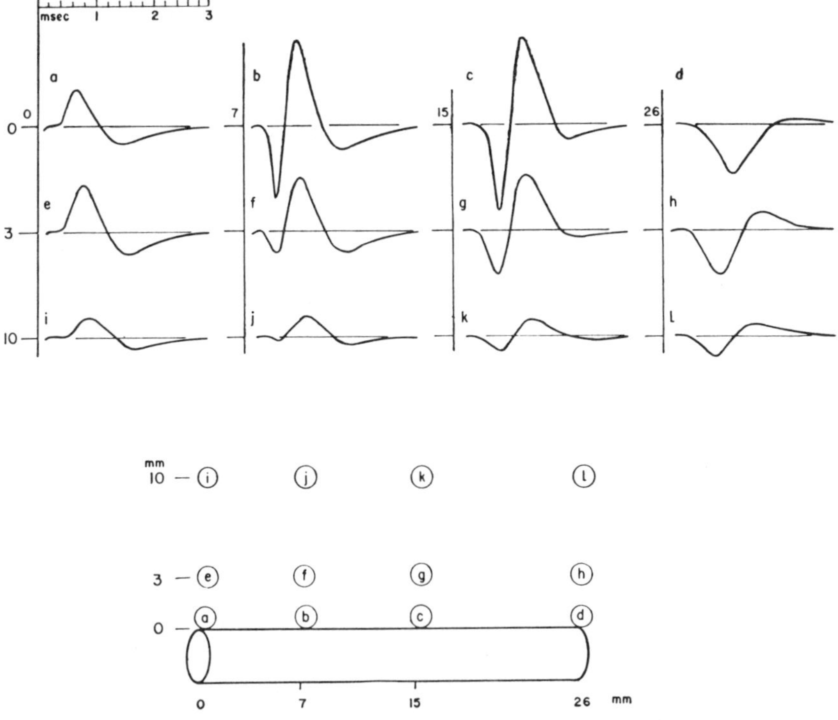

FIG. 3.5. Extracellular potentials recorded at different points along the nerve (*a*, *b*, *c*, *d*) and at various distances from it; *e*, *f*, *g*, and *h* are 3 mm from nerve, and *i*, *j*, *k*, and *l* are 10 mm from it. Impulse is initiated at point *a*. (Adapted from R. Lorente de Nó: *A Study of Nerve Physiology, Studies from the Rockefeller Institute of Medical Research*, vol. 132, p. 466. The Rockefeller University Press, New York, 1947.)

from Figure 3.5 that electrode movement of only a few millimeters may alter the shape and amplitude of the recorded potential.

In electromyography as well as electrocardiography and electroencephalography, the potential source is embedded in a volume conductor, and potential measurements are made by placing electrodes within or on the surface of the conducting medium. The electrodes are usually at a distance from the source of activity, and the interpretation of the recorded potentials is very difficult. As seen in the above illustrations, the shape, amplitude, and duration of the observed waveform are dependent on many factors. Because the system normally examined is closed, these factors must be treated as unknowns. Interpretation of the recorded responses requires an understanding of the physiology and anatomy of the system as well as fundamental understanding of volume conduction.

REFERENCES

1. Beranek, R.: Intracellular electromyography in man. Physiol. Bohemoslov., *10:* 94–96, 1961.
2. Bolte, H. D., Riecker, G., and Rohl, D.: Messungen des Membranpotentials an einzelnen quergestreiften Muskelzellen des Menschen in situ. Klin. Wochenschr., *41:* 356–359, 1963.
3. Goodgold, J., and Eberstein, A: Transmembrane potentials of human muscle cells in vivo. Exp. Neurol., *15:* 338–346, 1966.
4. Norris, F. H., Jr.: Unstable membrane potential in human myotonic muscle. Electroencephalogr. Clin. Neurophysiol., *14:* 197–201, 1962.
5. Rosenfalck, P.: Intra- and extracellular potential fields of active nerve and muscle fibres. Acta. Physiol. Scand., *Suppl. 321*, 1969.
6. Lorente de Nó, R.: *A Study of Nerve Physiology, Studies from the Rockefeller Institute of Medical Research*, vol. 132, pp. 384–477. The Rockefeller University Press, New York, 1947.
7. Brazier, M. A. B.: *The Electrical Activity of the Nervous System*, chap. 7. Pitman Medical and Scientific Publishing Co., Ltd., London, 1968.

chapter 4

Instrumentation for Electromyography; Electrical Safety

This chapter is intended to acquaint workers in the field of electrodiagnosis with the specific requirements as well as the limitations of the apparatus which is employed. The specifications and performance of the instrumentation influence the accuracy of measurement, so that meaningful recording of electrical activity can only be performed with properly designed equipment. It is essential that the electromyographer have a working familiarity with the components which make up the recording system and understand thoroughly the requirements necessary to ensure a valid recording. This familiarity obviously need not be as intensive as that of an engineer but should be sufficient to understand the specifications of apparatus as presented by different manufacturers, to appreciate the basic function of each component which comprises the whole system, and to realize when the system is not functioning within the proper limits. We have seen physicians just entering this field with excellent physiological and clinical experience having difficulty deciding which commercial system to buy because of their inability to understand and compare specifications; similarly, measurements are performed and results are obtained which are valueless because of improper settings of the recording apparatus. In this chapter we attempt to correct these deficiencies by describing the function and electrical characteristics of the electromyograph in the simplest possible terms. It is assumed that the reader has a general acquaintance with basic electricity; if not, he is referred to the text by Offner (1).

To gain some concept of the complexity of recording electrical activity from nerve and muscle, we compare the voltage range and frequency

TABLE 4.1. Required Electrical Characteristics of EEG, ECG, and EMG Recording Systems

Recording System	Voltage Range (mV)	Frequency Response (Hz)
EEG	0.001–0.10	0.02–100
ECG	0.02–5.0	0.1–30
EMG	0.003–5.0*	2–10,000

* Includes sensory nerve action potentials.

response of potentials observed in electrocardiography and electroencephalography with those obtained in electromyography. In Table 4.1 it is clearly shown that the range of voltage and frequency encountered in electromyography (EMG) is much greater than that observed in electroencephalography (EEG) and electrocardiography (ECG). Whereas EEG and ECG recording systems must handle biopotentials which may vary approximately 100-fold in amplitude and up to 100 Hz* in frequency range, the EMG apparatus must be designed to respond to voltages varying 1000-fold in amplitude and about 10,000 Hz in frequency range. It is obvious from these factors alone that one may not use an amplifier designed for EEG or ECG to record accurately single motor unit action potentials.

The objective in recording is to obtain a faithful reproduction of the physiological event; that is, the wave forms picked up by the electrodes should be amplified and presented to the observer without distortion and free from any interference which may obscure the signal. These objectives are secured by constructing the amplifier to satisfy certain conditions of input impedance, common mode rejection, and frequency response. Display and recording equipment must also meet certain specifications.

THE ELECTROMYOGRAPH

The block diagram in Figure 4.1 shows the basic features of a typical electromyograph. Action potentials are picked up by either a needle electrode or surface electrodes and then amplified by the amplifier. The output of the amplifier is connected to different monitoring devices: (a) an oscilloscope, to permit immediate display and visual monitoring of the potentials; (b) an audioamplifier and speaker, to allow acoustic monitoring of the potentials; and (c) a recorder, to make a permanent record of the displayed potentials. The recorder may be one of several available magnetic tape, film or fiberoptic photographic paper readout devices.

For conduction speed measurement, a stimulator generating rectangular pulses is usually included as part of the equipment. Besides the stimulus

* In accordance with recommendations of the International Organization for Standardization, the unit of frequency is called Hertz (Hz) instead of cycles per second.

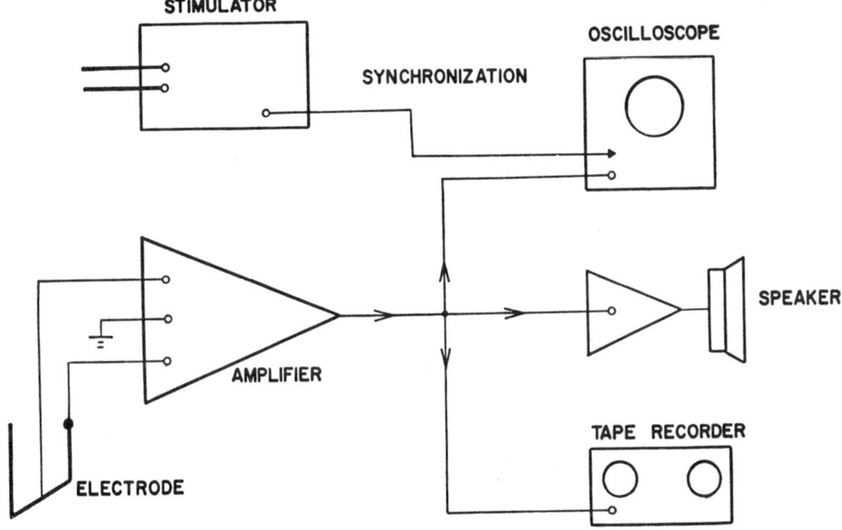

FIG. 4.1. Block diagram showing basic components of typical electromyograph.

output which is connected to the electrodes located on the patient, a synchronization pulse from the stimulator triggers the horizontal sweep of the oscilloscope. This serves to synchronize the response with the stimulus pulse and simplifies observations of the response on the oscilloscope.

The equipment shown in Figure 4.1 may be purchased as an integrated unit, available commercially from several different companies, or individually, and then interconnected into a single system. In either case, it is important that the electrical characteristics of the total system be evaluated. Nowadays there is no problem obtaining audio equipment, oscilloscopes, or recorders which demonstrate satisfactory performance; the correct choice of an amplifier which satisfies the rigorous requirements of electromyography is more difficult. The requirements which must be met by the amplifier will now be summarized. To avoid any misunderstanding, it is emphasized that we shall discuss the amplifier into which the recording or pickup electrodes are connected.

The Amplifier

The potentials picked up by the electrodes are usually very small in amplitude and consequently must be amplified to a level that can be conveniently handled by the other apparatus. The amplifier designed for this purpose should have the following characteristics: (a) high and uniform voltage gain for all frequencies within its stated range, (b) a frequency range of 2 to 10,000 Hz, (c) differential input, (d) high input impedance and low input capacitance, (e) high common mode rejection, and (f) low inherent noise.

Input Impedance

The input impedance of the amplifier is determined by the resistance of the amplifier input to the flow of current and is measured in the same units as resistance, ohms. In most applications, it is desirable to have the input impedance many times greater than the impedance of the electrode. This ensures that very little current is drawn from the source of the potential to be amplified, and there is minimal drop of voltage at the electrode. If the input impedance is lower than the electrode impedance, a condition known as "loading," a large current will flow from the source through the electrode and amplifier impedance, causing a comparatively large voltage loss across the electrode and a reduced voltage available for the amplifier. This condition results in distortion of the potential wave shape.

The distortion of the action potential is not simply limited to a loss of amplitude, but the shape of the potential changes as well. This is clearly seen in Figure 4.2. For an electrode of a given area, say 2000 μ^2, it is seen that as the input impedance decreases, the EMG potential decreases in amplitude and the wave shape changes; this is especially obvious for the square wave potential. Because the exposed surface area of a concentric EMG needle electrode is about 70,000 μ^2, it appears from Figure 4.2 that the input impedance of the EMG amplifier should be well over 2 megohms to ensure distortion-free recording. The change in wave shape, as well as amplitude, is attributed to the resistive and reactive components of the electrode impedance (2).

It is thus apparent that the input impedance of the amplifier must be high compared to impedance of the electrode to eliminate any distortion of the action potentials. A high input impedance is necessary for another reason: high input impedance effectively increases the common mode rejection ratio of the amplifier. This is important in the rejection of certain types of noise, such as hum, by the amplifier. Common mode rejection is discussed in the following section.

Differential Input

When an electrode is inserted into a muscle it picks up action potentials; however, it may also pick up 60-Hz hum potentials from power supplies or poor grounding or other sources. The latter potentials, if passed through an ordinary single-ended amplifier, would be amplified along with the muscle potentials. In this type of recording the quality of the amplifier output, especially if the action potentials are low amplitude, would be very poor.

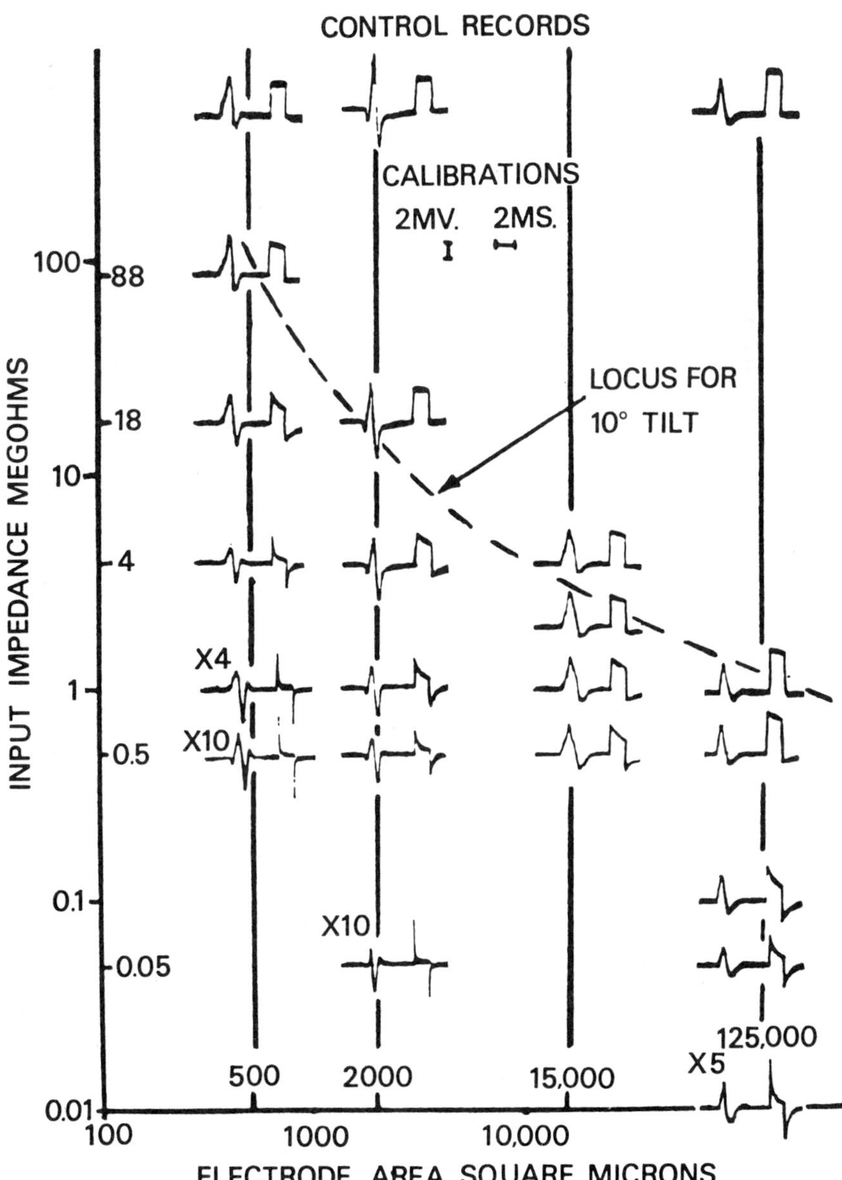

FIG. 4.2. The effect of amplifier input impedance on a typical action potential and a rectangular wave. The input or "control" is shown at the *top*, and the resulting outputs recorded with electrodes having surface areas ranging from 500 to 125,000 μ^2 are given below for various input impedances. The locus of points representing the conditions for 10% tilt on top of the rectangular wave is plotted as the *dashed line*. At 10% tilt, minimal distortion was detectable in the muscle action potentials. (From L. A. Geddes, L. E. Baker, and M. McGoodwin: The relationship between electrode area and amplifier input impedance in recording muscle action potentials. Med. Biol. Engin., *5:* 565, 1967.)

To improve the quality of the recording, extensive shielding could be used, or, alternatively, a differential amplifier could be used for the first stage of amplification. (In some cases, it is necessary to use both shielding and differential amplification.) The method of choice is to use a differential amplifier because it has the added advantage that the electrodes connected to the input need not be grounded and thus may be used to measure potential differences at any point.

The differential amplifier is simply a *difference* amplifier; that is, it amplifies the *difference* in *voltage* that exists at every instant between signals applied to the two inputs. In Figure 4.3 this corresponds to the voltage difference between signals applied to input *1* and input *2*. For example, two voltages identical in amplitude and phase that are applied to the differential amplifier cause no output voltage. One can now see the advantage of this type of device. In-phase signals arising from power lines or from sources outside the electrode field which would normally interfere with the desired action potentials will be rejected by the amplifier.

The ability of a differential amplifier to reject identical signals is called *common mode rejection.* The degree of common mode rejection of the amplifier depends primarily on the symmetry of the amplifier inputs. It is practically impossible to construct the two inputs to be exactly symmetrical in electrical characteristics. Slight variations in resistance and capacitance of the input transistors (or tubes) result in an imbalance of the two inputs, so that a difference signal is observed at the output even for identical input signals. The amount of difference signal obtained for identical inputs is specified by the common mode rejection ratio (CMRR). CMRR is defined as the ratio between a voltage common to the inputs of the amplifier and that difference in voltage between the two inputs which develop the same output voltage. For example, a differential amplifier that produces a 0.001-V output when driven by a 1.0-V signal common to both inputs has a CMRR of 1.0/0.001 or 1000/1.

A high CMRR is a necessary condition for eliminating interference from the recording. Restating the above example, if an amplifier has a CMRR of 1000/1, then a common 1.0-V input will cause an output of 1.0/1000, or

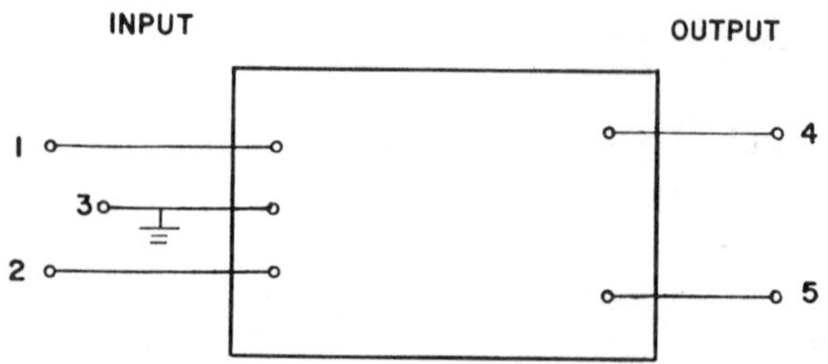

FIG. 4.3. Differential amplifier showing input and output connections; *1* and *2* are input (to recording electrodes), *3* is ground, and *4* and *5* are output terminals.

0.001 V. The higher the CMRR, the lower the output voltage resulting from voltages common to the two inputs.

It is very important that the determination of CMRR be made under actual operating conditions, that is, with an electrode connected to the amplifier and in situ. A simple technique for making this measurement is given in the paper by Guld et al. (3). The CMRR of the amplifier considered by itself may be extremely high (around 100,000); however, if the electrodes are considered part of the amplifier input, this figure falls precipitously (ranging from 5 to 2000). The reason is that the electrode and amplifier input impedances form a voltage divider which reduces the actual voltage applied to the input terminals (Fig. 4.4*A*). Also, because impedances of electrodes are rarely equal (different surface area or contact resistance between tissue and electrode surface), the signal voltages existing at the two terminals differ and the effective CMRR of the amplifier is reduced.

If the impedance of the electrodes is low compared to the input impedance of the amplifier, a fairly high CMRR will be obtained. This is seen in Figure 4.4*A* and corresponds to the use of surface or monopolar electrodes. If the impedances of the electrodes are unequal (Fig. 4.4*B*), then the CMRR is greatly reduced. This is the case with concentric needle electrodes, where the tissue-to-core impedance is greater than the tissue-to-cannula impedance. Likewise, a low amplifier input impedance and high electrode impedance severely reduces the CMRR (Fig. 4.4*C*). Thus, to obtain a high CMRR with high impedance electrodes such as concentric needle electrodes, a high input impedance differential amplifier is essential.

Unfortunately, the CMRR decreases as the frequency of the signal decreases. The rejection ratio may be maintained at a high level throughout the required frequency range by using an amplifier with very high input impedance (200 megohms or more).

Frequency Response

Thus far we have discussed two characteristics of the amplifier which are required to minimize distortion and interference: differential input and high input impedance. Another factor of considerable importance in our quest for faithful reproduction of source potentials is the ability of the apparatus to follow reliably any changes in potential with time. In electromyography the apparatus must be designed to follow fairly rapid changes in potential amplitude; for example, when fibrillation potentials are recorded with concentric needle electrodes, a variation of 100 μV may occur in less than 1 msec. If the apparatus cannot follow the fast changes, then both the amplitude and duration of the recorded signals will be inaccurate.

The response of the amplifier can be easily determined by comparing the amplitude of the output with that of the input for sine waves of varying frequency. As with measurement of the CMRR, the frequency response

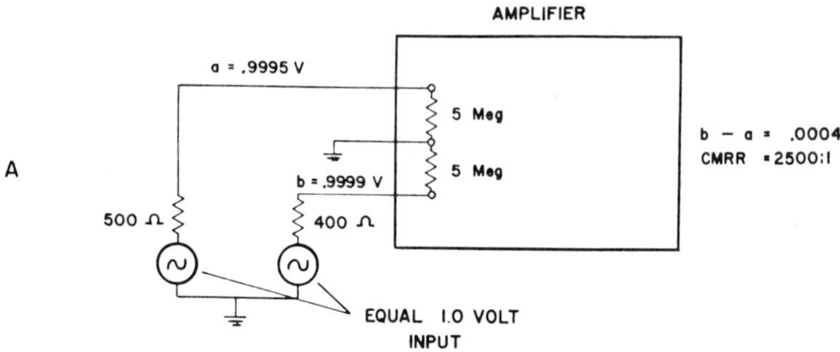

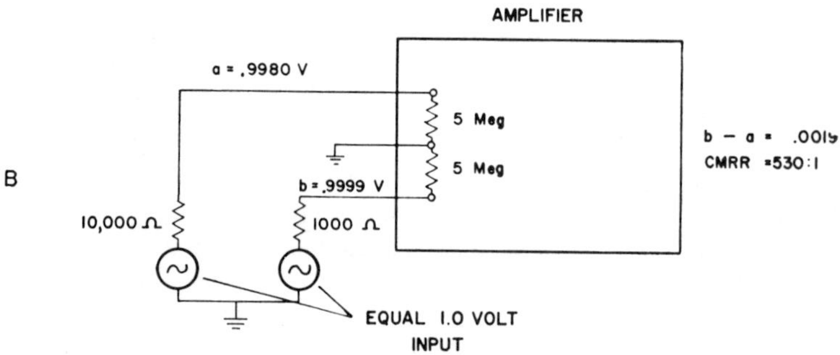

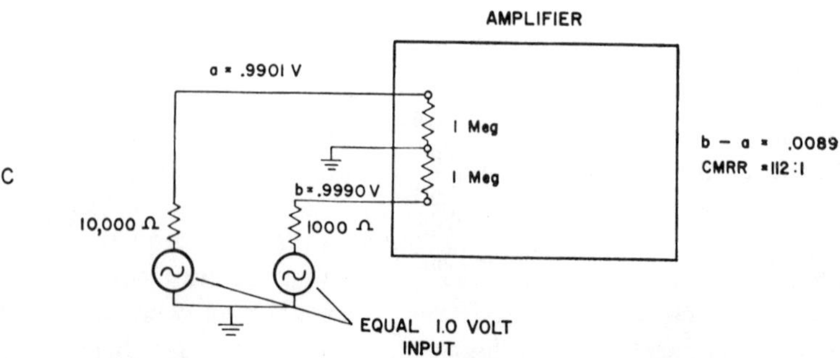

FIG. 4.4. Common mode rejection ratio (*CMRR*) of electrode and amplifier calculated for different conditions. Input impedances of input *a* and *b* are 5 megohms in *A* and *B*, 1 megohm in *C*. Electrode impedances are 500 and 400 ohms in *A*, 10,000 and 1000 ohms in *B*, and 10,000 and 1000 ohms in *C*. Actual voltage applied to each input terminal is shown.

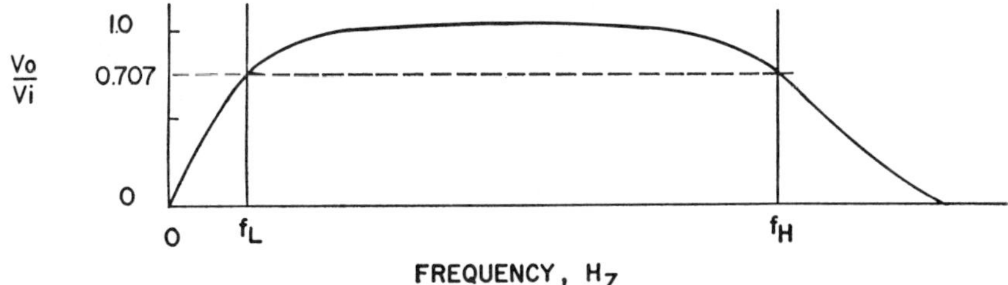

FIG. 4.5. A frequency response characteristic for an amplifier. f_H is high frequency cutoff, f_L is low frequency cutoff; and Vo/Vi is ratio of voltage output to input.

should be determined with electrodes connected to the amplifier. The "Report of the Committee on EMG Instrumentation" (3) discusses methods of measuring the frequency response of the amplifier with unipolar electrodes or a concentric needle electrode.

The frequency response of electrodes and amplifier is similar to that illustrated in Figure 4.5. The output voltage remains constant or "flat" for a portion of the frequency spectrum and decays at both ends of the curve, the low and high frequency ranges. The points on the curve designated f_L and f_H represent frequencies for which the voltage response is 0.707 of the midband value. The amplifier power output is reduced to one-half of the midfrequency value at these points so that the frequencies f_L and f_H are designated the "half-power" or "3 dB" points.† Stated another way, at the low and high cutoff frequencies f_L and f_H, the response is down 3 dB.

In selecting the best frequency response for the EMG amplifier, two factors must be considered: (a) no distortion of any recorded potentials and (b) noise voltages maintained as low as possible. If we choose a wide frequency range to ensure distortion-free recording, we may also allow noise, which is introduced via the electrode or amplifier wiring, to pass through the amplifier. Consequently, the frequency response is carefully chosen on the basis of the frequency content of the EMG potentials and the elimination of potentials of all other frequencies.

Tests with potentials of different shapes and duration (4) showed that for general electromyography a frequency response with f_L at 2 Hz and f_H at 10,000 Hz will provide sufficiently accurate reproduction of all potentials, and the noise level will be acceptably low. Properly stated, the frequency response of the amplifier (including the electrode) should be flat with 3 dB points at 2 Hz and 10,000 Hz.

† Because it is conventional to use logarithmic scales to plot gain and frequency characteristics, a unit convenient to handle the log of a ratio was defined. Called the decibel, abbreviated dB, it is

$$\text{dB} = 20 \log Vo/Vi$$

where Vo/Vi is the ratio of voltage output to input or the "gain."

There are occasions when it is desirable to reduce the frequency response in order to increase the signal-to-noise ratio. When recording evoked potentials, movement of the electrode or wires may cause a low frequency shifting of the base line. This may be reduced by increasing the lower cutoff frequency from 2 to around 20 Hz. In recording low amplitude voltages, as from sensory nerves, for conduction velocity measurements, the signal-to-noise ratio may be improved by decreasing the noise. One possible solution is to decrease the upper cutoff frequency to perhaps 2000 Hz, thereby reducing high frequency noise components still further. The measurement accuracy of the sensory nerve voltage is not appreciably affected by the narrowing of the frequency response because no steep change in potential is involved.

It should be obvious that the frequency response of oscilloscopes and recording equipment, such as tape recorders, connected to the amplifier should be at the very least 2 to 10,000 Hz. A pen recorder with a frequency response of 0 to 500 Hz, even if connected to the best EMG amplifier, severely distorts most of the potentials. Oscilloscopes and recorders with wide frequency ranges are fairly easy to obtain and satisfactory to use because most of the noise is reduced by the input amplifier.

Input Capacitance and Noise

Stray and wiring capacitances in parallel with the input resistance are termed the amplifier input capacitance. Cable capacitance is due to capacitance to ground of the electrode leads and is additive to the input capacitance (see Fig. 4.6*A*).

All circuits have a certain amount of inherent capacitance due to the physical placement of wires and components. Stray capacitance situated at the input of the amplifier and capacitance of the electrode and their cables contribute to attenuation and distortion of the incoming signal. Because the capacitance of the electrode cables is added to the amplifier input capacitance, the resulting input capacitance may be very high.

The effect of the input capacitance is to reduce the high frequency components of the incoming signal. For example, if the input capacitance of an amplifier is 500 pF (500×10^{-12} Farads), the equivalent impedance of the capacitance at 1000 Hz is about 300,000 ohms ($X_c = 1/2\pi fC$). If the electrode impedance is about 300,000 ohms, then the 1000 Hz component will be reduced by nearly 50%. At progressively higher frequencies the voltage is reduced still further. Thus, it is important to keep the input capacitance as low as possible to maintain a good frequency response. A high input capacitance also reduces the CMRR at the higher frequencies.

Most EMG amplifiers are carefully designed to have low input capacitance, so the presence of appreciable input capacitance may be attributed to electrode cable capacitances. The magnitude of the cable capacitance de-

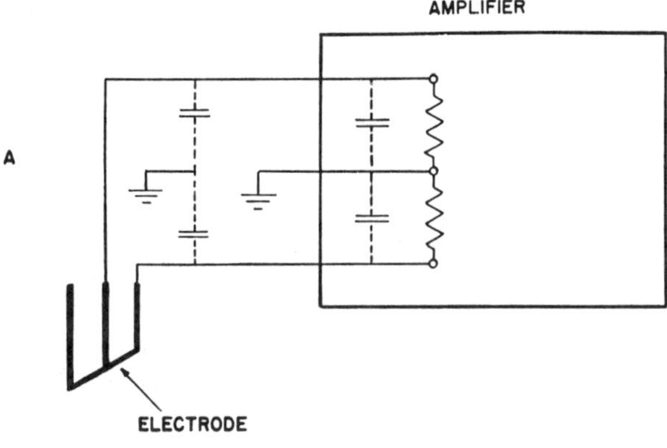

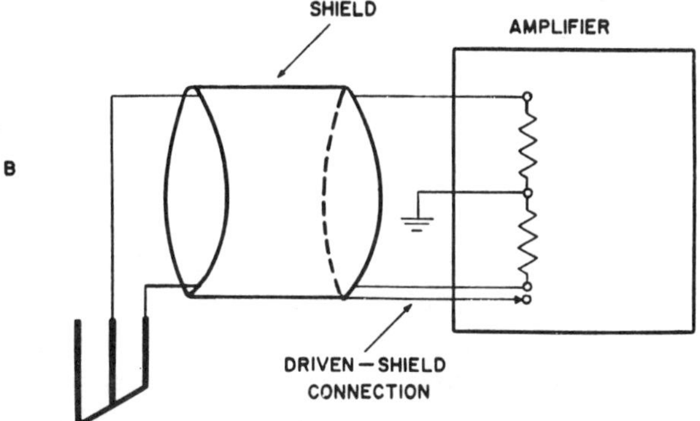

FIG. 4.6. *A*, schematic drawing illustrating input capacitance of amplifier and capacitance to ground of electrode leads; *B*, arrangement of driven shield around electrode leads. Shield is not grounded.

pends on the construction of the electrodes. Two types of concentric needle electrodes are currently marketed, one with a shielded cable and the other without. The shield (which is connected to ground) surrounding the wires reduces the pickup of electrical interference; however, it adds considerable capacitance to the amplifier input. The nonshielded cable has the disadvantage of being exposed to possible noise voltages; however, it has low cable capacitance, especially if the length is kept short. The shielded cable capacitance may be reduced by using either short cables or a "driven shield" arrangement. In the driven shield method the shield is not connected to ground but rather to a point in the specially designed amplifier circuit such that a voltage is impressed on the shield which varies in time with the input potential (Fig. 4.6*B*). As a result, the shield and the inner wires are approximately at the same potential, and no current flows through the capacitor formed by the shield and inner wires. Thus, the effect of the cable capacitance is minimized and the high frequency response is restored.

A carefully designed EMG amplifier has an input capacitance of 100 pF or less.

Undesired random voltage fluctuations appearing in the amplifier output, not related to the input or source voltage, are called amplifier noise and may limit the accuracy of the recording. The noise arises from various sources within the amplifier: random motions of electrons due to thermal agitation in resistors, random motion of electrons flowing between cathode and plate in vacuum tubes, and semiconductor noise. The noise, superimposed on the desired action potentials, is obvious at the higher levels of amplification, that is, when the weaker signals are being recorded.

Although it is impossible to eliminate all noise inherent in an amplifier, noise effects can be minimized by the careful selection of tubes, resistors, and transistors and proper circuit design. Amplifiers for electromyographic use are, therefore, constructed with great care and can be obtained with noise levels less than 10 μV peak to peak for the full frequency range, as measured with shorted input.

ELECTRODES USED IN ELECTROMYOGRAPHY

Surface or Skin Electrodes

Gross muscle electrical activity may be recorded without penetrating the skin or muscle tissue by applying electrodes on the surface of the skin directly over the muscle of interest. These electrodes usually consist of two square or circular metal (tin or silver) plates with attached leadoff wires (Fig. 4.7*A*). The impedance between the plates and skin is reduced by carefully scraping the skin or cleansing it with ether and applying electrode paste. They are affixed with adhesive tape. Dimensions may vary, although they usually are about 1 by 2.5 cm.

A new type of skin electrode has been developed which minimizes movement artifacts and is excellent for long term monitoring of activity such as exercise (Fig. 4.8).

The disadvantages of skin electrodes as compared to needle electrodes are (a) the difficulty of recording from a deep muscle without interference from nearby muscles, (b) the inability to observe single motor unit activity, and (c) the loss of high frequency components. In Figure 4.9 the frequency spectrum is compared as recorded with skin and needle electrodes from the biceps brachii. At about 100 Hz the frequency content of the electrical activity starts to differ, the surface electrode showing much less energy in the high frequencies than the needle electrode.

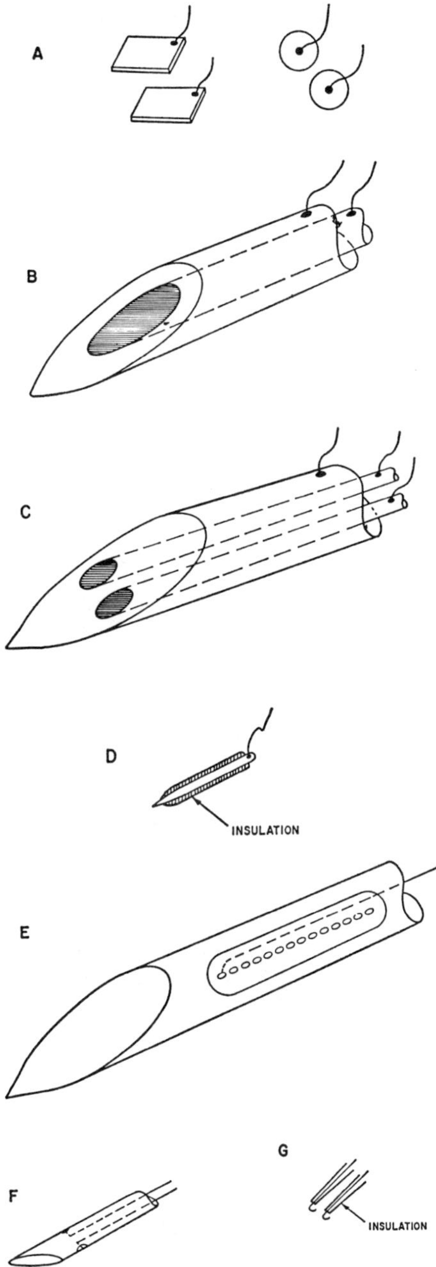

FIG. 4.7. *A*, surface electrodes. Dimensions vary, usually are about 1 by 2.5 cm. *B*, concentric needle electrode. Hypodermic needle (no. 26), diameter of inside wire 0.1 mm. *C*, bipolar needle electrode, no. 23 hypodermic needle with 0.1 mm diameter wires. *D*, monopolar electrode. Diameter, approximately 0.8 mm. *E*, multielectrode. Fourteen electrodes, 0.1 by 1 mm in size, in a cannula 1 mm in diameter. *F*, Janus electrode. Needle about 0.6 mm in diameter with 2 leads 25μ in diameter. *G*, flexible wire electrodes.

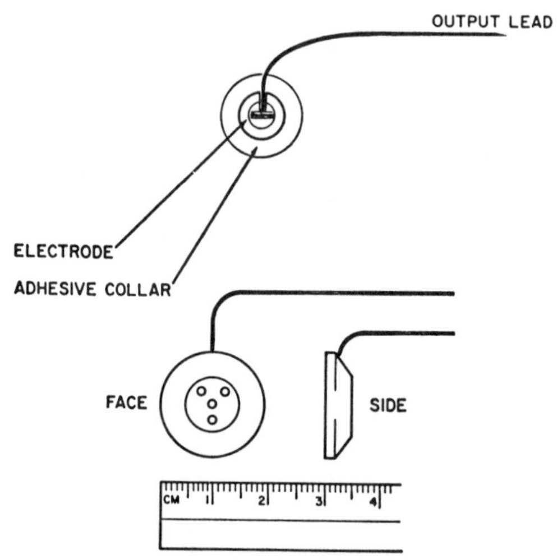

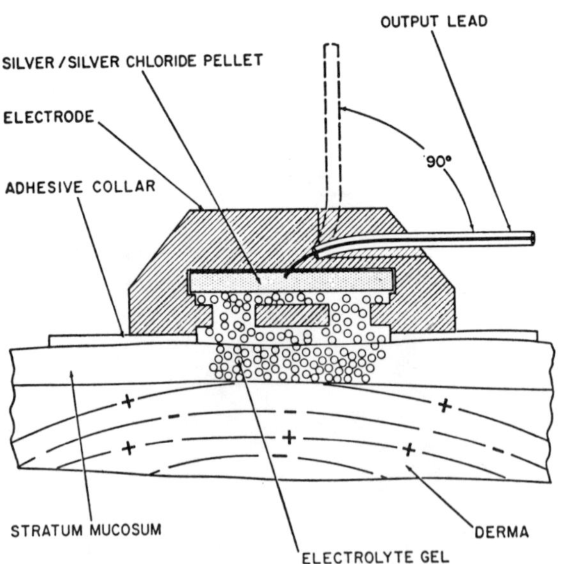

FIG. 4.8. Skin electrode, (From *Beckman Biopotential Skin Electrode Instruction Manual*, O-TB-002, pp. 0, 4. Spinco Division of Beckman Instruments, Inc., Palo Alto, Calif., 1965.)

Concentric Needle Electrode

The most common electrode used for recording directly from the muscle is the concentric needle electrode (Fig. 4.7*B*). It consists of a platinum wire located centrally inside a hypodermic needle but completely insulated from it. Typical electrodes may vary from 0.3 to about 1 mm in outside diameter

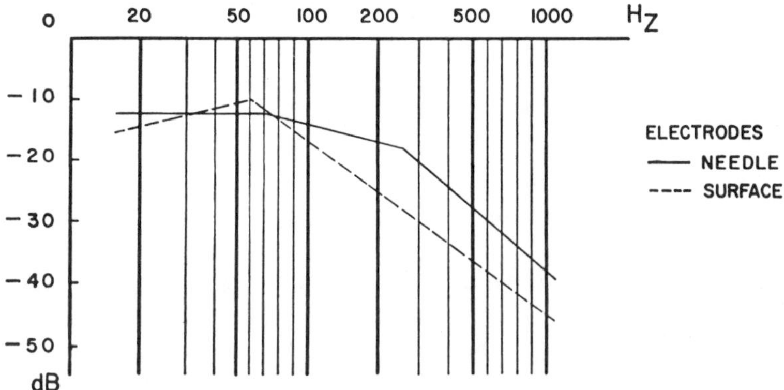

FIG. 4.9. Comparison of frequency spectrum recorded from biceps brachii with needle and surface electrodes. (From R. Kadefors, E. Kaiser, and L. Petersen: Dynamic spectrum analysis of myo-potentials with special reference to muscle fatigue. Electromyography, *8:* 53, 1968.)

with a center wire of 0.1 mm diameter. The average impedance of this electrode may be around 50,000 ohms. Both the inside wire and the outside cannula are connected to the amplifier input terminals. Ground is a large plate electrode affixed to the skin and connected to the amplifier.

Bipolar Needle Electrode

The bipolar electrode is similar to the concentric electrode except that two platinum wires are embedded in the hypodermic needle, necessitating large diameter cannulas if the same size platinum wire is used. Each inside wire is connected to the amplifier input and the cannula is grounded. Thus, no separate ground plate is necessary. The bipolar electrode is limited to detecting potentials from a smaller volume than the concentric electrode (Fig. 4.7*C*).

Monopolar Electrode

The monopolar electrode is usually constructed from a stainless steel wire sharpened to a pointed tip and then insulated except for the very tip. The diameter of the wire averages around 0.8 mm, and the insulating sleeve is usually Teflon if it is to be sterilized. Teflon-coated electrodes appear to be less painful in passing through the skin. It is common practice to insert one such electrode into the muscle and to use a surface electrode as the indifferent electrode. A monopolar electrode inserted under the skin may also be used as the indifferent electrode. A separate metal plate placed on the skin is the ground electrode.

Multielectrode

This is a special purpose electrode developed by Professor Fritz Buchthal (5) for the determination of motor unit territory. As shown in Figure 4.7*E*,

14 platinum wires, each insulated from each other and from the cannula, are exposed through the side of the cannula, not from the end. Action potentials are recorded between each lead of the multielectrode and the indifferent electrode. The indifferent electrode is one of the outer leads of the 14, and not the cannula. The cannula is connected to ground. Recording is made by switching each lead and the indifferent electrode to an amplifier, or, if more than one amplifier is available, simultaneous recording may be performed from several leads.

The outside diameter of the cannula is 1 mm, and the spacing between the leads depends on its application. For measurement of motor unit territory in diseases of myogenic origin, the leads (each 0.1 by 1 mm in size) are spaced 0.5 mm apart, whereas for diseases of neurogenic origin the leads (each 0.1 by 1.5 mm in size) are 1 mm apart.

"Janus" Electrode

Another special purpose electrode, designated the Janus electrode, is illustrated in Figure 4.7*F*. Its construction is similar to that of the bipolar electrode except that the two platinum wires are brought out of two openings at opposite sides of the cannula instead of the tip (6). Thus, simultaneous recordings may be made from muscle fibers separated by the diameter of the needle, an aid in elucidating motor unit organization.

Flexible Wire Electrodes

Flexible wire electrodes are useful when one wishes to record intramuscularly during kinesiological examinations. The flexibility of the wires permits freedom of movement without any painful sensation to the subject. The number of motor units actually recorded depends on the diameter of the wire. Single unit activity has been recorded with a 27-μ diameter Karma alloy wire with liquid nylon insulation (7). The more common wire electrodes are about 0.1-mm diameter insulated platinum wires.

The procedure for placing the wires in the muscle involves inserting them first in a hypodermic needle, introducing needle and wires through the skin into the muscle, and then carefully withdrawing the cannula. The wires remain positioned within the muscle (8).

HAZARDS OF ELECTRODIAGNOSTIC EQUIPMENT

In recent years electrical safety in hospitals has become a matter of increasing concern. It has become apparent not only that electrocution takes place with currents in the order of a few milliamperes (60 Hz AC) flowing through surface tissue (macroshock) but that under certain circumstances currents as low as a few microamperes (60 Hz AC) can also be fatal (microshock).

An external transthoracic current of 20 ma can cause ventricular fibrillation, especially if it is delivered at the phase of the cardiac cycle which corresponds to the beginning of the "T" wave of the ECG; a leakage current of 10 to 20 μa applied directly to the myocardium by a cardiac catheter may also be sufficient to induce ventricular fibrillation, precipitating the need for immediate adequate resuscitation.

The circumstances which give rise to the serious episodes do not appear solely as inadvertent laboratory accidents, but frequently the potentially lethal problem commences on the day the manufacturer delivers his equipment or on the day that the hospital's electrical wiring is installed. In reviewing the inadequacy of safety standards in medical instrumentation, Ben-Zvi (9) noted that approximately 40% of newly delivered mechanical and electronic equipment to the New York Downstate Medical Center over a 2-year period was defective or outright rejectable.

The dangerous circumstances which arise are generally due to faults in the grounding system which cause the flow of "leakage current" through the cardiac region. Small undesirable current, known as leakage current, is present in almost all electrical equipment, such as motors, lamps, instruments, and the wiring itself. Leakage current may occur even if the switch is turned off. It is produced by the direct leakage of electricity or the capacitive action between two current-carrying conductors separated by insulating material. If the grounding system is properly installed, leakage current is minimal—leakage current caused by defective equipment is shunted harmlessly to ground or sets off an appropriate alarm.

The grounding system is made up of low resistance conductors connected to a common terminal which acts as a uniform reference point for the development of electrical potentials. The ideal ground is everywhere and at all times at the same potential. Under normal circumstances, one terminal of the common power outlet is at ground potential and the other is at the line voltage (the "hot" lead) with respect to the ground. The modern laboratory is usually provided with outlets having a third grounding terminal connected to the building ground which includes the metallic structure of the building, the plumbing, air conditioning, electrical fixtures, etc.

As a safety factor, the exposed metal surfaces of electrical equipment are connected to ground. This protects against the possibility that the equipment, not being properly grounded (e.g., a separate equipment grounding cable is clipped to a "painted" pipe, or a hidden break in the grounding connection occurs), becomes electrically hot owing to some defect, while at the same time a patient simultaneously touches the apparatus and ground (or the patient may be intentionally grounded by an attached electrode during electromyographic examination) and completes a circuit through which lethal current may flow.

It is important that all grounded laboratory equipment be routinely checked to verify that ground connections are intact, ground loops are not present, and leakage current is limited. Ground loops may be avoided by connecting the equipment to a common point. Also, the ground should be at the same potentials as all of the exposed conductive materials in the room.

Manufacturers of electrical equipment are careful to provide good electrical insulation and low capacitance between the exposed surfaces and power line connections to ensure that very little leakage current flows through a grounded patient or operator. Properly designed equipment notwithstanding, the leakage current should be routinely measured with a leakage meter between exposed metal surfaces and ground, between input and output terminals and ground, and between adjacent grounding conductors. These values indicate the current which will flow through the patient or operator if contact is made between the two points. Acceptable leakage current should be in the low 10's of microamperes.

A potential shock hazard are small appliances which have ungrounded metal cases, such as radios, televisions, and lamps. These appliances may satisfy Underwriter Laboratory (UL) specifications if leakage current to the case is less than 5000 μa. Thus, a grounded patient reaching for one of these devices could be shocked, or, more seriously, if the heart is directly exposed to this current via a grounded pacemaker lead, ventricular fibillation could be induced. As a rule, all metal surfaces, grounded or ungrounded, should be kept out of reach of the patient. It is also recommended that the examining table be made of wood or else removed from contact from all conducting devices.

Electrically operated equipment which presents a "tingling" sensation when touched should be investigated and repaired. The sensation represents a leakage current of about 1 ma at 60 Hz AC, which, under most circumstances, is not dangerous but may become a hazard or at least frighten the patient. It is well to remember that the investigator himself may be a link between a current source and the patient by touching an ungrounded power line-operated device and the grounded patient.

A technique which offers some protection against macroshock is the use of a power line isolation transformer. With an isolation transformer, instruments connected to a grounded patient cannot be the source of harmful current even if a defect causes contact with either side of the line (i.e., secondary of transformer). However, leakage currents are still present and may capacitatively accumulate on the ungrounded equipment, thereby becoming potentially hazardous. When this system is used, careful attention must be given to ground connections and the occurrence of electrical faults. Bruner (10), who wrote an excellent review of hazards of electrical apparatus, stated that neither transformer isolation nor battery-operated apparatus is necessary if careful consideration is given to circuit design and grounding.

Shock-interrupting devices are designed to limit exposure time and, therefore, the energy delivered by the shock, rather than to reduce the ground fault current to safe levels. This is a means of meeting only the problem of macroshock due to faults to ground by detection of excessive current flow in the ground circuit. It automatically breaks the circuit so that only a maximal current flow of 5 ma through the patient can take place. However, it must be pointed out that only one-thousandth of this value, 5 μa, when applied directly to the myocardium may be sufficient to induce ventricular fibrillation.

The danger of electrocution is a function of the current pathway as well as current density and frequency. In conduction velocity studies, for example, perfectly innocuous pulses of 0.1 to 0.5-msec duration at 70 ma can be delivered to the extremity. It is possible to avoid a transthoracic current pathway by restricting the location of stimulating electrodes, patient ground, and recording electrodes to the same extremity.

There is no doubt that maximal safety to staff and patient ensues from careful initial planning of the electrodiagnostic laboratory, careful checkout of all newly purchased and fabricated instrumentation, and periodic, thorough inspection of the entire electrical system.

REFERENCES

1. Offner, F. F.: *Electronics for Biologists.* McGraw-Hill Book Co., Inc., New York, 1967.
2. Geddes, L. A., Baker, L. E., and McGoodwin, M.: The relationship between electrode area and amplifier input impedance in recording muscle action potentials. Med. Biol. Engin., *5:* 561–569, 1967.
3. Guld, C., Rosenfalck, A., and Willison, R. G.: Report of the Committee on EMG Instrumentation. Electroencephalogr. Clin. Neurophysiol., *28:* 399–413, 1970.
4. Buchthal, F., Guld, C., and Rosenfalck, P.: Action potentials parameters in normal human muscle and their dependence on physical variables. Acta Physiol. Scand., *32:* 200–218, 1954.
5. Buchthal, F., Guld, C., and Rosenfalck, P.: Volume conduction of the spike of the motor unit potential investigated with a new type of multielectrode. Acta Physiol. Scand., *38:* 331–354, 1957.
6. Ekstedt, J.: Human single muscle fiber action potentials. Acta Physiol. Scand., *61 (Suppl. 226):* 19, 1964.
7. Clamann, H. P.: Activity of single motor units during isometric tension. Neurology (Minneap.), *20:* 254–260, 1970.
8. Basmajian, J. V., and Stecko, G.: A new bipolar electrode for electromyography. J. Appl. Physiol., *17:* 849, 1962.
9. Ben-Zvi, S.: The lack of safety standards in medical instrumentation. Trans. N.Y. Acad. Sci., *31:* 737–750, 1969.
10. Bruner, J. M. R.: Hazards of electrical apparatus. Anesthesiology, *28:* 396–425, 1967.

chapter 5

The Normal Electromyogram

Electromyography developed into a useful technique for clinical examination after the introduction of the concentric needle electrode by Adrian and Bronk in 1929 (1). The electrode made possible the intramuscular sampling of different regions of each muscle suspected of abnormal behavior. Its importance may be gauged by considering the patchy involvement of muscles in some neuromuscular diseases. Along with this development, the refinement of electromyographic instrumentation during the past 20 years permitted accurate observation and recording of electrical activity and simplified practical diagnostic procedure. Current procedures permit muscle action potentials to be detected, amplified, and permanently recorded so that the state of the muscle and activity of the motor nerves may be defined.

Unfortunately, standardization of the electromyographic examination cannot be as complete as, for example, an electrocardiographic examination. Skeletal muscle is not localized to one area, so that standard electrode positions are not applicable. Instead the muscles are dispersed; in the course of an examination, several muscles may be tested and each one may be sampled many times. Furthermore, the sampling of a muscle involves not only changing the position of the electrode, but also detecting potentials under different conditions of muscle activity: relaxed, mild and strong contraction. The recorded potentials for the different conditions are dissimilar in amplitude and frequency. It is thus necessary to discuss the electromyographic examination not only in terms of the patient as a whole, but also as a complete examination of each skeletal muscle.

SPONTANEOUS ACTIVITY IN THE RELAXED MUSCLE

The examination begins with the introduction of the electrode into the muscle. Because most investigators use the concentric needle electrode for routine electromyography, the present discussion assumes that this electrode is used unless stated otherwise. As the electrode penetrates into the muscle, fibers are mechanically stimulated as well as cut and injured, giving rise to a "spontaneous" burst of potentials. This discharge is also observed when the electrode is shifted from one point to another within the muscle. The spontaneous activity is called *insertion activity* and, in normal muscle, is of short duration, averaging less than 300 msec (Fig. 5.1). Diminished insertion activity is difficult to gauge but approaches zero in fibrotic atrophic muscles.

Insertion activity should not be confused with spontaneous activity detected *after* cessation of needle movement. For example, in myotonia, activity is observed after insertion activity has disappeared and there is no volitional activity. Spontaneous activity usually refers to potentials recorded after insertion activity has subsided. Of course, it is difficult to judge accurately when insertion activity ends and spontaneous activity begins; however, the distinction is unimportant when spontaneous firings are observed in disease.

Normal muscle at rest is electrically silent. This indicates that the neuromuscular system is completely relaxed and no electrical activity can be detected after the brief burst of insertion activity. In practice, it is difficult at times to obtain a completely relaxed muscle. Nervousness or improper positioning of the patient may contribute to a low frequency of firing which is *not* indicative of disease. Electrical silence in a relaxed muscle is a significant finding and should be carefully considered in the evaluation of the muscle.

An exception to the statement that a relaxed normal muscle is electrically silent are the spontaneous discharges which can be detected by a needle electrode in the end-plate region. High frequency, low amplitude spontaneous potentials are one type of discharge frequently recorded (Fig. 5.2). Ranging from 10 to 100 μV in amplitude, short in duration (1 to 2 msec), and negative in deflection, they resemble amplifier noise and over the loudspeaker have the characteristic sound of a seashell held to the ear. They also disappear with slight movement of the electrode. Buchthal and Rosenfalck (3) suggested that these potentials, commonly referred to as *end-plate noise*, represent the summated activity of nonpropagated potentials and correspond to the miniature end-plate potentials first recorded with micro-

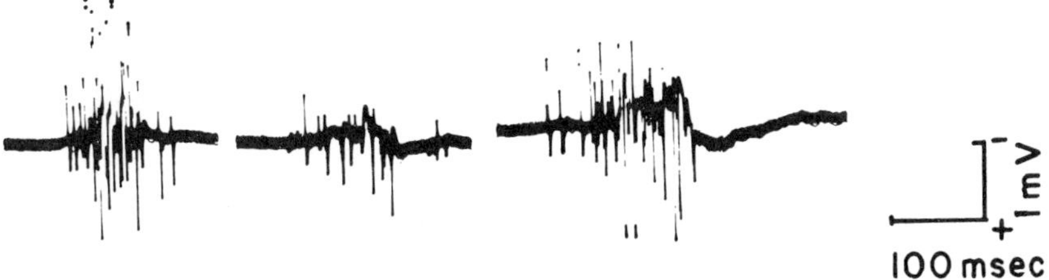

FIG. 5.1. Insertion activity recorded in normal muscle.

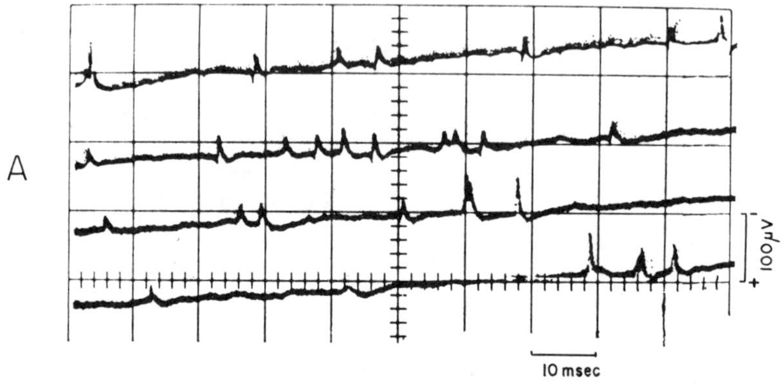

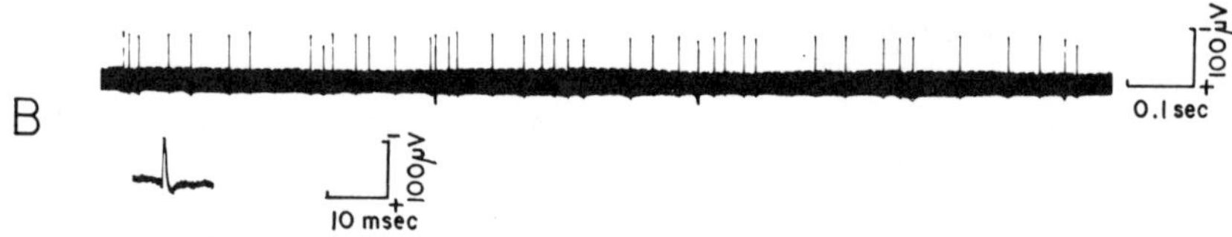

FIG. 5.2. *A*, end-plate noise. Spontaneous activity recorded in region of end-plate. *B*, another type of end-plate noise.

electrodes by Fatt and Katz (4) in amphibian muscle. Miniature end-plate potentials are nonpropagated subthreshold depolarizations and have a negative polarity when recorded extracellularly with microelectrodes. Wiederholt (5) has presented histological, electrophysiological, and pharmacological evidence which supports the hypothesis that end-plate noise recorded with EMG electrodes represents miniature end-plate potentials.

Also detected in the end-plate region are spike potentials firing at a rapid but irregular rate (Fig. 5.2). They are short duration (3 to 5 msec), low amplitude (up to 200 μV peak to peak), with a negative initial phase followed by a positive deflection. These potentials most likely originate in the muscle fibers stimulated by mechanical activation of nerve terminals (3). These potentials should not be confused with fibrillation potentials. Fibrillation potentials have an initial positive phase when recorded outside the end-plate zone.

Generally associated with these potentials may be the complaint by the patient of distinct pain; slight withdrawal of the needle causes disappearance of both potentials and pain.

THE MOTOR UNIT

With a very weak voluntary contraction, activity from single motor units may be recorded and studied. Usually several units may be seen firing together; however, delicate manipulation of the electrode and a carefully controlled volitional effort by the subject will succeed in the detection of a single motor unit action potential (Fig. 5.3). If it is recorded with a "fast" sweep on the oscilloscope or with rapidly moving paper, both amplitude and duration may be measured. During the past 20 years, Professor Fritz Buchthal and his associates have probably made the most comprehensive study of the single motor unit action potential and established useful criteria for both normal and diseased muscle (6).

For a weak volitional effort, the frequency of firing of motor units will be between 5 and 15 per sec. The parameters defining the single motor unit action potential (amplitude and duration) cannot be rigorously established because of their dependence on the type and size of the recording electrodes, the distance between electrode and the active unit, and the number of active fibers lying close to the tip of the electrode. Variation in any of these alters the amplitude or the duration (or both) of the recorded potential. Although the size and type of electrodes might be controlled, the distance between electrode and the active fibers and the exact number of active fibers are unknowns and can only be inferred from the shape of the recorded potential. At a distance of 0.12 mm from the active fibers, the peak-to-peak amplitude of the spike potential has decreased 50%, and at 0.38 mm it has fallen 90% (7). At a distance of 1 mm from the active fibers, the voltage is only about 1% of the maximal recorded spike potential and its shape has changed considerably; i.e., the positive-to-negative deflection is no longer steep. It is thus obvious that the recorded voltage amplitude is highly dependent on the distance between the electrode and the source of the action potentials.

The concentric needle electrode is the most suitable for recording single motor unit action potentials. Very gentle movement or rotation of the electrode in the muscle will certainly detect a single unit potential. Monitoring these potentials may be simplified by using a "delay line" (8). The principle of the delay line is that a single potential first triggers the oscillo-

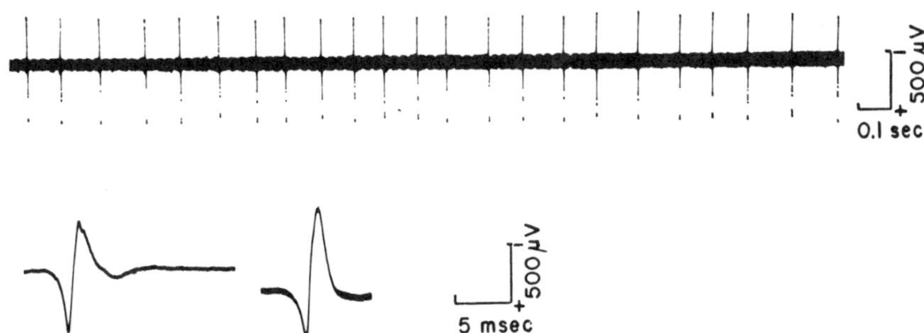

FIG. 5.3. Single motor unit action potentials recorded from biceps brachii.

scope sweep; then after a selected time delay (about 5 to 10 msec), it is displayed on the screen. When this is combined with a storage oscilloscope, amplitude and duration measurements may be easily performed. In normal muscle, the single unit action potential may be seen as a diphasic or triphasic wave. The duration of the positive-to-negative deflection should be very short, around 100 to 200 μsec. The amplitude ranges from 300 μV to 5 mV, and the total duration ranges from 3 to 16 msec. The "spike" of the action potential denotes the fast positive-to-negative phases of the potential wave shape.

The duration is measured as the time interval between the first deflection from the base line to the point at which the deflection finally returns to the base line. The duration of single motor unit action potentials may vary considerably from point to point within the same muscle and also from muscle to muscle. The mean duration should be determined by recordings of 20 to 40 different motor unit potentials within the same muscle. It should be understood that the motor unit action potential may result from the summation of action potentials from several muscle fibers of the unit, the contribution from each fiber depending on its distance from the electrode. Potentials from fibers at a distance of more than 1 mm contribute to the low amplitude slow initial and terminal phases of the motor unit potential and add to its total duration. Thus, motor unit potentials recorded with bipolar concentric electrodes tend to be shorter in duration than those from monopolar concentric needles because the distant potentials arrive simultaneously at each pickup electrode and cancel each other. The dispersion of arrival times at the monopolar electrode is determined by the spatial distribution of motor end-plates for the different fibers of the motor unit and the variation in conduction velocity. In the normal biceps brachii, for example, 67% of all nerve endings are localized within a band equal to 10% of its total muscle length (9). The *different points of origin* of the impulses may account for the spread of arrival times at the electrode and for the total duration of the unit action potential. It follows that differences in summated potential durations may be attributed to differences in the width of the zones of innervation.

Motor unit potential duration will also vary with age. For example, in the biceps brachii at age 3 the mean duration is 7.3 msec and at age 75 it is 12.8 msec. In the tibialis anterior, it is 9.2 msec at age 3 and 15.9 msec at age 75. The facial muscles normally show a much shorter mean duration: 4.3 and 7.5 msec at ages 3 and 75, respectively (10). In our laboratory we have observed the lower range to be 1 to 2 msec in normal orbicularis oris.

Finally, it should be mentioned that polyphasic potentials are observed in normal muscle. A polyphasic potential is one containing more than four phases. In some limb muscles, approximately 10% of the units may be polyphasic (11).

The Origin of the Single Motor Unit Action Potential

It is generally agreed that a fibrillation potential represents the activity of a single muscle fiber. Does the spike potential of the single motor unit also originate from a single fiber or is it the summated response of several fibers? This question has troubled electromyographers for many years, and only suggestive evidence has been available to answer it. An accurate picture of the spatial arrangement of the muscle fibers in a single motor unit would help immensely in solving this problem. Unfortunately, this knowledge is very difficult to obtain in human skeletal muscle. However, attempts have been made to infer the spatial distribution of the single unit from available histological and electrophysiological examination.

The first indication of the spatial arrangement of muscle fibers belonging to one motor unit came from the observation of patches of atrophic muscle fibers in motor neuron disease. Wohlfart (12) observed that the number of atrophic fibers *in a group* was smaller than the calculated number of fibers belonging to a single unit. Buchthal et al. (7) found, in examination of biopsies from patients with mild motor neuron disease, that the average number of muscle fibers *per atrophic field* was 10.2 ± 6.7 fibers and interpreted these findings to indicate that the single unit consists of several nonadjacent fiber groups. Buchthal called the closely packed groups "subunits" and suggested that the fibers of each motor unit are divided into such subunits, each containing an average of 10 fibers.

Buchthal devised a needle electrode containing 14 closely spaced leads (the multielectrode) which permits one spike potential to be recorded at different transverse distances (13). Results of studies performed in human skeletal muscle indicated that a maximal number of 10 to 30 fibers contributes to the spike of a single motor unit potential. This number, which represented the fibers in a subunit, was determined by noting the decrease in the motor unit spike potential with increasing distance from the source of the potentials. The single motor unit potential thus represents the completely synchronized firing of the fibers within a subunit.

Other investigators have questioned the existence of subunits in human muscle and whether the single motor unit potential actually represents the synchronized discharge of several fibers. Krnjevic and Miledi (14) investigated the distribution of single motor units in the rat phrenic-hemidiaphragm preparation by isolating and stimulating single motor nerve fibers and recording the electrical potentials of active muscle fibers with extracellular and intracellular electrodes. They presented evidence that in the rat diaphragm each motor unit extends over a relatively large area of the muscle and conjectured that, in human muscle, the potential spikes recorded electromyographically represent not more than one or two muscle fibers. Similarly, Norris and Irwin (15) found the fibers of a motor unit to be widely scattered in rat peroneus longus muscle. Ekstedt (16), in a detailed study of voluntary action potentials in human muscle with a specially constructed multielectrode and also with the Janus electrode, presents evidence that *single* muscle fiber action potentials can be recorded in the normal human electromyogram. He also observed nonsimultaneous action potentials from closely adjacent fibers belonging to the same motor unit. Ekstedt concluded that the concept of the subunit as a group of tightly packed fibers with perfectly synchronized action potential conduction was inconsistent with his results.

Stålberg et al. (17) studied the motor unit in normal extensor digitorum communis and biceps brachii muscles with a multielectrode which permitted recording from 44 sites, 300 μ apart. They demonstrated that in these muscles the muscle fibers in a single motor unit are scattered like those in animals in glycogen-depletion experiments. There was no evidence of grouping and never more than three fibers over one recording electrode in the 101 motor units studied.

Rosenfalck (18) presented an excellent mathematical analysis of the spread of action currents within nerve and muscle fibers and through the volume conductor surrounding the fibers. His calculations show that motor unit spike potentials (as well as high voltage fibrillation potentials) of human muscle can be derived from the activity of a single muscle fiber, as suggested by Krnjevic and Miledi and by Ekstedt. Rosenfalck points out that this conclusion is not incompatible with the existence of subunits. It differs, however, from the view previously held by Buchthal et al., in that Rosenfalck's analysis shows that the interaction between the action potentials of adjacent muscle fibers does not result in complete synchrony between the fibers. The absence of complete synchrony does not mean that the summated potentials from several adjacent fibers will be polyphasic; but, depending on the temporal dispersion of the action potentials, the motor unit potential may contain only small irregularities in its shape.

From this evidence, Buchthal and Rosenfalck (19) concluded that the concept of the motor subunit in normal human muscle should be abandoned.

THE INTERFERENCE PATTERN

With a minimal effort, one or two spike potentials may be clearly distinguished (discrete activity). With increased effort, the rate of discharge increases and additional motor units are recruited (reduced interference pattern). This results in a recording of many spike potentials firing asynchronously, but individual potentials can still be discriminated. As greater tension is developed, a pattern is obtained in which the many potentials, firing at a high frequency, interfere with one another so that single potentials can no longer be discriminated. This type of a record is commonly called a *full interference pattern*, and for normal muscle it is clearly observed during strong contractions (Fig. 5.4). It is usually recorded at a slow sweep speed, around 10 msec per cm.

During maximal effort the single motor units are innervated at frequencies ranging from 25 to 50 per sec. The smoothness of the contraction is due largely to the asynchronous discharge of the motor units. During muscle fatigue, grouping of motor unit potentials (decrease in frequency and increase in amplitude) has been observed and interpreted as synchronization of potentials. This synchronization is considered to be a pure chance occurrence without any physiological significance (20).

Analysis of the Interference Pattern

Attempts are constantly being made to derive more significant information from the interference pattern. After all, the interference pattern does represent the activity of many muscle fibers firing at relatively high frequencies, and it is to be expected that intensive analysis should contribute toward an accurate definition of the state of muscle. Three procedures stand out as the most interesting: (a) integration of the interference pattern, (b) frequency analysis, and (c) counting the number of spikes in the recording.

Integration of the Interference Pattern

Originally, the electromyogram was integrated by time-consuming direct measurement. The area underneath the photographed potentials was meas-

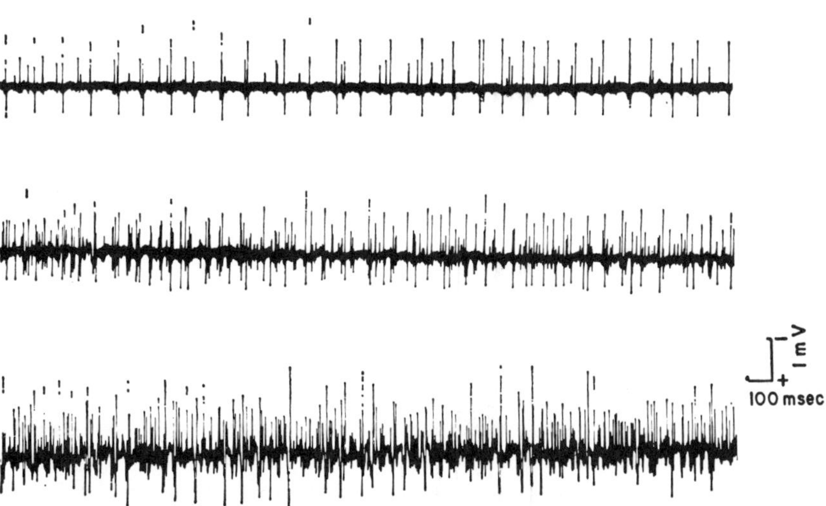

FIG. 5.4. Interference patterns. Discrete activity is shown in *top* recording. With increased effort, frequency of discharge increases and additional motor units are recruited (*middle* and *bottom* recordings).

ured with a planimeter. Today, electronic devices are available which permit integration to be performed swiftly, accurately, and over varying time intervals. The integration is accomplished by first full-wave rectifying the potentials; i.e., all negative potentials are converted to identical positive deflections so that the pattern consists of positive deflections only. The rectified potentials are then passed through a circuit which accumulates the area underneath the potentials so that the amplitude of the output at any time represents the total area summed from a given starting time. The integrator may be reset to zero at fixed time intervals or when the output reaches a predetermined level. The amplitude of the integrated activity is proportional to the amplitude, the duration, and the frequency of the potentials.

The purpose of integrating the electromyogram is to obtain a measurement which is a function of the mechanical activity of the muscle, which is very difficult to measure directly. With increasing effort, both the discharge frequency of the single motor units and the number of active units increase, so that one might expect the integrated electromyogram to increase likewise. A considerable amount of work has accumulated which defines the relationship between the muscle tension and the electrical activity. Lippold (21) recorded the electrical activity of human calf muscles with surface electrodes while simultaneously measuring the isometric tension with a dynamometer. He found a linear relationship between isometric tension and the integrated electromyogram for a submaximal contraction. Other investigators (22, 23) have demonstrated this relationship with more advanced electronic systems (Fig. 5.5). Similarly, it has been shown (24) that the integrated electrical activity increased linearly with the velocity of shortening when the muscle contracted with constant tension. At constant velocity of shortening, the integrated potentials were proportional to the tension. It is evident from these studies that integration of the interference pattern provides a measure of the number of active fibers and their rate of discharge.

In a study involving abduction of the little finger, Mason and Munro (25) concluded that the amplitude of the action potentials, either maximum or mean, is not a reliable indicator of muscle tension. Instead, they consider the frequency of electrical activity a better estimate of isometric tension.

Frequency Analysis

An analysis of the electromyogram for the various frequency components was first introduced as a convenient method for determining changes in the duration of the action potential. Because the action potential duration appears to change most consistently with different neuromuscular disorders and may also be a good indicator of the early stages of disease, it was felt that their determination would enhance electromyographic diagnosis. However, the procedure for recording and measuring these durations is time

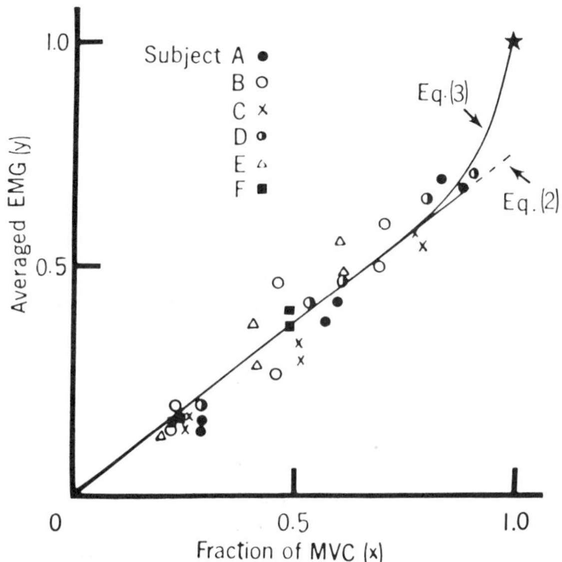

FIG. 5.5. Plot of the magnitude of force exerted (fraction of maximal voluntary contraction (*MVC*)) and the averaged EMG activity for six subjects. *Line* through data points represents the best fit as calculated from two curve-fitting equations. Both the force value and the averaged EMG activity have been normalized, as a proportion of the subject's maximal force and of the EMG value corresponding to that force, respectively. The EMG activity increases almost linearly with the force in the submaximal force range but increases more sharply near the maximal force. (From E. Kuroda, V. Klissouras, and J. H. Milsum: Electrical and metabolic activities and fatigue in human isometric contraction. J. Appl. Physiol., *29:* 360, 1970.)

consuming. In 1951 Richardson (26) described a simple technique for the instantaneous frequency analysis of an electromyogram which could detect the desired changes and replace the measurement of individual fiber action potentials. In 1965 Kaiser and Petersen (27), using their own technique of frequency analysis, demonstrated a good correlation between actual measurement of potential duration and that derived from frequency analysis. Essentially, frequency analysis was used by some electromyographers to provide a more objective method of discriminating normal from pathological activity. However, this technique has not gained wide acceptance in clinical electromyography.

A complex muscle action potential pattern may be considered as a summation of many simple waveforms, each of which has a frequency and an amplitude. Frequency analysis determines the amplitude of these waveforms at each frequency. Frequency analysis has been performed by passing an interference pattern through several electronic filters and plotting the result as a histogram of frequency distribution (28). Another method involves first digitizing the data, then using a digital computer to perform the analysis and to present a smoothed spectrum over a given frequency range (29). Analysis may be performed from either needle or surface electrode recording. The basic difference between frequency spectra of the two types of electrodes is the lower high frequency content of the surface electrodes (Fig. 4.9).

Walton (28), using needle electrodes, investigated the potential amplitude variation between 40 and 16,000 Hz for a large group of normal subjects and patients with neuromuscular diseases. He found in most cases single peaked curves with occasional double peaked variations. During maximal effort of normal muscles against resistance, the spectra peaks were between 100 and 200 Hz, falling off rapidly to zero at about 800 Hz. In patients with myopathy, a significant shift of the peak frequencies to higher values (greater than 400 Hz) was reported. This shift was related to the presence of polyphasic potentials. Richardson (30) and Fex and Krakau (31) also observed a shift to higher frequencies in myopathy. The latter authors found in patients with anterior horn cell lesions a shift of the peak frequencies to the opposite direction, toward the lower values.

More recently, Cosi and Mazzella (32) reported that the frequency spectrum of voluntary effort using a needle electrode varies from one point to another in the same muscle and even at the same point, depending upon the amount of effort. With surface electrodes, the spectrum changed very little with different degrees of effort. In normal tibialis anterior muscle, the peak frequency was between 185 and 228 Hz. They recommend examining at least three to five points of each muscle with needle electrodes.

Even with the added sensitivity of frequency analysis of EMG potentials, diagnosis of the early stages of neuromuscular disease is difficult. Although shifts from normal peak frequency are observed for both myopathic and neuropathic disorders, the difficulty is deciding at which point the shift to the right or left is significant. A better definition of the peak frequencies obtained from normal muscle under fixed conditions is required.

Frequency analysis of EMG potentials has been applied extensively to the study of muscle fatigue. Kadefors et al. (33), using both needle and surface electrodes, reported the following modifications of the frequency spectrum from a fatigued normal muscle: (a) a total increase in the EMG level, (b) an increase in the amplitude of the low frequency components, and (c) a decrease in the high frequency components. They considered that the increase in EMG level was due to synchronization and recruitment of new motor units. In later work, Kadefors et al. (34) indicate that interruption of the blood flow through the muscle may cause changes in the frequency spectrum.

In our own study of muscle fatigue attributable to prolonged isometric contraction, we also observed an increase in low frequencies and a decrease in high frequencies (Fig. 5.6). A narrow band frequency analyzer was used to determine the spectrum from an interference pattern recorded with surface electrodes.

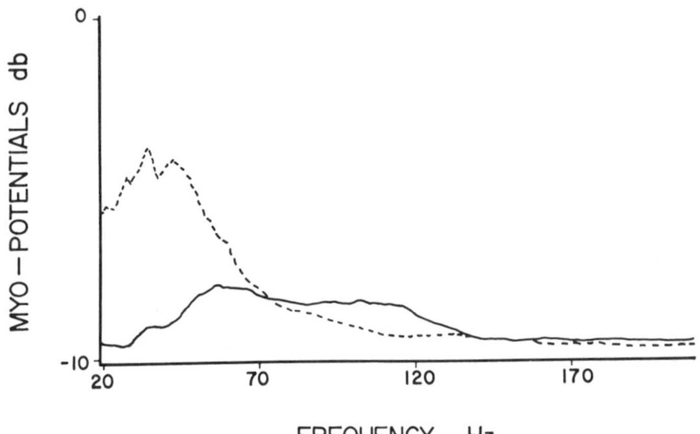

FIG. 5.6. *Solid line*, frequency spectrum obtained from biceps brachii with surface electrodes before fatiguing contraction. *Dashed line*, response obtained after 2 min of holding a 20-lb weight.

Willison Procedure

Another approach to characterize the pattern of activity during volitional effort has been the determination of the number of spikes occurring in the interference pattern. Willison (35) devised an excellent technique which circumvents some of the problems associated with simple counting of spikes with a pulse counter. Instead of counting spikes from a fixed base line, this technique uses the point of change in phase of potential variations (turns) as the reference point for determining the amplitude of the following potential. Every change of potential greater than 100 μV was counted. This threshold level was selected to avoid counting small random oscillations and noise. Thus, changes in direction of the potential are counted and not the individual motor unit action potentials. The mean amplitude of these potentials was also computed.

Interference patterns were recorded during voluntary contraction at standard tensions with a concentric needle electrode. Willison (35) found, in patients with muscle disease, counts of potential changes up to 3 times the highest observed in normal subjects. The mean amplitude of the potential changes was also abnormal.

Automatic methods have since been devised which permit the interference pattern to be converted into two pulse trains which represent increments of voltage and changes of phase. Finally, a special purpose digital computer analyzes the pulse trains and presents data describing the EMG activity. These include the total number of reversals of potential occurring in a preset period of time, histograms of the intervals between potential reversals, and the accumulated amplitude of all potentials in a preset period (36).

Fuglsang-Frederiksen and Månsson (37) analyzed the method of Willison

(35) and found that during repeated contractions the number of turns and mean amplitude were reproducible within 10 to 25%, suggesting that the same motor units are activated during repeated contractions. In their study, the electrical activity during different degrees of voluntary effort was recorded and analyzed both on-line and off-line in flexors and extensors of the arm at the elbow. For adequate representation of activity it was necessary to record from 10 sites evenly distributed over the muscle. Fuglsang-Frederiksen and Månsson also demonstrated that when a fixed force of 2 kg was exerted at the wrist (35), the number of turns decreased by 30 to 40% with increasing maximum force of different adult subjects, whereas when the force was adjusted relative to the maximum force, the number of turns was the same in different subjects. Reproducibility was best when 30% of maximum was used, although the variation from subject to subject was the same whether the force was 10, 20, or 30% of maximum. The shape of the histograms of time intervals and of amplitudes between turns varied considerably. The percentage of short time intervals (less than 0.75 msec) and of small amplitudes (less than 0.4 mV) was best suited to compare with findings in patients.

AUTOMATIC ANALYSIS: COMPUTERS

Present criteria for the evaluation of the electromyograph are based on study of the duration, amplitude, shape, and variation in the discharge pattern of the muscle's electrical potentials. Measurements of these parameters are usually performed manually, if and when they are actually determined. Too often, evaluation is dependent on the examiner's subjective observations, with the result that important but subtle changes in mild, early cases or variations in the course of the disease may be missed. It has become more and more apparent that quantitative and objective assessment of the electromyographic data is essential if the state of the art and our capabilities are to be improved. Enhancement of accurate interpretation of the data, less time spent per examination in laborious manual calculation, and increased diagnostic accuracy are some of the benefits which are to be derived from quantification of electromyography.

To attain these goals, various approaches employing either analog or digital techniques have been explored. The major effort in recent years has been to automate measurement of motor unit potential durations, the significance of which is obvious when one considers the importance of this information and the difficulty of manual determinations. However, the procedure is not simple. Variations in wave shape, base line noise, and overlap of two or more potentials impose requirements on the automaticity of the procedure which are not easily remedied even with a high speed digital computer. Measurement of the potential duration requires, essentially, recognition of the fluctuations as true motor unit potentials, reliable determination of the base line, and definition of the start and end of the potentials.

Rathjen et al. (38), one of the first to apply the digital computer to analysis of the duration of motor unit potentials, used a Digital Equipment Corporation PDP-8. Basically, their system involved the detection of myopotentials with a double coaxial needle electrode, amplification, analog-to-digital conversion, and analysis. A preset voltage "window" eliminated low amplitude noise and base line drift, and wave shape recognition and selection were performed visually from a monitor oscilloscope by the investigator. When acceptable motor units were observed, the automated analysis was initiated so that each potential was processed.

At about the same time, Kunze and Erbslöh (39) and Kopec and Hausmanowa-Petrusewicz (40) independently developed an automatic analyzer of electromyograms which operated on-line using a digital computer. In the former system, action potential duration, polarity of the first phase, number of phases, and integrated amplitude were some of the parameters measured and printed out (41). Using a Polish digital computer ANOPS, Kopec and Hausmanowa-Petrusewicz measured the duration of single motor unit potentials at a level of 20 μV above the base line and the number of phases in the potential by counting the changes of polarization above 40 μV. Only motor unit potentials with peak-to-peak amplitude greater than 100 μV were accepted and analyzed by the computer. Two independent histograms showing potential durations and number of phases of the chosen potentials were simultaneously displayed.

Mean values obtained by conventional manual measurement techniques were compared with the data obtained from digital analysis of the same electromyographic examination of the biceps brachii of 115 patients (34 controls, 68 patients with myopathy, and 13 patients with neurogenic atrophy). There were only insignificant differences between the two methods in the control group. In myopathy the mean duration value obtained from the automatic analysis was about 20% shorter than those measured conventionally, whereas in neurogenic atrophy the automatically derived mean value was 50% longer. The authors consider the automatic analysis to be sufficiently accurate to differentiate between pathological (myogenic and neurogenic) and normal activity. In addition, the numerical determination of phases and the mean values of duration are helpful in distinguishing borderline pathology (42).

Bergmans (43) developed two different programs for a Digital Equipment Corporation PDP-12 computer, one where recognition of the different motor unit potentials was made automatically by the computer and another where recognition was made by the operator who interacted with the computer with push buttons. The program proceeded as follows: the computer was instructed to isolate a single potential from an electromyograph record and to compare it with other sequential potentials. A given potential was considered a single motor unit potential when the program detected its occurrence twice under identical form. The computer was programmed to continue seeking a "first" potential until this criterion was satisfied.

When a single motor unit potential was identified, duration, amplitude (peak-to-peak), number of phases, and number of peaks of the potential were then measured and stored. After this, the potential was displayed to enable the operator to determine whether it was to be accepted or rejected (e.g., if an artifact was present or if the given motor unit potential was seen to recur). If it was accepted, the various measured parameters were directed in core memory to areas where histograms could be generated and later displayed. In the automatic mode of operation, each identified motor unit potential was subjected to a point-to-point comparison with all potentials already stored and, if different, was placed in storage for measurement of the parameters.

Duration measurements were performed by detecting the beginning and end of the motor unit potential with a process of identification which eliminated potentials superimposed on slow potential shifts, and in which superimposed noise was reduced by summation of the motor unit potentials. The elimination of the noise before the duration measurement permitted the threshold to be maintained at a low level and reduced to a minimal amount the possible errors attributable to loss of the initial and final components of the motor unit potential.

The program using operator recognition proved to be faster and more efficient with respect to the amount of core memory occupied by the program. Parameters of 100 different motor unit potentials could usually be determined in less than 1 hr.

Recently, Hirose et al. (44) compared quantitation of the interference pattern as determined manually with that obtained by digital computer analysis. The number of potentials, the mean amplitude, and the mean interval (not measured manually) were calculated from an electromyogram recorded during maximal volitional effort for a period of 1 sec. The results established that computer analysis was more accurate and efficient and that information could be obtained more easily from each muscle, diminishing sampling bias.

As an alternative to measurements performed with the aid of a digital computer, Moosa and Brown (45) devised an automatic method of detecting changes in motor unit action potential duration using simple analog computer techniques. Recorded at maximum strength of contraction, the potentials were passed through an analog analyzer which computed an index corresponding to the reciprocal of the amplitude-weighted mean phase duration of the signal. This index is closely related to the index used by Van den Bosch (46), which is the ratio of the mean number of phases per potential to the mean potential duration, except that the Moosa and Brown index is weighted according to the relative amplitude of the EMG signals and obtained automatically. Moosa and Brown found that their analog analysis gave excellent discrimination between normal and abnormal electromyographic patterns.

The results of the various laboratories demonstrate the successful applicability of computer analysis to the evaluation of electromyographic data. It is apparent, however, that the general format and procedure are still in the developmental stage. Further exploration combined with modern technology, encouraged by the low cost of computer hardware, and improved software will ultimately permit the generalized employment of automatic online analysis and quantitative evaluation.

ESTIMATION OF THE NUMBER OF MOTOR UNITS WITHIN A MUSCLE

An accurate assessment of the number of active motor units within a muscle would be of inestimable value in the investigation and detection of neuromuscular disease. Procedures based on the analysis of the interference pattern, although presenting valuable information, provide only approximations of the intact motor unit content. A method was recently described which, although restricted to particular muscles, presumes to provide an estimate of the number of functioning motor units (47). The principle is relatively simple: the amplitude of the muscle action potential generated by a single motor unit of average size divided into the potential sum of all of the motor units in the whole muscle equals the number of motor units within the muscle. In practice, the procedure is a quantal one: to grade carefully the strength of an electrical stimulus applied to an appropriate motor nerve, to recruit successive single motor units, and then to calculate the mean motor unit potential amplitude; the response of the total population of units is evoked by a maximal stimulus to the nerve.

The majority of observations were made with the extensor digitorum brevis (EDB) muscle. A pair of stimulating electrodes was positioned over the EDB so as to completely cover the end-plate zone (Fig. 5.7). The stimulus, consisting of rectangular voltage pulses of 50-μsec duration, was gradually increased from a subthreshold value until 11 increments in the EDB muscle response were recorded (Fig. 5.8*a*). The increments appeared to be quantal, inasmuch as intermediate responses were never observed; therefore, each was attributed to activation of an additional motor unit. The muscle response after supramaximal motor nerve stimulation was also recorded (Fig. 5.8*b*). In the example shown in Figure 5.8 for a normal subject, the mean motor unit potential was 40 μV, the total muscle response was 8 mV, and the number of motor units was calculated to be 200.

The authors themselves acknowledge that the method is a gross one, with the difficulty of investigating a sample of units that is representative of the entire population, and that some of the increments may not correspond to

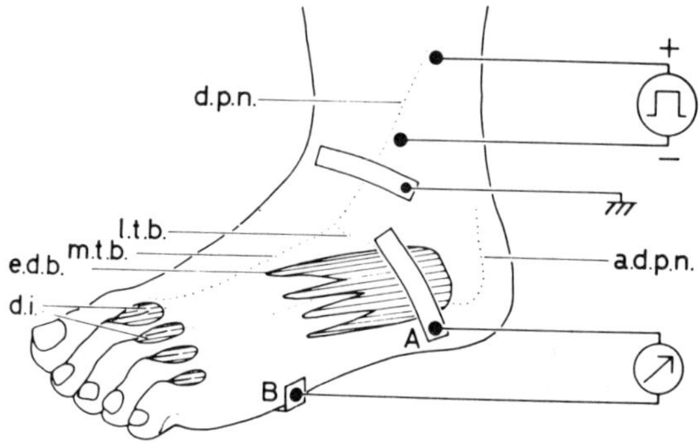

FIG. 5.7. Termination of the deep peroneal nerve on the dorsum of the foot and arrangement of stimulating and recording electrodes. *A*, recording electrode over end-plate zone of EDB; *B*, reference electrode; *a.d.p.n.*, accessory deep peroneal nerve; *d.i.*, first and second dorsal interosseus muscles; *d.p.n.*, deep peroneal nerve; *e.d.b.*, extensor digitorum brevis; *l.t.b.* and *m.t.b.*, lateral and medial terminal branches of deep peroneal nerve. (From A. J. McComas, P. R. W. Fawcett, M. J. Campbell, and R. E. P. Sica: Electrophysiological estimation of the number of motor units within a human muscle. J. Neurol. Neurosurg. Psychiatry, *34:* 123, 1971.)

additional single unit responses. In spite of these reservations they found that the reproducibility of the results in any subject was acceptable, and the experimental results agreed reasonably well with calculations based on counts of axons in postmortem specimens of the peroneal nerve (47, 48).

The procedure was subsequently applied by McComas and his colleagues to the study of patients with various types of neuromuscular disorders. The results, particularly those observed in the different forms of muscular dystrophy, and conclusions drawn therefrom have not conformed with classical concepts and, hence, have become highly controversial. McComas and his associates found a reduction in the number of functioning motor units of the EDB muscle in each of the following disease states: Duchenne's muscular dystrophy (49), myotonic dystrophy (50, 51), limb girdle and facioscapulohumeral dystrophies (52), Kugelberg-Welander disease (53), motor neuron disease (53), atrophy after upper motor neuron lesions (54), McArdle's disease (55), and thyrotoxicosis (56).

Likewise, a progressive decrease in the number of functioning motor units was established to occur in healthy individuals beyond the age of 60 years (57). Extending the study to other muscles, the same investigators also found a selective loss of motor units in the thenar, hypothenar, and soleus muscles of patients with muscular dystrophy (58). This could not have been due to nerve trauma, because there was no evidence of sensory axon involvement in the median, ulnar, and sural nerves. It was noted, however, that in any one patient, the EDB muscle is likely to be more involved than the thenar or hypothenar muscles.

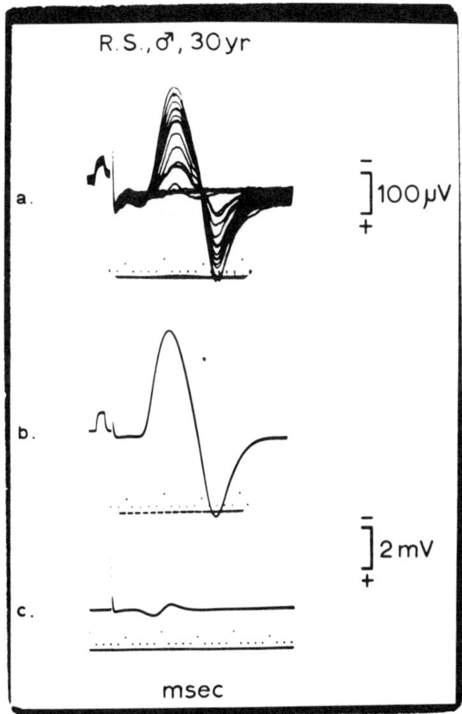

FIG. 5.8. Incremental responses of EDB after excitation of deep peroneal nerve with threshold and slightly suprathreshold stimuli (*a*) and maximal stimuli (*b*). In *a*, several traces have been superimposed for each size of response. In the lowest trace (*c*), surface electrodes on the dorsum of the foot were used to excite selectively the first dorsal interosseus muscle, and the electrotonically conducted potentials were recorded by the standard electrodes over EDB and the sole. (From A. J. McComas, P. R. W. Fawcett, M. J. Campbell, and R. E. P. Sica: Electrophysiological estimation of the number of motor units within a human muscle. J. Neurol. Neurosurg. Psychiatry, *34:* 124, 1971.)

To explain their unique observations, McComas et al. introduced the concept of "sick" motor neurons (48, 59). Their hypothesis defined three stages of motor neuron function (Fig. 5.9): "healthy," "sick," or "dead." A motor neuron was regarded as healthy if it conducted impulses at normal rates along the axon, transmitted excitation effectively across the neuromuscular junctions, and maintained all of the muscle fibers of the motor unit in a healthy condition. A sick motor neuron, a result of disease, had difficulty maintaining satisfactory synaptic connections with its muscle fibers. Thus, conduction velocity along the axon could be normal but the ability to acquire previously denervated muscle fibers was impaired. Dead motor neurons are those which have ceased to exert any influence on the muscle fibers. In Duchenne's and myotonic dystrophy the surviving motor neurons were

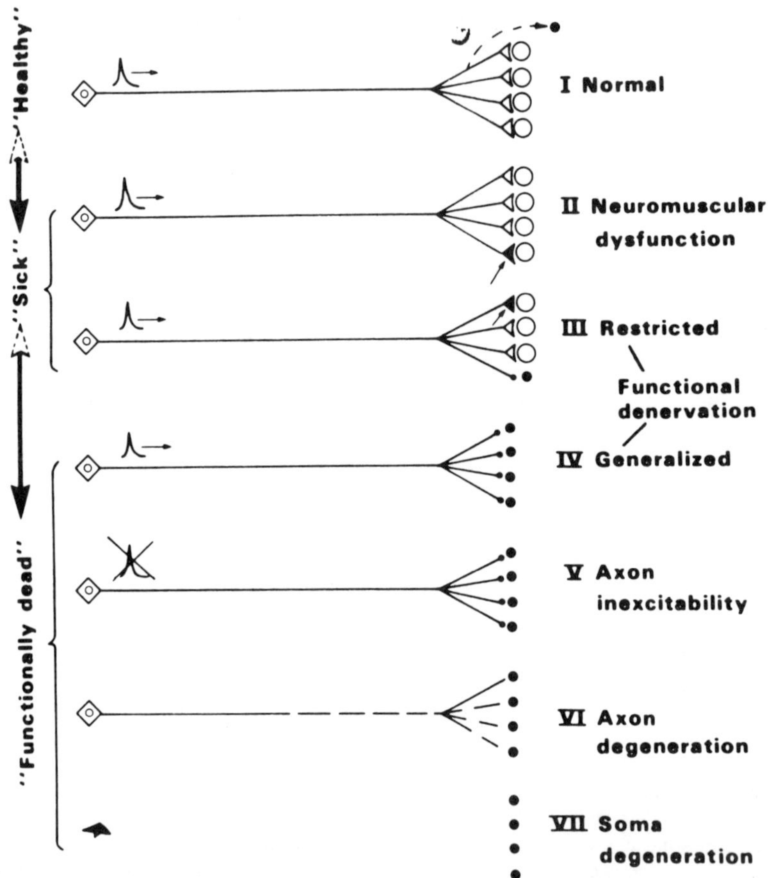

FIG. 5.9. Stages of motor neuron dysfunction. Muscle fibers are shown at *right*, atrophied ones indicated by *filled circles*. In phase *I* the ability of a healthy motor neuron to adopt a denervated muscle fiber by axonal sprouting is evident. In phases *II* and *III* the *arrows* signify impaired neuromuscular transmission. Completely nonfunctioning axon terminals are represented by *small filled circles*. Phase *II* signifies the onset of motor neuron dysfunction; phase *III* occurs when the denervated muscle fibers undergo degeneration; in phase *IV* all of the muscle fibers have become functionally denervated; phase *V* represents impulse propagation failure, and degeneration of the axon is phase *VI*. Functioning units which are normal or slightly reduced in size, as seen in the dystrophies, are represented by phases *II* and *III*. (From A. J. McComas, R. E. P. Sica, A. R. M. Upton, and F. Petito: Sick motoneurons and muscle disease. Ann. N. Y. Acad. Sci., *228:* 276, 1974.)

regarded as sick because the relatively normal sizes of their units indicated that the cells had failed to innervate muscle fibers relinquished by the dead motor neurons. In the limb girdle and facioscapulohumeral dystrophies, a neurogenic process was indicated as well, because the presence of enlarged motor units meant that potentially healthy muscle fibers had lost their original nerve supply and had been reinnervated by healthy neurons. It was thus concluded that diseases long considered primary disorders of muscle may actually be the result of abnormal motor neuron function.

The above proposal, representing the strongest support for the neurogenic hypothesis of muscle disease, has not received universal acceptance. The method has been criticized on the grounds that the noise level of the recording system was high enough to obscure motor unit action potentials of small amplitude which are expected in the dystrophies and indicated by the electromyographic findings of small amplitude and short duration motor unit action potentials (60). Another criticism was based on findings in the thenar and EDB muscles that demonstrated single motor units of much larger size than those few close to the motor threshold on which the average unit potential size is based (61). This suggests that the motor unit estimates based on an average unit potential size of the first few motor units excited above the motor threshold may not be valid but, in fact, may lead to an overestimate of the true motor unit population.

Independent investigations using variations of the McComas procedure have reported results disparate with the original findings. In one recent study, estimations of the number and size of motor units in the EDB muscle showed no significant difference between patients with Duchenne's muscular dystrophy and controls, whereas the size of the motor unit action potentials was significantly reduced in the patient group (60). Similarly, the same authors found no loss of functioning motor units in limb girdle muscular dystrophy but a decreased number in chronic spinal muscular atrophy (62).

New results were recently reported by Ballantyne and Hansen (63, 64) whose novel system utilized on-line computer analysis. The basic procedure was similar to that of McComas et al. (47) except that data processing was handled on-line by a PDP-12 computer. Successive motor units recruited singly by application of finely graded stimuli to the anterior tibial nerve were displayed and recognized by an operator, who then instructed the computer to store the potential. In this manner, the electrical responses of the first evoked motor unit, the first and second, the first, second, and third, and so on were each stored sequentially in up to 15 computer memory stores. Finally, the supramaximally evoked muscle action potential was sampled and stored. The number of motor units was calculated by dividing the average absolute area of a motor unit potential into the absolute area of the supramaximally evoked muscle action potential. This contrasts with the McComas et al. procedure, where peak-to-peak amplitudes of the evoked potentials were measured to calculate the number of motor units. It is interesting to note that the same on-line computer analysis can be used to isolate the electrical responses of individual motor units from the muscle compound action potential (i.e., by serial subtraction of the memory stores), and latencies, amplitudes, and durations can be measured (65). Ballantyne and Hansen found that the number of motor units in the EDB muscle was within the normal range in patients with myasthenia gravis and Duchenne, limb girdle, and facioscapulohumeral muscular dystrophies, but it was significantly reduced in myotonic muscular dystrophy (63, 64). They consider the computer-assisted method to be considerably more advantageous than the amplitude method of McComas et al., and they question the validity of the latter's results and concepts.

Brown and Milner-Brown (66, 67) presented evidence that two of the most critical assumptions made in estimating the number of motor units were not correct—namely, that (a) fluctuations in electrical excitability and overlap in firing thresholds are inherent properties of motor axons, and that (b) motor units whose voltages are much larger than the incremental steps evoked by nerve stimulation can be recruited at high isometric contraction and by the F recurrent discharge method. It follows that any estimate of the motor unit number which excludes these properties can generally lead to erroneous conclusions. The authors devised an independent method to eliminate the problem of fluctuation in the number of potential steps at constant stimulus intensity and to produce a large and more representative sample of motor units. With the aid of a laboratory computer (on-line Hewlett-Packard 2100), multiple point electrical stimulation along peripheral nerves was used to isolate 10 to 30 motor units from the thenar and hypothenar muscles of normal subjects and patients with entrapment neuropathy (68). They found with this method that (a) motor units were recruited in an orderly pattern from small to large and from longer to shorter latencies by graded electrical stimulation in both normal and pathological cases, and that (b) axonal branching can occur in the forearm 200 mm more proximal to the motor point in intrinsic hand muscles. One consequence of axonal branching could be that stimulation at points distal to the branching would excite fractions of single motor units and could account in part for the apparent exclusion of large motor units by nerve stimulation. As a result, the authors state that no method to quantitate the number of motor units in muscles has been found to be entirely acceptable.

McComas and his associates have attempted painstakingly to answer the various criticisms leveled at their observations (58, 69, 70). To date, the issue has not been settled objectively and remains controversial. The current state of affairs concerning the neurogenic theory of myopathic disorders is best summarized in the words of McComas et al., who stated (69): "further contributions for, or against, the neurogenic hypothesis are welcome, and we assure followers of the controversy that the matter is far from settled."

SINGLE FIBER ELECTROMYOGRAPHY

In 1963, Ekstedt and Stålberg (71) described a novel method of recording extracellular *single* muscle fiber action potentials in voluntarily activated human muscle, and 1 year later, after an extended study, Ekstedt (72) reported that when recording from two single muscle fibers belonging to the same motor unit, the time interval between the two fiber action potentials showed a variability (of the order of 10 to 30 μsec) at consecutive discharges. This variability was designated "action potential jitter" and was interpreted to be primarily due to variation in the synaptic delay of the two motor endplates (Fig. 5.10). Recording the jitter was found to be useful for research and diagnostic purposes and subsequently was utilized in the investigation of a gamut of neuromuscular disorders as well as in the measurement of fiber propagation velocity, muscle fiber density within the motor unit, activity in the terminal nerve tree, and single motor neurons (73). The technique is now called "single fiber electromyography" and is considered complementary to the conventional electromyographic examination on the grounds that additional information is acquired.

In single fiber electromyography, single muscle fiber action potentials are deliberately sought and discerned by studying their shape at consecutive discharges. The use of special electrodes and recording technique increases selectivity and facilitates the possibility of recording action potentials consistently from individual muscle fibers. The single fiber action potentials

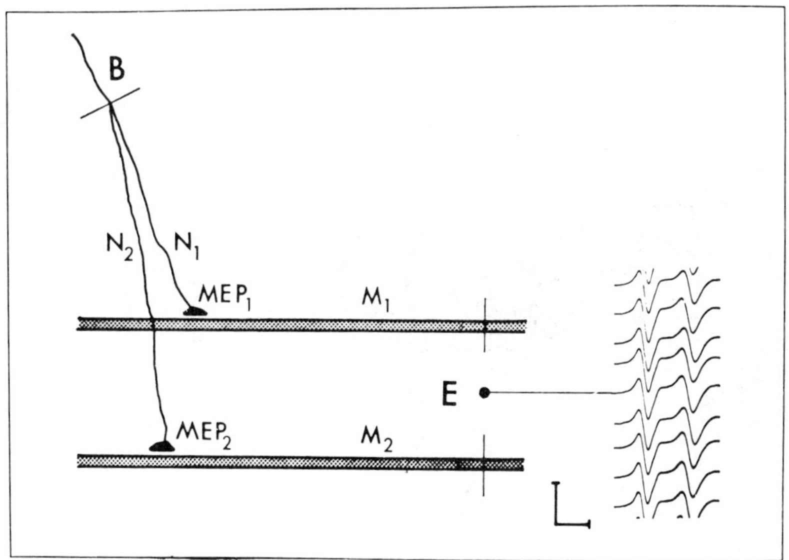

FIG. 5.10. Recording conditions. Two muscle fibers (M_1 and M_2) are innervated by an axon, dividing at point B into the terminal nerve fibers N_1 and N_2. The electrode, E, records action potentials from both M_1 and M_2, a potential pair. The time interval between the two fiber potentials varies at consecutive discharges (the jitter) because of differences in the transmission time between B and E for the two pathways. Calibration: 2 mV and 500 μsec. (From L.-O. Dahlback, J. Ekstedt, and E. Stålberg: Ischemic effect on impulse transmission to the muscle fibers in man. Electroencephalogr. Clin. Neurophysiol., *29:* 580, 1970.)

recorded with the special electrodes have a shorter duration, faster rise time, and considerably higher amplitude than those recorded with conventional concentric needle electrodes. Ekstedt and Stålberg (74) have defined important prerequisites for an optimal single fiber recording:

Small Electrode Surface

For a highly selective recording it is essential to have a maximal ratio between the amplitude of recorded action potentials from near and from distant fibers. The electrode should be small enough so that there is no decrease in the amplitude of the action potential or distortion of the potential shape when recording close to a muscle fiber. An electrode diameter of 25 μ has been shown to be optimal (75).

The electrode construction best suited for single fiber electromyography has been found to be a needle with electrode surfaces mounted in the side, similar to the Buchthal multielectrode (76) except that the former has a smaller diameter cannula and leading-off surfaces. Electrodes have been used with up to 14 platinum recording surfaces. For routine investigation, simple needle electrodes have been constructed with only one or a few leading-off surfaces, resembling the electrodes designed by Fleck (77) (Fig. 5.11). Recordings are usually made relative to a reference electrode, either

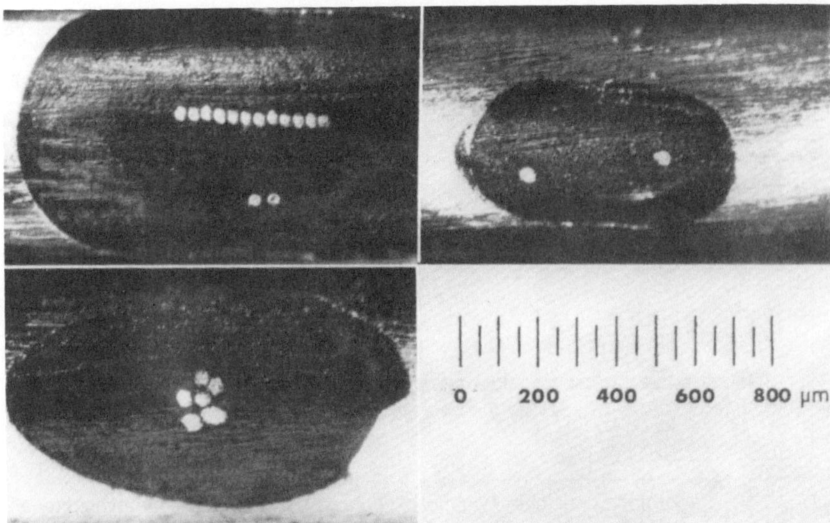

FIG. 5.11. Photomicrographs of the arrays of leading-off surfaces of some needle electrodes used for single fiber electromyography. The lower electrode can also be used for selective bipolar stimulation of intramuscular nerve twigs. The diameter of the leading-off surface is 25 μm. (From J. Ekstedt and E. Stålberg: Single fibre electromyography for the study of the microphysiology of the human muscle. In *New Developments in Electromyography and Clinical Neurophysiology*, vol. 1, p. 96. S. Karger, Basel, 1973.)

a cutaneous or a subcutaneously placed needle electrode, which is located near the muscle under investigation and electrically silent.

Small Electrode-Fiber Distance

Because the potential amplitude decreases steeply with increasing distance from the active fiber, the electrode should be as close as possible to the fiber surface. In this position, remote fibers of the motor unit do not contribute significantly to the recorded action potential.

Potential-triggered Sweeps

It is essential to have a potential-triggered oscilloscope display and a fast sweep speed (100 μsec per division). This permits the consecutive action potentials to be superimposed on the oscilloscope screen and examined for any variability.

Stable Action Potentials

To be classified a single muscle fiber action potential, the shape of consecutive action potentials must be identical at consecutive discharges provided that the recording system has a time resolution of at least 10 μsec. It is important, therefore, to have an amplifier of high electrical stability and a stable position of the electrode with respect to the muscle fiber to eliminate movement artifact. Hand-held electrodes have been found to be superior to any mechanical arrangement. Much of the interference can be reduced by setting the lower frequency limit to a value between 100 and 1000 Hz.

Single fiber electromyography is performed preferably during slight voluntary activation of the muscle, but electrical stimulation can also be used. Any muscle in which a slight contraction can be maintained for over 3 min can be employed; Ekstedt and Stålberg used the extensor digitorum communis muscle for many investigations. Owing to the random distribution of muscle fibers within a motor unit, activity from only one fiber is usually recorded. Occasionally, activities from two or sometimes more muscle fibers are recorded, as a potential pair or multiple potentials, respectively. At consecutive discharges the interpotential interval shows a random variation called "jitter." Triggering the sweep with the first action potential in the pair produces the second potential at different positions on the oscilloscope screen.

In normal muscle the jitter is due to a variable transmission time in the motor end-plate and, to a minor degree, variation in propagation velocity along the muscle and nerve fibers. Increased jitter outside the normal range is an indication of abnormal conduction in some part of these anatomic structures. In normal muscles, the jitter expressed as "mean consecutive difference" is of the order of 5 to 50 μsec, varying slightly with different muscles.

Myasthenia Gravis. Some of the motor end-plates of patients with myasthenia gravis show normal jitter; others show increased jitter with or without partial neuromuscular block within the same muscle. In addition, motor end-plates belonging to the same motor unit have different jitter. The minimal functional disturbance is an increased jitter; in more severe transmission defects, the jitter is further increased and impulse blockings occur. The degree of blocking increases during activity and is reduced after intravenous injection of Tensilon in untreated or undertreated patients, and the jitter decreases but does not become normal. In overtreated patients, a small dose of Tensilon increases the degree of blocking.

Single fiber electromyography can reveal a disturbed neuromuscular function before any transmission block appears, that is, before clinical symptoms are present and when other conventional neurophysiological investigations are normal. If the jitter is normal in all motor end-plates studied in a muscle with weakness, myasthenia gravis can be excluded. The procedure was recently expanded to include repetitive stimulation of the nerve to the muscle being investigated with single fiber recording techniques. The new method allows an improved evaluation of the patient who is minimally affected as well as the one severely involved (78–80).

Muscular Dystrophy. In muscular dystrophy of proximal distribution, the jitter is usually normal but occasionally can be slightly increased and show some blocking (73).

Dystrophia myotonica. Jitter and fiber density are usually increased.

Myotonia congenita. Jitter is usually normal.

Lower motor neuron. During reinnervation the recorded action potentials are successively more complex. The spike components initially show a large jitter and blocking, but, after some months, the complexes are more stable and show less jitter and little or no impulse blocking. This is a sign of functional improvement and can serve as a guide estimating the age of reinnervation potentials in different neuropathies. In amyotrophic lateral sclerosis, "giant potentials" are found to be composed of action potentials with up to 5 to 15 components as a sign of increased fiber density in the motor unit. The jitter is considerably increased and shows blocking. Fiber density and duration of the action potentials were also increased in progressive muscular atrophy, familial spinal muscular atrophy, and syringomyelia (73, 81).

In *polyneuropathy* due to uremia and diabetes, the fiber density within the motor unit and impulse transmission were mainly normal. In alcoholic polyneuropathy, fiber density was significantly increased and impulse transmission was impaired in a number of action potential complexes, which are signs of reinnervation (82).

MACROELECTROMYOGRAPHY

Both the concentric needle electrode and the monopolar electrode detect only a fraction of the total number of fibers that make up a motor unit. This point is illustrated in the biceps brachii muscle where the motor unit has at least 200 fibers, but only two to 12 fibers contribute to the spike component of the motor unit potential (83). To detect activity from more fibers of the motor unit and thereby gain more information, Stålberg (84) devised a special electrode to record what he called the "macro EMG."

The electrode is a 5.0-cm long steel cannula with a 25-μm diameter platinum wire exposed through a side port 1.0 cm from the tip. The cannula is insulated except for a 2-cm length from the tip. The small wire electrode with the cannula as a reference is connected to one channel; the cannula and a separate needle electrode inserted at least 30 cm away are connected to a second channel (Fig. 5.12).

The recording procedure involves averaging the activity detected on one channel, and the potentials on the other channel serve as the triggers for the averager. The procedure can be described briefly as follows. After insertion into a muscle, the cannula is positioned to record a single fiber action potential during a slight voluntary contraction. These potentials, which should be firing at a fairly regular rate, trigger an averager. The potentials

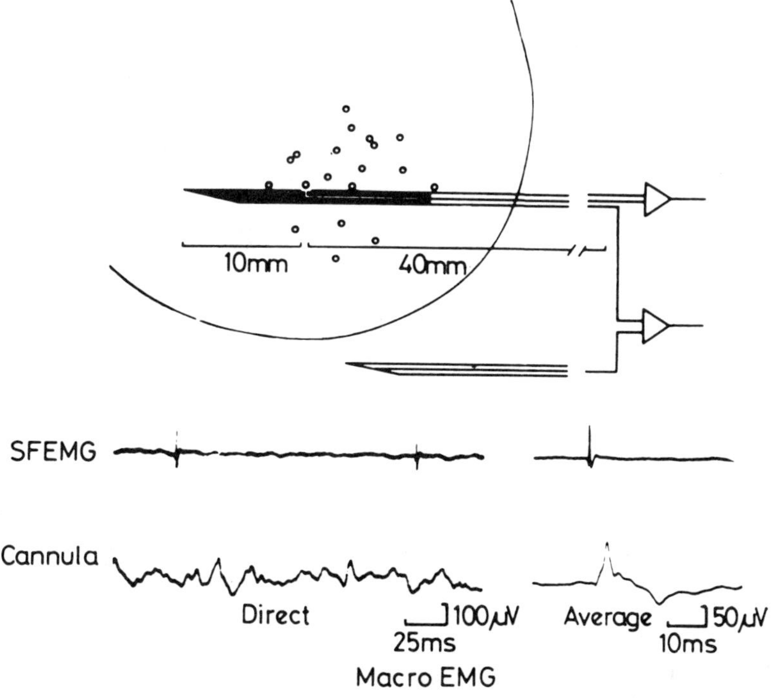

FIG. 5.12. Drawing illustrating the recording principle of macro EMG. The cannula with the small diameter electrode (*top*) is positioned to record action potentials from one muscle fiber (*SFEMG*). Activity detected by the cannula is averaged and the synchronous motor unit potential extracted after 128 to 512 averaged discharges. (From E. Stålberg: Macro EMG, a new recording technique. J. Neurol. Neurosurg. Psychiatry, *43:* 475–482, 1980.)

detected by the cannula (channel 2) are directed to the averager and averaged, usually for 128 to 512 impulses. The signal from the cannula is delayed for a short period after the trigger to permit any early components to be detected (Fig. 5.13).

In a study of normal subjects, Stålberg (84) measured the amplitude and area of the averaged motor unit potentials. Duration was not measured because of background noise on the base line and difficulty in locating the start and end of the potential. Area and peak amplitude showed considerable variation among the subjects, but there was a positive and significant correlation between the area and the amplitude. The shape of the motor unit potential is determined by the spatial distribution of the muscle fibers and also by the temporal distribution of the individual action potentials.

This technique is in the early stages of development and requires more investigation in normal and pathological conditions. The large size of the cannula allows the whole normal unit to be penetrated, and a large number of muscle fibers in the motor unit are close to the recording surface. Stålberg (84) feels that because of this, macro EMG records information about the whole motor unit and can be used as a measure of the motor unit size, including the number of fibers and their individual size.

FIRING RATES OF SINGLE MOTOR UNITS

Motor neurons and the muscle fibers they innervate are recruited into activity in a definite orderly manner during a gradually increasing voluntary contraction. The sequence of recruitment is, in general, determined by the neuron diameter. This idea was formulated by Henneman et al. (85, 86) and has come to be known as the "size principle." They found that the order of recruitment of motor units was inversely proportional to the size of the motor neuron; i.e., within a neuron pool of the spinal cord, the small motor neurons have a lower threshold of excitation than the larger ones. Conversely, the lower threshold motor units have smaller anterior horn cells and smaller axons and contain fewer muscle fibers. Consistent with the size principle is the fact that the conduction velocity of axons innervating low threshold motor units is slower than the velocity of axons innervating high threshold units (87).

The smaller motor neurons are, therefore, more easily recruited than the larger ones. This pattern is generally followed for a slowly contracting muscle (88). However, under certain conditions the order of recruitment can be altered. For example, in a rapid contraction, the large motor neurons may be recruited before the smaller ones (89).

The pattern and firing frequencies of normal units have been studied by many investigators (90–98). In one of the earlier studies performed in the abductor digiti minimi muscle, Bigland and Lippold (90) demonstrated the

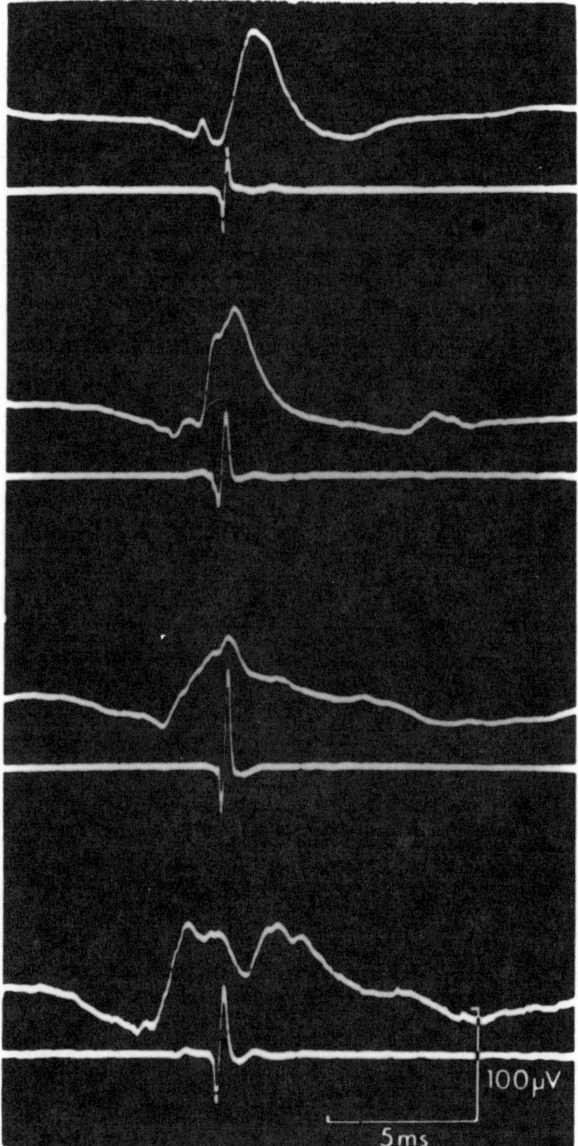

FIG. 5.13. Examples of actual recordings showing the average macro EMG (*first line*) and the triggering action potential (*second line*). The triggering action potential does not necessarily occur in the earliest part of the motor unit potential. The contribution of the macro EMG from the triggering action potential is usually not seen. Recording from tibialis anterior muscles in a healthy subject. (From E. Stålberg: Macro EMG, a new recording technique. J. Neurol. Neurosurg. Psychiatry, *43:* 475–482, 1980.)

increase in firing frequency of single motor units with increasing muscle tension and that the frequency varied mostly between 10 to 30 impulses per sec. Recordings were made with pairs of fine wire electrodes during increasing levels of contraction. The firing frequency increased nonlinearly with tension and was between 40 to 50 impulses per sec only during very strong contractions. Dasgupta and Simpson (91) observed a range of firing frequency of 8 to 20 impulses per sec in the first interosseus muscle; Tanji and Kato (98) found the range to be 3.4 to 24.9 impulses per sec in the abductor digiti minimi muscle; and Clamann (92) reported a similar range in the brachial biceps muscle, 7 to 24 impulses per sec. In the latter work, low threshold units had a wider range of firing frequencies compared to that of high threshold units.

Grimby and Hannerz have performed extensive electromyographic studies of the two types of motor units in the short extensor muscle of the big toe and the anterior tibial muscle with regard to firing rates, recruitment order, axonal conduction velocity, and contraction time (99–103). One type of motor unit had a firing range of 10 to 30 impulses per sec, and the lower frequency could be maintained apparently for an indefinite period of time. During rapid contractions, frequencies of 60 impulses per sec were observed. The conduction velocities of the axons innervating these units ranged from 30 to 45 m per sec and contraction times from 60 to 90 msec.

The firing rate of the other motor unit type ranged from 20 to 40 impulses per sec and discharged intermittently for short intervals only. Increased intensity of contraction produced firings up to 100 impulses per sec. The conduction velocities of the axons varied from 40 to 55 m per sec and contraction times from 40 to 55 msec. During prolonged maximal contraction, firing rates and the number of active motor units diminished. Those units initially discharging at 30 impulses per sec decreased to a rate of 15 to 20 impulses per sec; while the units firing at 60 impulses per sec became inactive but could be reactivated phasically during an increase in effort after a short period of relative relaxation.

In a contracting muscle maintaining constant tension, the firing rates are constant with no evidence of rotation of motor units (92, 94–96). Furthermore, at low or moderate efforts, there is no synchronous firing of different motor units; whereas, at maximum levels of contraction, the units may fire synchronously.

The studies of discharge patterns in normal muscle have been accompanied by similar investigations in various disorders. In patients with mild to moderate degrees of involvement, firing rates were found by Petajan to be increased in both neuropathy and myopathy, but normal rates were also observed (104). A more recent report also demonstrated an increase in firing frequency in myopathy and neuropathy (105). No significant difference was detected in one study between mean firing rates of units from normal and partially denervated muscle at comparable levels of relative force (106), whereas a different study reported a decrease in firing rate for this disorder (107).

It should be pointed out that the recording of single motor unit action potentials at intermediate and high levels of contraction is difficult. Synchronous firing and superposition of potentials make the following and analysis of single unit activity a complex undertaking. Furthermore, the methodology of recording can vary from one investigator to another so that comparison of results is questionable. Nevertheless, with increased interest and research, the recording of motor unit firing may become a valuable tool in differential diagnosis.

REFERENCES

1. Adrian, E. D., and Bronk, D. W.: The discharge of impulses in motor nerve fibers. Part II. The frequency of discharge in reflex and voluntary contractions. J. Physiol. (Lond.), *67:* 119–151, 1929.
2. Jones, R. V., Lambert, E. H., and Sayre, G. P.: Source of a type of "insertion activity" in electromyography with evaluation of a histologic method of localization. Arch. Phys. Med., *36:* 301–310, 1955.
3. Buchthal, F., and Rosenfalck, P.: Spontaneous electrical activity of human muscle. Electroencephalogr. Clin. Neurophysiol., *20:* 321–336, 1966.
4. Fatt, P., and Katz, B.: An analysis of the endplate potential recorded with an intracellular electrode. J. Physiol. (Lond.), *151:* 320–370, 1951.

Wiederholt, W. C.: "End-plate noise" in electromyography. Neurology (Minneap.), *21:* 214–224, 1970.

6. Buchthal, F., and Rosenfalck, P.: Electrophysiological aspects of myopathy with reference to progressive muscular dystrophy. In *Muscular Dystrophy in Man and Animals,* edited by G. H. Bourne, pp. 194–262. Hafner, New York, 1963.
7. Buchthal, F., Guld, C., and Rosenfalck, P.: Volume conduction of the spike of the motor unit potential investigated with a new type of multielectrode. Acta Physiol. Scand., *38:* 331–354, 1957.
8. Nissen-Petersen, H., Guld, C., and Buchthal, F.: A delay line to record random action potentials. Electroencephalogr. Clin Neurophysiol., *26:* 100–106, 1969.
9. Buchthal, F., Guld, C., and Rosenfalck, P.: Innervation zone and propagation velocity in human muscle. Acta Physiol. Scand., *35:* 174–190, 1955.
10. Buchthal, F.: *An Introduction to Electromyography,* p. 40. Scandinavian University Books, Copenhagen, 1957.
11. Caruso, G., and Buchthal, F.: Refractory period of muscle and electromyographic findings in relatives of patients with muscular dystrophy. Brain, *88:* 29–50, 1965.
12. Wolfart, G.: Muscular atrophy in diseases of the lower motor neuron. Contribution to the anatomy of the motor units. Arch. Neurol. Psychiatry (Chicago), *61:* 599–620, 1949.
13. Buchthal, F.: The general concept of the motor unit. Neuromusc. Dis., *38:* 3–30, 1961.
14. Krnjevic, K., and Miledi, R.: Motor units in the rat diaphragm. J. Physiol. (Lond.), *140:* 427–439, 1958.
15. Norris, F. H., and Irwin, R. L.: Motor unit area in rat muscle. Am. J. Physiol., *200:* 944–946, 1961.
16. Ekstedt, J.: Human single muscle fiber action potentials. Acta Physiol. Scand., *61* (Suppl. 226): 1–96, 1964.
17. Stålberg, E., Schwartz, M. S., Thiele, B., and Schiller, H. H.: The normal motor unit in man. J. Neurol. Sci., *27:* 291–301, 1976.
18. Rosenfalck, P.: Intra- and extracellular potential fields of active nerve and muscle fibers. Acta Physiol. Scand., Suppl. *321:* 1–168, 1969.
19. Buchthal, R., and Rosenfalck, F.: On the structure of motor units. In *New Developments*

in EMG and Clinical Neurophysiology, edited by J. E. Desmedt. pp. 71–85. S. Karger, Basel, 1973.
20. Taylor, A.: The significance of grouping motor unit activity. J. Physiol. (Lond.), *162:* 259–269, 1962.
21. Lippold, O. C. J.: The relation between integrated action potentials in a human muscle and its isometric tension. J. Physiol. (Lond.), *117:* 492–499, 1952.
22. Lenman, J. A. R.: A clinical and experimental study of the effects of exercise on motor weakness in neurological disease. J. Neurol. Neurosurg. Psychiatry, *22:* 182–194, 1959.
23. Kuroda, E., Klissouras, V., and Milsum, J. H.: Electrical and metabolic activities and fatigue in human isometric contraction. J. Appl. Physiol., *29:* 358–367, 1970.
24. Bigland, B., and Lippold, O. C. J.: The relation between force, velocity and integrated electrical activity in human muscles. J. Physiol. (Lond.), *123:* 214–224, 1954.
25. Mason, R. R., and Munro, R. R.: Relationship between EMG potentials and tension in abduction of the little finger. Electromyography, *9:* 185–199, 1969.
26. Richardson, A. T.: Newer concepts of electrodiagnosis. St. Thomas Hosp. Rep., *7:* 164–174, 1951.
27. Kaiser, E., and Petersen, I.: Muscle action potentials studied by frequency analysis and duration measurement. Acta Neurol. Scand., *41:* 213–236, 1965.
28. Walton, J. H.: The electromyogram in myopathy: Analysis with the audio frequency spectrometer. J. Neurol. Neurosurg. Psychiatry, *15:* 219–226, 1952.
29. Scott, R. N.: Myo-electric energy spectra. Med. Biol. Engin., *5:* 303–305, 1952.
30. Richardson, A. T.: Electromyography in myasthenia gravis and other myopathies. Am. J. Phys. Med., *38:* 118–124, 1959.
31. Fex, J., and Krakau, C. E. T.: Some experiences with Walton's frequency analysis of the electromyogram. J. Neurol. Neurosurg. Psychiatry, *20:* 178–184, 1957.
32. Cosi, V., and Mazzella, G. L.: Frequency analysis in clinical electromyography: A preliminary report. Electroencephalogr. Clin. Neurophysiol., *27:* 100, 1969.
33. Kadefors, R., Kaiser, E., and Petersen, I.: Dynamic spectrum analysis of myopotentials with special reference to muscle fatigue. Electromyography, *8:* 39–74, 1968.
34. Kadefors, R., Magnusson, R., Nilsson, N. J., and Petersen, I.: Effects of ischemia on the myoelectric signal spectrum. Acta Physiol. Scand., Suppl. *330:* 110, 1969.
35. Willison, R. G.: Analysis of electrical activity in healthy and dystrophic muscle in man. J. Neurol. Neurosurg. Psychiatry, *27:* 386–394, 1964.
36. Dowling, M. H., Fitch, P., and Willison, R. G.: A special purpose digital computer (Biomac 500) used in the analysis of the human electromyogram. Electroencephalogr. Clin. Neurophysiol., *25:* 570–573, 1968.
37. Fuglsang-Frederiksen, A., and Månsson, A.: Analysis of electrical activity of normal muscle in man at different degrees of voluntary effort. J. Neurol. Neurosurg. Psychiatry, *38:* 683–694, 1975.
38. Rathjen, R., Simons, D. G., and Peterson, C. R.: Computer analysis of the duration of motor-unit potentials. Arch. Phys. Med., *49:* 524–527, 1968.
39. Kunze, K., and Erbslöh, F.: Automatic EMG analysis, a new approach. Electroencephalogr. Clin. Neurophysiol., *25:* 402, 1968.
40. Kopec, J., and Hausmanowa-Petrusewicz, I.: Histogram of muscle potentials recorded automatically with the aid of the averaging computer "ANOPS." Electromyography, *9:* 371–381, 1969.
41. Kunze, K.: Quantitative-electromyographic measurement of muscular contraction. Pfluegers Arch., *300:* 77–78, 1968.
42. Kopec, J., and Hausmanowa-Petrusewicz, I.: Application of automatic analysis of electromyograms in clinical diagnosis. Electroencephalogr. Clin. Neurophysiol., *36:* 575–576, 1974.
43. Bergmans, J.: Computer assisted on line measurement of motor unit potential parameters in human electromyography. Electromyography, *11:* 161–181, 1971.
44. Hirose, K., Unono, M., and Sobue, I.: Quantitative electromyography comparison between manual values and computer ones on normal subjects. Electromyography, *14:* 315–320, 1974.
45. Moosa, A., and Brown, B. H.: Quantitative electromyography: A new analogue technique

for detecting changes in action potential duration. J. Neurol. Neurosurg. Psychiatry, *35:* 216–220, 1972.

46. Van den Bosch, J.: Investigations of the carrier state in the Duchenne type dystrophy. In *Proceedings of the Second Symposium on Current Research in Muscular Dystrophy*, pp. 23–30. Pitman Medical and Scientific Publishing Co., Ltd., London, 1963.
47. McComas, A. J., Fawcett, P. R. W., Campbell, M. J., and Sica, R. E. P.: Electrophysiological estimation of the number of motor units within a human muscle. J. Neurol. Neurosurg. Psychiatry, *34:* 121–131, 1971.
48. McComas, A. J., Sica, R. E. P., Upton, A. R. M., and Petito, F.: Sick motoneurons and muscle disease. Ann. N. Y. Acad. Sci, *228:* 261–279, 1974.
49. McComas, A. J., Sica, R. E. P., and Currie, S.: An electrophysiological study of Duchenne dystrophy. J. Neurol. Neurosurg. Psychiatry, *34:* 461–468, 1971.
50. McComas, A. J., Campbell, M. J., and Sica, R. E. P.: Electrophysiological study of dystrophia myotonica. J. Neurol. Neurosurg. Psychiatry, *34:* 132–139, 1971.
51. McComas, A. J., Sica, R. E. P., and Campbell, M. J.: Numbers and sizes of human motor units in health and disease. In *New Developments in Electromyography and Clinical Neurophysiology*, edited by J. E. Desmedt, vol. 1, pp. 55–63. Karger, Basel, 1973.
52. Sica, R. E. P., and McComas, A. J.: An electrophysiological investigation of limb-girdle and facioscapulohumeral dystrophy. J. Neurol. Neurosurg. Psychiatry, *34:* 469–474, 1971.
53. McComas, A. J., Sica, R. E. P., Campbell, M. J., and Upton, A. R. M.: Functional compensation in partially denervated muscles. J. Neurol. Neurosurg. Psychiatry, *34:* 453–460, 1971.
54. McComas, A. J., Sica, R. E. P., Upton, A. R. M., and Aguilera, N.: Functional changes in motoneurones of hemiparetic patients. J. Neurol. Neurosurg. Psychiatry, *36:* 183–193, 1973.
55. Upton, A. R., McComas, A. J., and Bianchi, A. F.: Neuropathy in McArdle's syndrome. N. Engl. J. Med., *289:* 750–751, 1973.
56. McComas, A. J., Sica, R. E. P., McNabb, A. R., Goldberg, W. M., and Upton, A. R. M.: Evidence for reversible motoneurone dysfunction in thyrotoxicosis. J. Neurol. Neurosurg. Psychiatry, *37:* 548–558, 1974.
57. Campbell, M. J., McComas, A. J., and Petito, F.: Physiological changes in ageing muscles. J. Neurol. Neurosurg. Psychiatry, *36:* 174–182, 1973.
58. McComas, A. J., Sica, R. E. P., and Upton, A. R. M.: Multiple muscle analysis of motor units in muscular dystrophy. Arch. Neurol., *30:* 249–251, 1974.
59. McComas, A. J., Sica, R. E. P., and Campbell, M. J.: "Sick" motoneurones, a unifying concept of muscle disease. Lancet, *1:* 321–325, 1971.
60. Panayiotopoulos, C. P., Scarpalezos, S., and Papapetropoulos, T.: Electrophysiological estimation of motor units in Duchenne muscular dystrophy. J. Neurol. Sci., *23:* 89–98, 1974.
61. Feasby, T. E., and Brown, W. F.: Variation of motor unit size in the human extensor digitorum brevis and thenar muscles. J. Neurol. Neurosurg. Psychiatry, *37:* 916–926, 1974.
62. Panayiotopoulos, C. P., and Scarpalezos, S.: Electrophysiological estimation of motor units in limb-girdle muscular dystrophy and chronic spinal muscular atrophy. J. Neurol. Sci., *24:* 95–107, 1975.
63. Ballantyne, J. P., and Hansen, S.: A new method for the estimation of the number of motor units in a muscle. J. Neurol. Neurosurg. Psychiatry, *37:* 907–915, 1974.
64. Ballantyne, J. P., and Hansen, S.: New method for the estimation of the number of motor units in a muscle. J. Neurol. Neurosurg. Psychiatry, *37:* 1195–1201, 1974.
65. Ballantyne, J. P., and Hansen, S.: Computer method for the analysis of evoked motor unit potentials. J. Neurol. Neurosurg. Psychiatry, *37:* 1187–1194, 1974.
66. Brown, W. F., and Milner-Brown, H. S.: Some electrical properties of motor units and their effects on the methods of estimating motor unit numbers. J. Neurol. Neurosurg. Psychiatry, *39:* 249–257, 1976.
67. Milner-Brown, H. S., and Brown, W. F.: New methods of estimating the number of motor units in muscle. J. Neurol. Neurosurg. Psychiatry, *39:* 258–265, 1976.

68. Kadrie, H. A., Yates, S. K., Milner-Brown, H. S., and Brown, W. F.: Multiple point electrical stimulation of ulnar and median nerves. J. Neurol. Neurosurg. Psychiatry, *39:* 973–985, 1976.
69. McComas, A. J., Upton, A. R. M., and Sica, R. E. P.: Myopathies: The neurogenic hypothesis. Lancet, *2:* 42, 1974.
70. McComas, A. J., Sica, R. E. P., and Upton, A. R. M.: Comparisons of motor unit populations in disease. Trans. Am. Neurol. Assoc., *98:* 76–79, 1973.
71. Ekstedt, J., and Stålberg, E.: A method of recording extracellular action potentials of single muscle fibers and measuring their propagation velocity in voluntarily activated human muscle. Bull. Am. Assoc. Electromyogr. Electrodiagn., *10:* 16, 1963.
72. Ekstedt, J.: Human single muscle fiber action potentials. Acta Physiol. Scand., *61* (Suppl. 226): 1–96, 1964.
73. Stålberg, E., and Ekstedt, J.: Single fibre EMG and microphysiology of the motor unit in normal and diseased human muscle. In *New Developments in Electromyography and Clinical Neurophysiology*, edited by J. E. Desmedt, vol. 1, pp. 113–129. Karger, Basel, 1973.
74. Ekstedt, J., and Stålberg, E.: Single fibre electromyography for the study of the microphysiology of the human muscle. In *New Developments in Electromyography and Clinical Neurophysiology*, edited by J. E. Desmedt, vol. 1, pp. 89–112. Karger, Basel, 1973.
75. Ekstedt, J., and Stålberg, E.: How the size of the needle electrode leading-off surface influences the shape of the single muscle fibre action potential in electromyography. Computer Prog. Biomed., *3:* 204–212, 1973.
76. Buchthal, F., Guld, C., and Rosenfalck, P.: Volume conduction of the spike of the motor unit potential investigated with a new type of multielectrode. Acta Physiol. Scand., *38:* 331–354, 1957.
77. Fleck, H.: Action potentials from single motor units in human muscle. Arch. Phys. Med., *43:* 99–107, 1962.
78. Ekstedt, J., and Stålberg, E.: Myasthenia gravis: Diagnostic aspects by a new electrophysiological method. Opuscula Med., *12:* 73–76, 1967.
79. Stålberg, E., Ekstedt, J., and Broman, A.: Neuromuscular transmission in myasthenia gravis studied with single fiber electromyography. J. Neurol. Neurosurg. Psychiatry, *37:* 540–547, 1974.
80. Schwartz, M. S., and Stålberg, E.: Single fibre electromyographic studies in myasthenia gravis with repetitive nerve stimulation. J. Neurol. Neurosurg. Psychiatry, *38:* 678–682, 1975.
81. Stålberg, E., Schwartz, M. S., and Trontelj, J. V.: Single fibre electromyography in various processes affecting the anterior horn cell. J. Neurol. Sci., *24:* 403–415, 1975.
82. Thiele, B., and Stålberg, E.: Single fibre EMG findings in polyneuropathies of different aetiology. J. Neurol. Neurosurg. Psychiatry, *38:* 881–887, 1975.
83. Thiele, B. and Boehle, A.: Number of single muscle fibre action potentials contributing to the motor unit potential. In *Fifth International Congress of EMG*, Rochester, Minnesota, 1975, p. 67.
84. Stålberg, E.: Macro EMG, a new recording technique. J. Neurol. Neurosurg. Psychiatry, *43:* 475–482, 1980.
85. Henneman, E., Somjen, G., and Carpenter, D. O.: Excitability and inhibitibility of motoneurons of different sizes. J. Neurophysiol., *28:* 599–620, 1965.
86. Henneman, E., Somjen, G., and Carpenter, D. O.: Functional significance of cell size in spinal motoneurones. J. Neurophysiol., *28:* 650–680, 1965.
87. Freund, H. J., Dietz, V., Wita, C. W., and Kapp, H.: Discharge characteristics of single motor units in normal subjects and patients with supraspinal motor disturbances. In *New Developments in Electromyography and Clinical Neurophysiology*, edited by J. E. Desmedt, vol. 3, pp. 242–250. Karger, Basel, 1973.
88. Henneman, E., Clamann, H. P., Gillies, J. D., and Skinner, R. D.: Rank-order of motoneurons within a pool: Law of combination. J. Neurophysiol., *37:* 1338–1349, 1974.
89. Grimby, L., and Hannerz, J.: Tonic and phasic recruitment order of motor units in man under normal and pathological conditions. In *New Developments in Electromyography and Clinical Neurophysiology*, edited by J. E. Desmedt, vol. 3, pp. 225–233. Karger, Basel, 1973.

90. Bigland, B., and Lippold, O. C. J.: Motor unit activity in the voluntary contraction of human muscle. J. Physiol. (Lond.), *125:* 322–335, 1954.
91. Dasgupta, A., and Simpson, J. A.: Relation between firing frequency of motor units and muscle tension in the human. Electromyography, *2:* 117–128, 1962.
92. Clamann, H. P.: Activity of single motor units during isometric tension. Neurology, *20:* 254–260, 1970.
93. Milner-Brown, H. S., Stein, R. B., and Yemm, R.: Changes in firing rate of human motor units during linearly changing voluntary contractions. J. Physiol. (Lond.), *230:* 371–390, 1973.
94. Stålberg, E., and Thiele, B.: Discharge pattern of motoneurones in humans: A single-fibre EMG study. In *New Developments in Electromyography and Clinical Neurophysiology*, edited by J. E. Desmedt, vol. 3, pp. 234–241. Karger, Basel, 1973.
95. Freund, H. J., Budingen, J. H., and Dietz, V.: Activity of single motor units from human forearm muscles during voluntary isometric contractions. J. Neurophysiol., *38:* 933–946, 1975.
96. Petajan, J. H., and Philip, B. A.: Frequency control of motor unit action potentials. Electroencephalogr. Clin. Neurophysiol., *27:* 66–72, 1969.
97. Monster, A. W., and Chan, H.: Isometric force production by motor units of extensor digitorum communis muscle in man. J. Neurophysiol., *40:* 1430–1443, 1977.
98. Tanji, J., and Kato, M.: Recruitment of motor units in voluntary contractions of a finger muscle in man. Exp. Neurol., *40:* 759–770, 1973.
99. Hannerz, J.: Discharge properties of motor units in relation to recruitment order in voluntary contraction. Acta Physiol. Scand., *91:* 374–384, 1974.
100. Grimby, L., and Hannerz, J.: Firing rate and recruitment order of toe extensor motor units in different modes of voluntary contraction. J. Physiol., *264:* 865–879, 1977.
101. Borg, J., Grimby, L., and Hannerz, J.: Axonal conduction velocity and voluntary discharge properties of individual short toe extensor motor units in man. J. Physiol., *277:* 143–152, 1978.
102. Grimby, L., Hannerz, J., and Hedman, B.: Contraction time and voluntary discharge properties of individual short toe extensor motor units in man. J. Physiol., *289:* 191–201, 1979.
103. Grimby, L., Hannerz, J., and Hedman, B.: The fatigue and voluntary discharge properties of single motor units in man. J. Physiol., *316:* 545–554, 1981.
104. Petajan, J. H.: Clinical electromyographic studies of diseases of the motor unit. Electroencephalogr. Clin. Neurophysiol., *36:* 395–401, 1974.
105. Halonen, J.-P., Falck, B., and Kalimo, H.: The firing rate of motor units in neuromuscular disorders. J. Neurol., *225:* 269–276, 1981.
106. Miller, R. G., and Sherratt, M.: Firing rates of human motor units in partially denervated muscle. Neurology, *28:* 1241–1248, 1978.
107. Dietz, V., Budingen, H. J., Hillesheimer, W., and Freund, H. J.: Discharge characteristics of single motor fibres of hand muscles in lower motoneurone diseases and myopathies. In *Studies on Neuromuscular Diseases*, edited by K. Kunze and J. E. Desmedt, pp. 122–127. Karger, Basel, 1975.

chapter

6

Spontaneous Activity

In the preceding chapter we discussed spontaneous activity, such as nerve potentials and end-plate noise, which is confined to the end-plate zone of normal muscle. Spontaneous activity detected away from the end-plate zone is usually significant and indicative of abnormality. The types of spontaneous activity which may be encountered from a muscle at rest are fibrillation potentials, positive waves, fasciculations, and high frequency discharges.

FIBRILLATION POTENTIALS

Spontaneous potentials of short duration and low voltage frequently observed in denervated muscle are called fibrillation potentials. They are not visible through the skin, although occasionally they may be seen in the tongue. Fibrillation potentials may be diphasic or triphasic in shape, with the initial deflection in the positive direction if recorded outside the zone of innervation (Fig. 6.1). The amplitude of the third positive phase is usually small compared to the total peak-to-peak amplitude. When detected within the end-plate zone, they are diphasic with an initial negative deflection, indicating that the electrode is near the source of the activity (1). In the end-plate zone, care must be exercised by the electromyographer to differentiate fibrillation potentials from normally occurring spontaneous activity. Evaluation of fibrillation potentials is facilitated by recording from areas outside the zone of innervation.

The duration of fibrillation potentials recorded with concentric needle electrodes is described as ranging from 1 to 5 msec with an average of 2.7 msec (1). The amplitude may vary from 20 to 300 μV. The frequency of firing is of the order of 1 to 30 per sec. Buchthal and Rosenfalck (1), in their study of 67 patients (64 with peripheral nerve involvement, three with signs

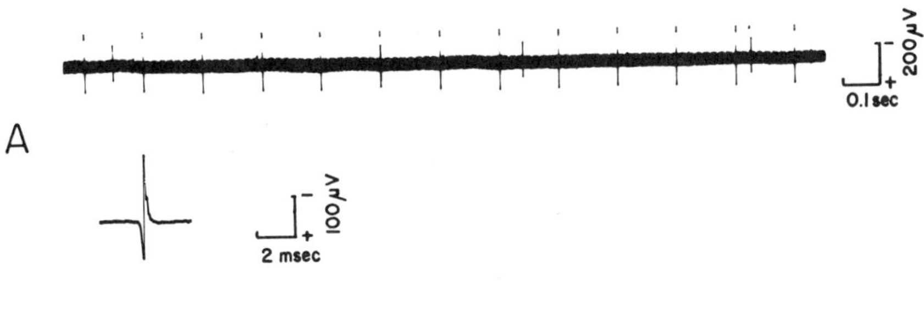

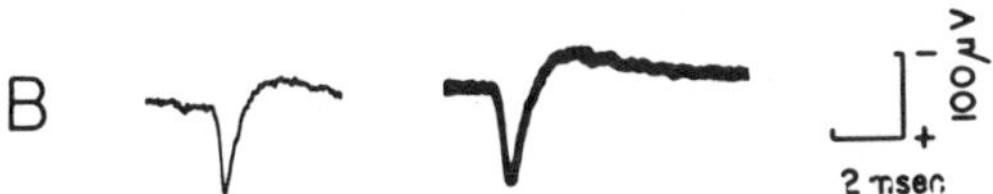

FIG. 6.1. *A*, fibrillation potentials recorded at slow and fast sweep speeds; *B*, typical positive sharp waves.

of anterior horn cell involvement), reported fibrillation potentials occurred at irregular intervals with an average frequency of 13 per sec and also at regular intervals with an average frequency of 1 to 10 per sec. These authors also demonstrated that the intramuscular electrode is not involved in the initiation of fibrillation potentials by recording them subcutaneously.

Fibrillation potentials are not exclusively observed in denervated muscle. They may be detected in patients with primary myopathic diseases. In a study of 76 patients with progressive muscular dystrophy, Buchthal and Rosenfalck (1) found fibrillations in 29 patients or in 34 of the 108 muscles examined in all of the patients. In our own experience we have also recorded fibrillation potentials in myopathies, but to a lesser extent—in about 25% of the cases examined.

The fibrillation potentials observed in dystrophic muscle are indistinguishable from those seen in denervated muscle. Fibrillation potentials have also been reported in patients with polymyositis (2), botulism (3), and hyperkalemic familial periodic paralysis (4). To be diagnostically significant, fibrillation potentials must be detected in at least two and preferably three different sites of the muscle outside the end-plate zone. Because fibrillation potentials are occasionally recorded in otherwise healthy muscle, the isolated appearance of these potentials cannot be considered as indicating nerve damage or other abnormality.

Do fibrillation potentials represent the discharge of a single muscle fiber or the synchronous firing of a small bundle of fibers? The small amplitude, short duration, and smooth shape of recorded potentials suggest that they arise from single muscle fibers. The theoretical analysis of Rosenfalck (5) showed that even "high voltage" fibrillation potentials (1 mV or more) may originate from a single muscle fiber lying in contact with the electrode. Buchthal and Rosenfalck (1) determined the volume conduction of fibrillation potentials with the multielectrode and found that high voltage fibrillations decline in amplitude along the electrode in the same way as single motor unit potentials, suggesting that these fibrillation potentials represent the spontaneous discharge of a subunit.

It is most likely that fibrillation potentials originate from a single muscle fiber. However, it is possible that fibrillations may also arise from the activity of small groups of fibers.

Denervation and Trophic Influence of the Nervous System

It is well known that transection of the motor nerve is followed by degenerative changes in the muscle. The most prominent electrical and physiological changes of denervated muscle are the development of spontaneous fibrillation potentials and the hypersensitivity to acetylcholine of the entire muscle fiber in contrast to the localized sensitivity at the end-plate zone of innervated muscle. To explain these changes, some investigators have assumed a specific "trophic" influence of the intact nervous system on the muscles. It is the deprivation of the trophic influence which leads to the observed alterations of the muscle. Whether the trophic influence is mediated via acetylcholine or some other neurohumoral agent or via motor nerve impulses is still unsettled. A considerable body of work has accumulated, especially in recent years, which attempts to explain the morphological and metabolic alterations of denervated muscle and also to define the nature of the trophic influence (for an excellent review of trophic influences, see reference 6).

Although still controversial, increasing evidence indicates that the lack of the neuromuscular transmitter, acetylcholine, is the cause of the spontaneous denervation potentials. Blocking acetylcholine release at mammalian motor nerve terminals with botulinum toxin produced both hypersensitivity and fibrillation (7, 8). Similarly, mercaine, a long acting local anesthetic, produced denervation-like effects including spontaneous fibrillations in rats after subcutaneous injections in a study by Sokoll et al. (9). They suggest that mercaine produces the denervation changes by rendering the muscle cell insusceptible to acetylcholine. More recently, Robert and Oester (10, 11) produced muscle paralysis in rabbits by blocking nerve conduction without injury or irreversible intervention and, after 14 days, did not observe spontaneous denervation potentials. Because the trophic influence is still operative, this study suggests that it is independent of nerve impulses and that prolonged nerve impulse deprivation does not cause hypersensitivity to acetylcholine or fibrillations.

In contrast to the above findings, Miledi (12) found that denervation of frog muscle produced increased sensitivity to acetylcholine but no spontaneous activity, a result indicating the lack of a direct relationship between acetylcholine and fibrillation.

Other mechanisms have been proposed to explain the occurrence of fibrillation potentials: spontaneous oscillations of the membrane potential of denervated muscle fibers trigger propagated spikes whenever the depolarization reaches threshold (13, 14); functional changes in the sarcoplasmic reticulum, as shown by the increased calcium binding by the sarcoplasmic reticulum in denervated guinea pig muscle, as well as alterations in the muscle fiber membrane, may be the cause of fibrillations in denervated muscle (15, 16).

It is obvious that the cause of spontaneous activity in denervated muscle is still unknown and requires further study.

POSITIVE SHARP WAVES

Positive sharp waves are diphasic potentials appearing spontaneously and at irregular intervals. They are distinguished by a sharp initial positive deflection followed by a slow decay into the negative direction (Fig. 6.1). The negative phase is much lower in amplitude than the positive deflection and prolonged in duration, sometimes continuing for 100 msec.

Positive sharp waves are not seen in normal muscle but are most frequently observed in denervated muscle, along with fibrillation potentials. They have been recorded in dystrophic muscle, particularly in myotonic dystrophy. The amplitude of positive sharp waves may vary anywhere from about 50 μV to 1 mV. Recording with a concentric needle electrode, Buchthal and Rosenfalck (1) found that the amplitude averaged 120 μV (standard deviation of 45) in 45 denervated muscles. The total duration is longer than that of fibrillation potentials, usually exceeding 10 msec. The frequency of discharge may range from 2 to 100 per sec but more commonly at about 10 per sec.

Positive sharp waves are considered to originate from single muscle fibers and are probably detected near a damaged region of the fibers. Frequently they are present only in the first few seconds after insertion of the needle electrode into the muscle and then abruptly disappear.

FASCICULATION

Fasciculation is the spontaneous nonvolitional twitching of a bundle of muscle fibers which may be visible if it occurs superficially and may cause movement of the skin but not the joints. It is not to be confused with fibrillation, the spontaneous contraction of single muscle fibers not normally visible to the eye, nor with tremor or myoclonus, gross twitching of a muscle or group of muscles. Fasciculation may or may not indicate disease, because this is also observed in normal individuals. Pathologically, it is most frequently encountered in active degenerative lesions of the anterior horn cell, such as motor neuron disease and spinal muscular atrophy. It also occurs in inflammatory or compressive nerve root lesions and thyrotoxicosis. Fasciculation is not observed in primary muscle diseases. Benign fasciculations are occasionally seen in normal subjects, particularly in the calf muscles and the small muscles of the hands and feet.

The wave shapes of fasciculation potentials are simple di- or triphasic or complex polyphasic waves. The duration and amplitude of the simple potentials are similar to single motor unit potentials and remain unchanged with repetition. The repetition frequency may vary from 1 to 50 per min, but irregularity of rhythm is characteristic. Attempts have been made to differentiate fasciculation potentials associated with motor neuron disease and those associated with benign neuromuscular disorders. Fasciculation action potentials accompanying motor neuron disease have been described as irregular in amplitude, grouping, and rhythm and of varying polyphasicity on repetition, whereas in benign disorders they are di- or triphasic in shape (17). Trojaborg and Buchthal (18) could not confirm this differentiation. They found that only 10 to 20% of fasciculation potentials were polyphasic in 10 patients with motor neuron disease. The only difference observed between "malignant" and "benign" fasciculations was the frequency of discharge. The average interval between successive fasciculation potentials in motor neuron disease was 3.5 sec (SD 2.5 sec, n = 481) as compared with 0.8 sec (SD 0.8 sec, n = 477) in benign fasciculation.

HIGH FREQUENCY DISCHARGES

High frequency discharges may be seen in any irritation lesion of anterior horn cells and peripheral nerves and in the myopathies. These bizarre discharges consist of extended trains of potentials of various forms whose identifying characteristic for diagnostic purposes is their frequency. In the myotonias, the discharge is characterized by a continuous increase and decrease in frequency, which may vary from as high as 150 per sec down to 20 per sec, producing a sound in the loudspeaker similar to that of a "divebomber." The potentials may be of short duration or approximate normal motor units and may also increase and decrease in amplitude. This type of high frequency discharge is called a "myotonic response" and may be initiated by needle movement, percussion, or volitional activity. These responses have also been recorded with the muscle seemingly at rest; however, it is not certain whether they are truly spontaneous or evoked by the increased mechanical excitability of myotonic muscle.

In contrast to the myotonic response, brief discharges at fairly constant frequency are observed occasionally in progressive muscular dystrophy and more frequently in polymyositis. In the latter disease, the potentials are usually polyphasic in form and may also be evoked by needle movement.

The burst of potentials starts and stops abruptly and, generally, is shorter in total duration than the equivalent activity occurring in myotonia.

REFERENCES

1. Buchthal, F., and Rosenfalck, P.: Spontaneous electrical activity of human muscle. Electroencephalogr. Clin Neurophysiol., *20:* 321–336, 1966.
2. Lambert, E. H., Sayre, G. P., and Eaton, L. M.: Electrical activity of muscle in polymyositis. Trans. Am. Neurol. Assoc., *79:* 64–69, 1954.
3. Peterson, I., and Broman, A. M.: Electromyographic findings in a case of botulism. Nord. Med., *65:* 259–261, 1961.
4. Morrison, J. B.: Electromyographic changes in hyperkalemic familial periodic paralysis. Ann. Phys. Med., *5:* 153–155, 1960.
5. Rosenfalck, P.: Intra- and extracellular potential fields of active nerve and muscle fibers. Acta Physiol. Scand., Suppl. 321, 1969.
6. Guth, L.: "Trophic" influences of nerve and muscle. Physiol. Rev., *48:* 645–687, 1968.
7. Thesleff, S.: Supersensitivity of skeletal muscle produced by botulinum toxin. J. Physiol. (Lond.), *151:* 598–607, 1960.
8. Josefsson, J. D., and Thesleff, S.: Electromyographic findings in experimental botulinum intoxication. Acta Physiol. Scand., *51:* 163–168, 1961.
9. Sokoll, M. D., Sonesson, B., and Thesleff, S.: Denervation changes produced in an innervated skeletal muscle by long-continued treatment with a local anesthetic. Eur. J. Pharmacol., *4:* 179–187, 1968.
10. Robert, E. D., and Oester, Y. T.: Electrodiagnosis of nerve-impulse deprived skeletal muscle. J. Appl. Physiol., *28:* 439–443, 1970.
11. Robert, E. D., and Oester, Y. T.: Nerve impulses and trophic influence: Absence of fibrillation after prolonged and reversible conduction block. Arch. Neurol. (Chicago), *22:* 57–63, 1970.
12. Miledi, R.: The acetylcholine sensitivity of frog muscle fibres after complete and partial denervation. J. Physiol. (Lond.), *151:* 1–23, 1960.
13. Li, C. L., Shy, G. M., and Wells, J.: Some properties of mammalian skeletal muscle fibers and particular reference to fibrillation potentials. J. Physiol. (Lond.), *135:* 522–535, 1957.
14. Bowman, W. C., and Rafer, C.: Spontaneous fibrillary activity of denervated muscle. Nature (Lond.), *201:* 160–162, 1964.
15. Brody, I. A.: Relaxing factor in denervated muscle: A possible explanation for fibrillations. Am. J. Physiol., *211:* 1277–1280, 1966.
16. Radu, H., Godri, I., Albu, E., Radu, A., and Robu, R.: Calcium uptake and bioelectrical activity of denervated and myotonic muscle. J. Neurol. Neurosurg. Psychiatry, *33:* 294–298, 1970.
17. Richardson, A. T.: Muscle fasciculation. Arch. Phys. Med., *35:* 281–286, 1954.
18. Trojaborg, W., and Buchthal, F.: Malignant and benign fasciculations. Acta Neurol. Scand., *41* (Suppl. 13): 251–254, 1965.

chapter 7

Motor and Sensory Nerve Conduction Measurements

Although the first determinations of nerve conduction velocity in man were performed about 100 years earlier (1), the first measurements of motor conduction velocity in patients was made by Hodes et al. in 1948 (2). They determined the conduction velocity in the median, ulnar, peroneal, and tibial nerves in normal subjects and in patients with peripheral nerve injuries or hysterical paralysis. After this, Lambert and his colleagues went on to develop the technique as a diagnostic tool and made valuable contributions regarding peripheral nerve conduction velocity in diseased states (3, 4).

Dawson and Scott (5) demonstrated in 1948 that it was possible to detect evoked potentials from the median and ulnar nerves with surface electrode stimulation and, in 1956, Dawson (6) recorded the first purely sensory action potentials in man. The clinical application of sensory nerve studies to patients with peripheral nerve lesions was advanced by the contributions of Gilliatt and his associates (7, 8). They demonstrated, for example, that in some disorders (e.g., carpal tunnel syndrome) sensory nerve conduction may indicate abnormality before motor nerve conduction.

The state of the art of nerve conduction as a diagnostic aid is still undergoing evaluation and improvement. This is true particularly in sensory action potential recording. A significant and detailed contribution toward improving the technique of sensory nerve conduction measurements and establishing norms was presented by Buchthal and Rosenfalck (9).

Problems of technique and interpretation notwithstanding, determination of nerve conduction velocity has progressed to a level where it is now used routinely as part of the electrodiagnostic examination. The clinical value of nerve conduction measurements has repeatedly been demonstrated in the examination of diseases or injuries which might be difficult to diagnose with electromyography alone. Localized neuropathy, Charcot-Marie-Tooth disease, and diabetic neuropathy are examples of abnormalities which primarily affect the nerve fibers. The procedure is especially useful in the diagnosis of compression neuropathies.

The actual clinical procedures are fairly simple to perform, are easily tolerated, and require little cooperation from the patient. Interpretation of the results, however, requires knowledge of the range of normal values and, of equal importance, the sources of error which may affect the finding.

INSTRUMENTATION

In electromyography, the recorded potentials are either spontaneous or volitional, whereas in nerve conduction measurements the potentials detected from muscles or nerves are evoked by nerve stimulation. Thus, appropriate instrumentation includes not only the conventional electromyograph but also a stimulator and stimulating electrodes. Rectangular pulse generators are the most common type of stimulators used because amplitude and duration of rectangular pulses can be easily changed and measured. The stimulator should be capable of delivering voltages up to 150 V in amplitude at durations of 0.1 to 3 msec and at variable frequencies at least up to 50 Hz. Guld et al. (10) recommend that the stimulation current output extend up to 100 ma.

To minimize the stimulus artifact, the stimulator should be isolated from ground. A shielded isolation transformer or an electronic isolation unit is available for this purpose; we prefer the isolation transformer.

Although technique varies from one laboratory to another, we prefer to record the complete artifact as well as the response so that we may measure from the beginning of the artifact. To accomplish this, the oscilloscope sweep is triggered by the stimulator before the actual stimulus to the patient. This delay permits first the artifact and then the response to be recorded.

Buchthal and Rosenfalck (9) recommended that in nerve stimulation the stimulating current intensity delivered to the patient be monitored to detect any distortion by the electrode and tissue. This measurement is now performed in our laboratory, and, in fact, the current amplitude is recorded (on a separate channel) along with the response. It is accomplished fairly simply by inserting a current transformer in one of the output leads connected to the stimulating electrodes.

Electrodes

Electrodes commonly used for nerve stimulation vary in size and shape, ranging from pipe cleaners soaked in saline to hand-held units containing a potentiometer in the handle. For most of our studies, we use the hand-held type which consists of two metal rods encased in a plastic handle. A small amount of electrode paste is placed on the tips, carefully avoiding any spread of the paste on the skin between the electrodes, which would short-circuit the stimulator. Small plastic or stainless steel blocks with protruding silver or felt plugs are convenient to use as a stimulating electrode unit because they can be fixed in place by straps wrapped around the limb. At times, as for sciatic nerve conduction studies, needle electrodes inserted through the skin may be used for stimulation.

For sensory nerve stimulation, strips of silver or strips of flannel soaked in saline wrapped around the finger tips may be used.

For recording the response to stimulation, either surface (most common) or needle electrodes may be used. In our laboratory, Beckman surface electrodes are the most frequently used in motor conduction measurements; however, silver discs about 1 cm in diameter are also satisfactory. When necessary, concentric needle electrodes inserted into the muscle are used for recording. Evoked sensory potentials can also be recorded with ring or disc electrodes. Buchthal and Rosenfalck (9) used specially designed needle electrodes inserted close to the nerve to increase the signal amplitude. The electrodes are Teflon-coated, stainless steel needles exposed at the tip and treated electrolytically. In addition, to improve the signal-to-noise ratio when recording action potentials of small amplitude, they used an *input transformer*, the electrodes connected to one side and the other side connected to the input amplifier.

PROCEDURE

Essentially, nerve conduction velocity measurements involve stimulating a nerve at one point and recording the response either at the muscle or at some distance along the nerve. The former applies to motor nerve and the latter to sensory nerve conduction rates.

Motor Conduction

The procedure is limited to those nerves which are accessible to stimulation. In the upper extremities these include the median, ulnar, radial, and axillary nerves; in the lower extremities they are the sciatic, femoral, tibial, and peroneal nerves. Conduction times have also been reported for the recurrent laryngeal nerve (11), the accessory nerve (12), and the phrenic nerve (13).

The actual technique for stimulating and recording may vary from one laboratory to another. Type, size, and position of the electrodes have not been standardized. We present the procedure followed in our laboratory, which can be performed easily and rapidly and gives useful information.

Whichever technique is used, it is recommended that each laboratory determine its own normal values for the various nerves and compare these with published normal standards to establish reliability.

Upper Extremities

The motor conduction velocity of the *ulnar* nerve is obtained by placing the active recording electrode over the belly of the abductor digiti quinti muscle and the reference electrode over its tendon at the base of the little finger. Before electrode placement, the hypothenar eminence and the back of the hand are lightly abraded with sandpaper and cleansed with ether to reduce electrical resistance between electrode and skin. The ground electrode (an alloy of tin and lead) is fixed in place under the dorsum of the hand.

At the wrist, the ulnar nerve may be stimulated percutaneously in the region of the flexor carpi ulnaris tendon (Fig. 7.1). Because stimulation is at the cathode, the stimulating electrodes are placed with the cathode nearest the recording electrodes. Starting with low intensity and short duration (about 0.1 msec) at a low repetition rate (1 pulse per sec), the intensity is slowly increased until a response is observed. The intensity is further increased until the amplitude of the muscle action potential no longer increases, at which time the stimulus is further increased about 25% to ensure that the stimulus intensity is supramaximal.

The stimulus artifact and the generated response can be displayed and photographed. A typical record of this kind is shown in Figure 7.2. A sharp deflection from the base line, which can usually be obtained by proper positioning of the active electrode, is essential for accuracy of measurement. The elapsed time between the start of the stimulus and the onset of the response represents the propagation of the impulse along the nerve, the

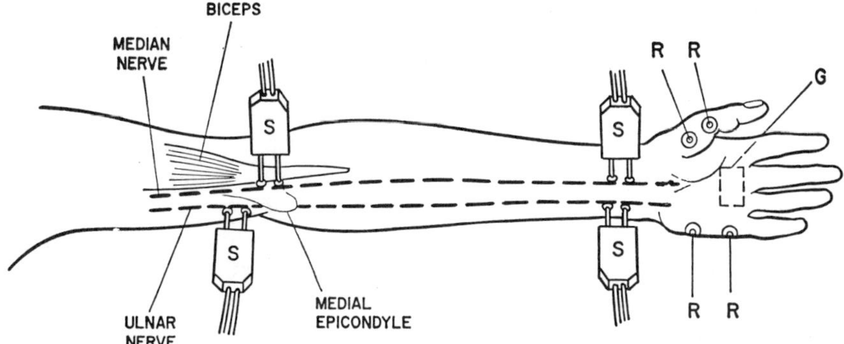

FIG. 7.1. Drawing of arm indicating relation of median and ulnar nerves and positions of stimulating electrodes (*S*) at the wrist and elbow. The recording electrodes (*R*) are shown in position for recording the responses to median and ulnar nerve stimulation. The ground electrode (*G*) is placed on the back of the hand.

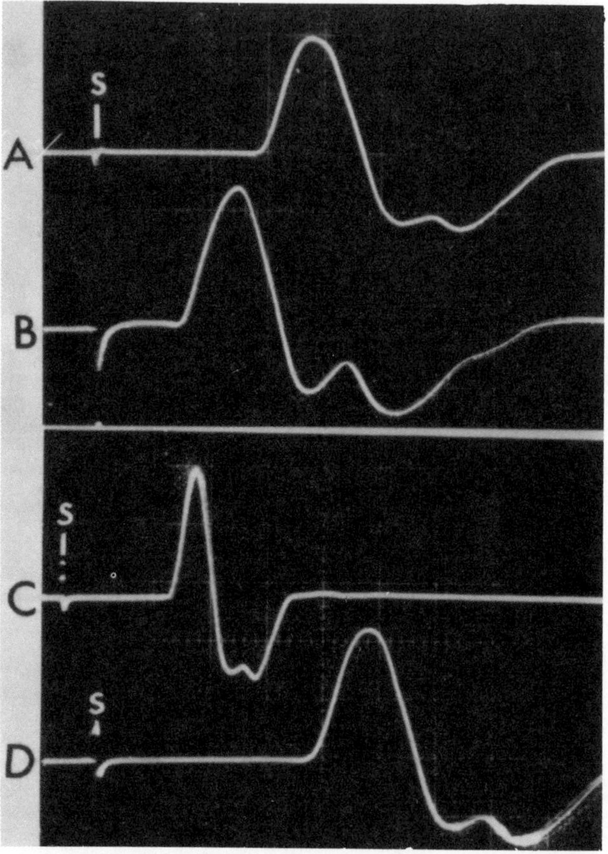

FIG. 7.2. Responses recorded over the abductor digiti quinti muscle after stimulation of the ulnar nerve below elbow (*A*), wrist (*B*), and axilla (*C*) and above elbow (*D*). Calibration: vertical, 5 mV per div; horizontal, 2 msec per div except in *C* (5 msec per div). Positive deflection is downward. *S* represents the stimulus.

transmission across the end-plate, and the depolarization of muscle fibers. This time is called the *latency* of response. By subtracting the latencies determined by stimulating the same nerve at two different points, the nerve conduction time for the segment between the two points is obtained. The latency obtained by stimulating at the most distal possible point along the nerve is called the terminal conduction time.

Residual latency refers to the difference between the measured terminal latency and an estimated time for conduction from the wrist to the motor end-plate, assuming that the velocity in the terminal nerve segments is the same as in the more proximal segments. The estimated time is calculated by dividing the distance from the point of stimulation (at the wrist) to the recording electrode by the conduction velocity of the nerve segment between wrist and elbow. The residual latency varies with: (a) accuracy of measurement and calculations; (b) nerve velocity; (c) slowing of impulses in terminal fibers; (d) synaptic delay, including depolarization at the end-plate; and (e) conduction time of an action potential through muscle tissue and skin pickup electrodes. Several investigators have calculated residual latencies for normal ulnar and median nerves. For example, Mavor and Libman (14) found the average residual latency in the ulnar nerve to be 1.5 msec (range 1.0 to 1.9). In the median nerve, the average residual latency was 2.1 msec (range 1.7 to 2.7).

An accurate measurement of nerve conduction velocity can be made by stimulating at two different points along the nerve and measuring the latency for each response. Thus, for the ulnar nerve, one can stimulate at the wrist and at the elbow. Obviously, at the elbow a longer latency will be recorded (Fig. 7.2). The conduction velocity is calculated by dividing the distance between the two points of stimulation (measured on the skin from cathode to cathode) by the difference between the latencies obtained by stimulating at the two points:

$$\text{conduction velocity} = \text{distance}/\text{latency (2)} - \text{latency (1)}$$

In this way the conduction velocity is determined between two points along the nerve and is always expressed in meters per second. Taking the records of Figure 7.2 as an example:

Latency: below elbow to abductor digiti quinti	5.7 msec
Latency: wrist to abductor digiti quinti	2.9 msec
Difference:	2.8 msec
Distance: between below elbow and wrist	19.5 cm

Conduction velocity = 19.5 cm/2.8 msec = 6960 cm/sec or 69.6 meters/sec

The ulnar nerve can also be stimulated above the elbow and at the axilla and the conduction velocities can be calculated from above to below elbow, axilla to above elbow, etc. With the recording electrode fixed in position, the latency changes but the shape of the response should be the same for the different points of stimulation along the nerve (Fig. 7.2). This is one way of preventing false results by ensuring that the same nerve is being stimulated at each point. When two nerves lie fairly close together, as, for example, the ulnar and median nerves at the wrist or the posterior tibial and common peroneal nerves at the popliteal fossa, errors may arise by the spreading of the stimulus from the region over which the electrode is placed to the neighboring nerve.

It should be noted that by measuring from the start of the stimulus to the initial deflection of the muscle action potential, we are determining the conduction velocity of the fastest conducting axons of the nerve. The nerve trunk is composed of axons conducting impulses at different rates. Some investigators measure from the stimulus to the peak of the first response to get a rough estimation of the varied conduction rates. The initial deflection obtained in motor conduction examinations, and measurements at this point are reliable; however, with the low amplitude responses observed especially in sensory nerve studies, the take-off point may not be obvious. By carefully adjusting the position of the stimulating electrode, fixing the ground between stimulating and recording electrodes, and firmly fixing the recording electrodes, the effects of the stimulus artifact may be minimized and a satisfactory signal and take-off point may be recorded.

In cases of weak muscle responses and when poor signals are observed with surface electrodes, needle electrodes inserted into the appropriate muscle are used for the motor conduction examination.

For examination of *median* nerve conduction, the same procedures are followed with appropriate placement of the electrodes. The active recording electrode is placed over the motor point of the abductor pollicis brevis muscle, and the reference electrode is placed near its tendon of insertion (Fig. 7.1). The thenar eminence, finger, and dorsum of the hand are prepared before electrode placement. The median nerve may be stimulated at the wrist in the area between the palmaris longus and flexor carpi radialis tendons. It may be also stimulated just below the elbow, above the elbow, and at the axilla.

The response to *radial* nerve stimulation may be recorded from the extensor indicis or extensor pollicis longus muscles with surface or needle electrodes. Better initial deflections of the action potentials are obtained with needle electrodes in these muscles, so that we tend to use this type of electrode for radial nerve studies. The radial nerve can be stimulated at the radial groove, at the upper forearm, and at Erb's point in the supraclavicular fossa.

Latency times can be measured for the axillary, musculocutaneous, and suprascapular nerves by stimulating at Erb's point and recording from the corresponding muscles about the shoulder girdle. A surface electrode placed over the most prominent portion of the middle deltoid records responses initiated at the axillary nerve. Mean latency was found to be 3.9 ± 0.5 msec in normal subjects lying in the supine position (15). With surface electrodes placed distal to the midportion of the biceps brachii, mean latency for the musculocutaneous nerve was measured by Kraft (15) to be 4.5 ± 0.6 msec. The mean suprascapular nerve latency to the supraspinatus muscle was determined to be 2.7 ± 0.5 msec, and to the infraspinatus muscle, 3.3 ± 0.5 msec. Evoked potentials were recorded from the supraspinatus muscle with a coaxial needle electrode inserted medial to the midpoint of the spine of the scapula and withdrawn several millimeters when the scapula was reached. Abduction of the arm, with the subject in a sitting position, identified correct placement of the electrode. For the infraspinatus muscle, a needle was inserted several centimeters lateral to the medial border of the scapula and several centimeters below the scapular spine, and it was withdrawn several millimeters when the scapular periosteum was touched. External rotation of the arm at the shoulder identified the muscle.

Lower Extremities

The same procedure is followed for determining the latency and conduction velocity for nerves in the lower extremities. The most commonly examined are the posterior tibial and the peroneal nerves, because they can be fairly easily stimulated percutaneously at two superficial points.

The *posterior tibial* nerve may be stimulated at the ankle behind the medial malleolus and at the knee at the medial aspect of the popliteal space. Recording electrodes are placed over the abductor hallucis or abductor digiti quinti muscle.

The *peroneal* nerve can be examined by stimulating at the lateral aspect of the fibula head and at the ankle lateral to the tendon of the anterior tibial muscle. The recording electrode is placed over the extensor digitorum brevis muscle (Fig. 7.3).

To study the sciatic nerve, needle electrodes must be used for stimulation. They are inserted proximally in the buttock or upper thigh, either between the greater trochanter of the femur and the tuberosity of the ischium or directly below the middle of this position on a line drawn downward to the apex of the popliteal fossa (16). Action potentials may be recorded from the abductor hallucis (for tibial portion) and/or extensor digitorum brevis (for peroneal portion).

Sensory Conduction

Conduction along the sensory fibers of the median or ulnar nerves can be tested by stimulating the digital nerves at the fingers and recording the response at the wrist, elbow, and axilla. A purely sensory potential conducted orthodromically is obtained in this manner. The stimulus is applied through silver strips wrapped around the base and middle of the index or little finger. In the former, the evoked potentials can be recorded over the median nerve at the wrist and elbow; the active recording electrode is placed distally and the ground is between the stimulus and recording electrodes. In the case of the median nerve, a greater response may at times be obtained by stimulating both the index and middle fingers together. Most investigators determine latency by measuring to the *peak* of the major negative deflection.

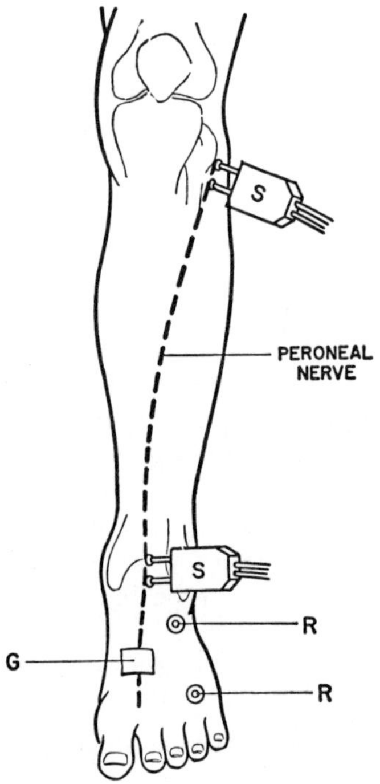

FIG. 7.3. Drawing of leg showing position of stimulating electrodes (*S*) at ankle and knee as well as the recording electrodes (*R*) for conduction velocity measurement of the peroneal nerve. *G* is ground plate.

Potentials evoked by stimulation of the little finger can be observed over the ulnar nerve at the wrist, elbow, and axilla.

Because impulses are propagated in both directions along the nerve from the point of stimulation, the stimulating and recording electrodes may be reversed. *Orthodromic* conduction denotes impulse propagation along an axon in the *normal* direction; for sensory fibers, this corresponds to impulse traveling from distal to proximal. *Antidromic* conduction refers to nerve impulses propagating in a direction *opposite* to normal, or from proximal to distal in the case of sensory conduction. The median and ulnar nerves are stimulated at the wrist and the responses are recorded with ring electrodes around the index and little finger, respectively. Both sensory and motor fibers are stimulated, but only the antidromically conducted sensory action potentials are recorded at the digits. Usually, a higher amplitude response is obtained with antidromic examination, most probably because the sensory nerves are closer to the skin in the fingers.

If the recording and stimulating electrode positions are kept constant, latencies measured orthodromically and antidromically are equal (Fig. 7.4).

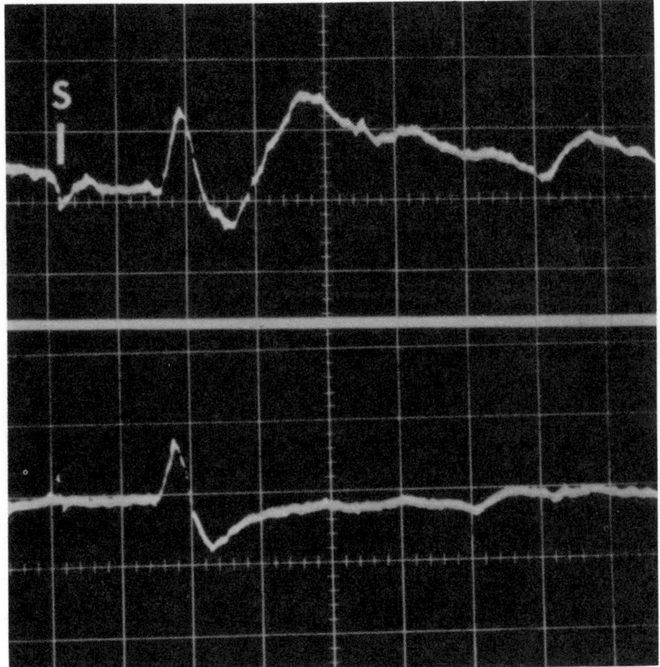

FIG. 7.4. Sensory nerve action potentials recorded from median nerve orthodromically (*top*) and antidromically (*bottom*). Orthodromic recording involved stimulating finger III and recording at wrist; antidromic recording consisted of reverse procedure. Calibration: vertical, 50 μV/div. Positive deflection is downward. *S* is the stimulus. Horizontal, 2 msec per div.

Stimulation of the digits, or orthodromic examination, appears to be more painful than stimulation of the nerve trunk.

Sensory potentials from the radial nerve can be evoked at the thumb and recorded over the radial nerve at the wrist, elbow, and axilla. Shahani et al. (17) describe a simple antidromic method for investigation of conduction in the most distal (sensory) segment of the radial nerve with surface electrodes. The radial nerve was stimulated on the dorsilateral aspect of the forearm, at the junction of the lower one-third and upper two-thirds where it pierces the deep fascia to lie subcutaneously. The recording electrodes were a pair of silver rings applied to the proximal phalanx of the digit. Both orthodromic and antidromic measurements were performed by reversing the position of the electrodes, but no essential difference in response was found between the two techniques. Downie and Scott (18) also describe a procedure for determining the velocity in the distal portion of the sensory division of the radial nerve.

In the lower limbs, sensory nerve action potentials can be obtained from the superficial peroneal, sural, and posterior tibial nerves. The procedure followed in our laboratory for sural nerve measurements involves the placement of the stimulation (surface) electrodes on the calf, slightly lateral to the midline of the leg, and recording with surface electrodes from the area between the lateral malleolus and heel cord. For the superficial peroneal nerve, surface stimulation is delivered at the junction of the middle and distal thirds of the leg, 3 to 4 cm lateral to the anterior crest of the tibia, and recording electrodes are placed on the anterior surface of the ankle. A study performed by DiBenedetto (19) of sensory conduction along these nerves produced the following results: superficial peroneal nerve, 53.1 ± 5.3 m per sec (mean conduction velocity) and 13.0 ± 4.6 μV (mean amplitude) for 1 to 15 years old; 47.3 ± 3.4 m per sec and 13.9 ± 4.0 μV for 15 years and older. Sural nerve, 52.1 ± 5.1 m per sec (conduction velocity) and 23.1 ± 4.4 μV (amplitude) for 1 to 15 years old; 46.2 ± 3.3 m per sec and 23.7 ± 3.8 μV for 15 years and older. Latencies of evoked potentials were measured from onset of stimulus artifact to the first negative deflection, and amplitude of response was measured from peak to peak.

Using electronic signal averaging, Lovelace et al. (20) determined sensory conduction velocities in peroneal and posterior tibial nerves in normal individuals and patients with peripheral neuropathies. In the latter group, velocities with potential amplitudes as low as 0.1 μV were computed. The peroneal nerve was stimulated with ring electrodes at the base of the first phalanx, and the response was recorded at the ankle and knee. The same stimulation point was used for the posterior nerve, recording over the nerve at the medial malleolus and popliteal fossa. The mean sensory nerve conduction velocity along the ankle to knee segment of the posterior tibial nerve in normal subjects (average age 30.3 years) was 49.7 ± 2.3 m per sec with a mean amplitude of 0.3 ± 0.8 μV. Sensory velocity along the ankle to knee segment of the peroneal nerve in normal subjects (average age 30.8 years) was 50.8 ± 5.5 m per sec with a mean amplitude of 0.33 ± 0.09 μV. Latencies were measured from the stimulus artifact to the peak of the initial negative evoked potentials.

Instead of recording evoked responses with surface electrodes over the nerve, Behse and Buchthal (21) used a needle electrode inserted near the nerve in their study of normal sensory conduction in the superficial peroneal, sural, and posterior nerves. The remote electrode, also needle, was placed about 2 to 4 cm from the near-nerve electrode. Recording close to the nerve combined with signal averaging permits sensory potentials of low amplitude (e.g., 0.05 μV) to be detected. The shortest latency of the sensory action potential was measured to the first positive peak. Stimulation was either with surface ring electrodes on the big toe or at other sites with near-nerve electrodes. The maximum sensory conduction velocity was 56.5 ± 3.4 m per sec in proximal and 46.1 ± 3.7 m per sec in distal segments of the nerves (subjects 15 to 30 years of age). Slowing of conduction with increasing age was the same proximally and distally: in 40- to 65-year-old subjects, proximally, 53.1 ± 4.6 m per sec and distally, 42.5 ± 5.5 m per sec. Behse and Buchthal noted the difference in findings between nerves of the lower and upper extremities: (a) the amplitude of the sensory potentials was 10 times smaller at the ankle than at the wrist; (b) potentials recorded between toes and ankle were split up into many components, whereas at the wrist they were smooth and triphasic and only split in old subjects; (c) the maximum velocity along the sensory fibers of the leg was 10 m per sec slower than in the arm; and (d) the maximum sensory velocity in the leg was 5 m per sec faster than the motor velocity, whereas there was no consistent difference between sensory and motor fibers in the arm.

Signal Averaging

The amplitude of the sensory nerve action potential in either the normal or pathological conduction may be quite low, in fact, approaching the noise level. Amplitudes less than 5 μV are not uncommon. Techniques are available which improve the perception of small signals so that they may be evaluated: photographic superimposition and electronic averaging.

Photographic superimposition was used by Dawson and Scott (5) in their study of sensory action potentials. This technique involves superimposing a number (10 to 100) of oscilloscope sweeps on film, each sweep containing the stimulus artifact and its response. The artifact and response, being fixed in time, appear brighter on the film, whereas the noise is dispersed in the background.

Instruments are now available which can recover repetitive small amplitude signals from random background noise. Some electromyographs currently on the market are equipped with this accessory. A large number of sweeps, each containing the evoked response, is applied to the averager. Each sweep is added to the previous ones so that the randomly occurring background noise tends to cancel, whereas the coherent signal reinforces itself. After a sufficient number of sweeps, the evoked response emerging from the noise can be displayed and measured. Singh et al. (22) were able to detect potentials as low as 0.03 μV by electronic averaging of 1000 signals.

NORMAL VALUES

A considerable volume of data has accumulated during the past 15 years. A complete list of published normal motor conduction velocity and terminal conduction times has been published by Sunderland (23). A compilation of motor and sensory conduction velocities and latencies for normal adults is presented in Tables 7.1 and 7.2. Meaningful comparisons of conduction velocity in peripheral nerves can be made only if segment, size, age, and temperature are known.

TABLE 7.1. Normal Motor Conduction Velocity and Distal Latency

Segment	Conduction Velocity Average and Range	Distal Latency	Reference
	m/sec	*msec*	
Ulnar nerve			
Axilla–wrist	60.0 (56.0–62.7)	2.8 (2.3–3.4)	14
Axilla–elbow	63.4 (SD 5.3)		
Elbow–wrist	56.4 (SD 4.8)		24
Axilla–wrist	59.4 (SD 4.1)		
Elbow–wrist	57.5 (49.5–63.6)	2.6 (2.0–3.4)	92
Median nerve			
Axilla–antecubital fossa	71.1 (60.3–86.4)	3.3 (2.8–4.2)	14
Antecubital fossa–wrist	60.1 (54.3–65.0)		
Axilla–wrist	64.3 (59.8–70.4)		
Axilla–elbow	67.9 (SD 7.7)		24
Elbow–wrist	56.1 (SD 5.3)		
Axilla–wrist	60.5 (SD 4.8)		
Axilla–elbow	66 (SD 8)		
Elbow–wrist	57 (SD 5)	3.9 (SD 0.4)	93
Axilla–wrist	62 (SD 5.5)		
Radial nerve			
Erb's point–above elbow	72.0 (56–93)		66
Above elbow–distal forearm	61.6 (48–75)		
Elbow–forearm	62 (SD 5.1)	2.4 (SD 0.5)	94
Posterior tibial			
Popliteal–above malleolus	51.2 (43.4–59.5)	2.1–5.6	95
Above–below malleolus	44.8 (21.0–67.0)		
Popliteal–medial malleolus	49.9 (37–57)		74
Peroneal nerve			
Capitulum fibula–ankle	50 (SD 3.5)	5.1 (SD 0.5)	93

TABLE 7.2. Normal Sensory Conduction Velocity and Latency

Segment		Conduction Velocity Average and Range	Latency, Average, and Range	Reference
		m/sec	*msec*	
Radial nerve				
Forearm–thumb		58.1 (50–68)	2.6 (2–3.3)	17
Thumb–wrist		58 (SD 6.0)		94
Median nerve				
Digits II and III–wrist	(ortho)	58.6 (SD 4.7)	3.0 (SD 0.25)	96
	(anti)	57.4 (SD 3.8)	3.2 (SD 0.25)	
Wrist–digit I		48 (SD 4.5)		93
Wrist–digits II and III		57 (SD 4.1)		
Ulnar nerve				
Digits IV and V–wrist	(ortho)	56.7 (SD 4.2)	3.0 (SD 0.20)	96
	(anti)	54.9 (SD 3.9)	3.2 (SD 0.30)	
Digit V–wrist (ortho)		51.9 (SD 5.6)	2.8 ± 0.2	14
Digit IV–wrist		54.8 (SD 4.9)	3.0 ± 0.2	

Despite variation in technique and the possibility of errors, the average velocities are remarkably consistent. In general, the motor conduction velocity in the upper extremities averages around 60 m per sec. The range that is accepted as normal is quite wide. Some investigators consider velocities between 45 and 75 m per sec as normal in the ulnar and median nerves and somewhat higher velocities, 45 to 80 m per sec, as normal in the radial nerves. The conduction velocity has been found, generally, to be faster in proximal segments of nerves than in distal segments. Explanations of this difference in velocity include the possibility that there is a temperature differential between the upper arm and forearm, and also that the diameter of the motor nerve fibers may gradually decrease distally (14, 24). It should be remembered that the conduction velocity of a nerve fiber is a function of the size of the fiber and the degree of myelination. In the lower extremities, the normal range is taken as 38 to 55 m per sec, with the mean in the mid-40's. The lower conduction rates in the lower extremities have been considered caused by the cooler temperature of the legs as compared to the arms.

Sensory nerve conduction velocities in the upper extremities between 45 and 75 m per sec are considered normal; there is an upper limit of 4 msec for normal distal latency. Normal range for latencies is about 2 to 4 msec. It is important to remember that an absent response is a positive finding and indicates significant abnormality. These values can only serve as a guide; each investigator should choose a technique and determine his own control values.

With surface electrodes, the amplitude of the sensory action potential may be 10 to 60 μV. Careful observation is necessary to discriminate the small sensory potentials from volume-conducted motor responses, a problem which is particularly significant in ulnar nerve examination but which can be corrected by proper placement of electrodes distally. The sensory potentials, the first response after the stimulus artifact, should show sharp deflections with short duration (about 2 msec or less), whereas the volume-conducted response is rounded and longer in duration.

Effects of Temperature and Age on Conduction Velocity

There are two factors which influence conduction velocity and are not related to pathology: temperature and age.

It has been demonstrated (9, 25, 26) that both motor and sensory conduction velocities are decreased as limb temperature is lowered. Temperature along the nerve can be measured with a thermistor needle probe inserted through the skin in the vicinity of the nerve. Studies indicate that the conduction velocity may be lowered 2 to 2.4 m per sec for each drop in temperature of 1°C. During an examination, a cold limb should be warmed and maintained at an even temperature with, for example, an infrared heater. Poliomyelitis is an example of a disease in which a lower conduction velocity as measured in an involved lower limb may be due to coolness of the limbs; almost normal velocity is observed when the limb is warmed.

In infants, young children, and the elderly, the conduction velocity is slower than in adults. Motor conduction velocity in the newborn is about one-half adult values (27–29) but proceeds to increase with age, the rate of increase being a function of the nerve. Gamstorp (28) found that the conduction velocity in the ulnar nerve increased rapidly during the first 3 years and then rose only slightly. For the median nerve, the rate increased slowly before 1 year of age, then increased rapidly, continuing to do so through adolescence. The peroneal nerve conduction velocity increased rapidly through infancy and then changed slightly after 1 year of age. Thomas and Lambert (29), measuring motor conduction velocity in the ulnar nerve, observed that almost all values were in the lower part of the adult range by age 3 years and not significantly different from adult values at 5 years of age. Baer and Johnson (27), in studies performed on 116 infants and children, found that the conduction velocity approaches 100% of the adult rate at slightly over 4 years of age and that from 4 to 16 years of age the conduction velocity slightly exceeds adult values.

Over 60 years of age, the motor conduction rate gradually slows with advancing age. Buchthal and Rosenfalck (9) found that in subjects 70 to 88 years of age the distal latency in sensory nerve fibers was slightly longer and the distal velocity slower than in young subjects. Similarly, Miglietta (30) demonstrated that sensory conduction velocity was slightly but significantly reduced with age.

Mixed Nerve Stimulation and Recording

Stimulating at the wrist and recording at the elbow, Dawson (6) and Dawson and Scott (5) found that sensory conduction time and threshold in the median and ulnar nerves were shorter and lower, respectively, than motor conduction time and threshold. The compound action potential recorded in this type of examination represents orthodromic sensory and antidromic motor conduction. Some investigators have taken advantage of the above findings for mixed nerves to determine proximal sensory nerve conduction with stimulation at the wrist. However, a controversy exists as to whether the faster conduction and lower threshold of sensory fibers are consistent findings. Gilliatt et al. (31) were unable to stimulate digital fibers in the ulnar nerve at the wrist without also exciting some motor fibers. In the median nerve, however, they were able to accomplish such differential stimulation. Buchthal and Rosenfalck (9) were able to confirm a lower threshold in sensory nerves only in the median nerve stimulated at the wrist in young subjects when recording from fingers I or II. Also, the difference in motor and sensory conduction times was not consistent, varying with age and nerve.

Mixed nerve stimulation and recording have also been used to measure the conduction velocity in the common peroneal nerves. Even though more information is not obtained with this technique compared to ordinary nerve conduction measurements, the ease of recording makes it useful when there is suspicion of abnormal nerve conduction.

CLINICAL FINDINGS

Peripheral Nerve Injury

Two methods of classification of nerve injuries in terms of the different types of localized lesions have been proposed, one by Seddon (32) and another by Sunderland (33). Seddon introduced a classification consisting of three categories: neurapraxia, axonotomesis, and neurotmesis. The term neurapraxia characterizes a transitory localized conduction block with no development of signs of denervation. In this type of injury, motor paralysis usually predominates, with little sensory or sympathetic fiber involvement. Complete recovery occurs within days or weeks.

Axonotmesis describes lesions that cause axonal interruption, in which the connective tissue and Schwann cell basement membrane remain intact (Fig. 7.5). Wallerian degeneration occurs distal to the injury. There is complete loss of motor, sensory, and sympathetic functions in the autonomous distribution of the injured nerve, including signs of denervation such as progressive atrophy in the affected muscles. Recovery takes place by axonal regeneration, and usually months are required for complete restoration of function.

Damage to the axon and connective tissue or complete transection of the nerve is denoted by the term neurotmesis. When the trunk is completely severed, Wallerian degeneration of the distal part of the nerve leads to complete dissolution of the myelin and the axis cylinder. Eventually the remaining hollowed tube of the Schwann's sheath becomes filled with cytoplasmic material formed by the Schwann cells. Muscle twitches may be clinically observed by stimulating the distal portion of the nerve for 3 or 4 days after nerve section, whereas evoked potentials may be recorded from the muscles for about 7 days after nerve section.

Within a few days after injury, the proximal stump of the nerve begins to develop a multitude of sprouts which represent the beginning of the nerve regeneration process. The sprouts grow from the proximal end and manage to continue into the sheaths of the distal degenerated portion of the nerve trunk. The tip of the regenerating fiber is unmyelinated, is small in diameter compared to the Schwann column in which it grows, and advances at a rate of 3 to 4 mm per day. The rate of regeneration appears to be faster proximally than distally. The increase in axon diameter and acquisition of myelin sheath gradually takes place over a period of 4 to 12 months and is called the process of maturation.

Approximately normal nerve conduction latencies along the distal segment

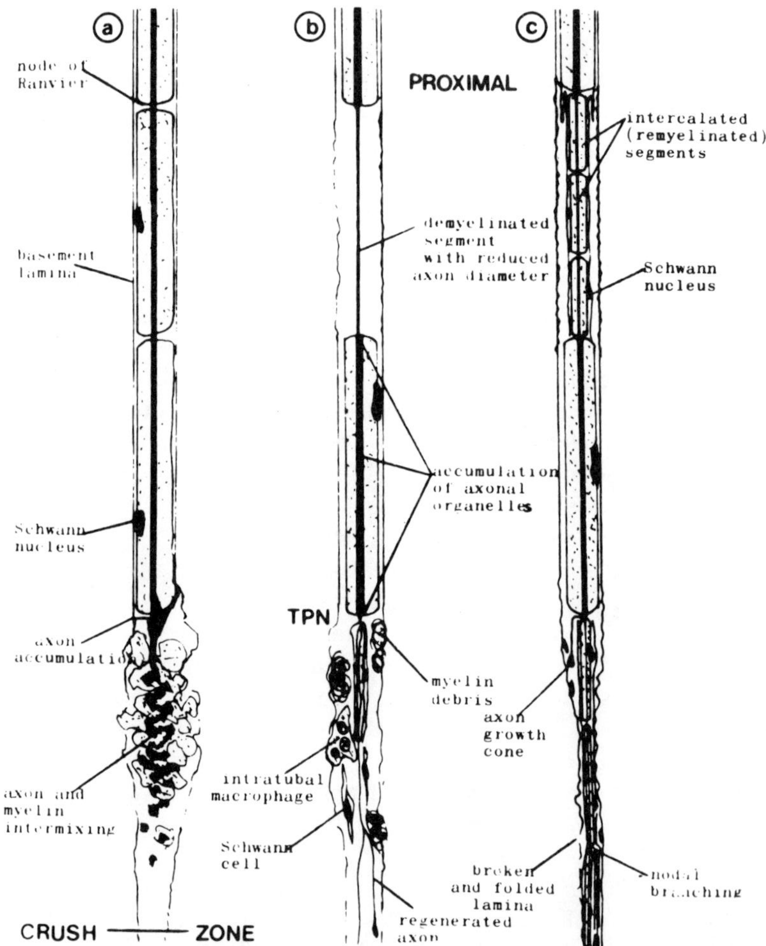

FIG. 7.5. Diagram summarizing the sequential events in the proximal region of a myelinated fiber which has undergone axonotmesis caused by localized nerve crush. (*a*) Immediately after trauma, the Schwann tube is vacated in the crushed zone as the separated nerve fiber recoils from the site of injury. (*b*) The severely interrupted zone has degenerated; Schwann cells are mitosed and form a band of Büngner. Regenerating axon sprouts are growing from the terminal node of Ranvier (*TPN*). Proximally an internode has demyelinated. (*c*) Several days after the injury, a cluster of regenerating axons is growing distally, within the confines of the old Schwann tube. The demyelinated internode has been replaced by three short remyelinating segments. (From M. Spinner and P. S. Spencer: Nerve compression lesions of the upper extremity. Clin. Orthop. Rel. Res., *104:* 58, 1974.)

may be observed for as long as conduction is possible, which is usually up to 7 days after nerve section. The amplitude of the evoked response, which decreases during this period, is more indicative of abnormality than the conduction velocity measurements. Fibrillation potentials may not appear in the denervated muscle for a period of approximately 10 to 21 days. Thus, nerve conduction and electromyographic studies do not present the earliest signs of denervation. One of the earliest indications of peripheral nerve lesion is an increase in the threshold of excitability of the nerve to electrical stimulation. Strength-duration measurements, a simple technique used to assess the presence or absence of denervation, can be very useful (34).

During the early phases of regeneration, stimulation at or below the nerve lesion results in no muscle response. If there has occurred only partial denervation, that is, if some of the fibers are degenerating and others are intact, then the muscle response to nerve stimulation does not disappear with time but is present, probably at a lower amplitude. Nerve conduction may return after nerve section long after recovery of voluntary movement. This is probably because the regenerating nerve has a higher threshold to external electrical stimulation than to normal voluntary stimulation. With electromyographic examination of the affected muscles, long polyphasic motor units may be observed before any clinical evidence of recovery. During the period of nerve regeneration, conduction velocity is extremely slow. According to Wynn Parry (34), nerve conduction is a poor index of reinnervation; strength-duration and electromyographic studies are more reliable.

It is helpful to remember that a partial injury may produce one or a combination of these gradations of injury to the individual nerve fibers within the trunk. In general, the severity of damage is determined by the location of the fiber in the nerve trunk, the force and velocity of the damaging agent, the duration of application, and the general health of the patient. Thus, some fibers may escape involvement, and others may suffer neurapraxia, axonotmesis, or neurotmesis.

Sunderland (33) defined five degrees of increasingly severe nerve injury. The first degree, involving interruption of conduction at the site of injury, is equivalent to neurapraxia. In second degree injury there is loss of continuity of the axons without breaching of the endoneurium; this corresponds to axonotmesis. The third degree injury results in axonal disintegration, Wallerian degeneration, and disorganization within the fascicles. Fourth degree injury includes the alterations of the previous categories as well as the rupture of the perineurium surrounding each fascicle, but there is no loss of continuity of the nerve. Fifth degree injury describes complete severance of the nerve trunk. The third to fifth degrees of injury are subdivisions of neurotmesis in Seddon's classification.

Median Nerve

Carpal Tunnel Syndrome

An entrapment neuropathy represents a localized injury of a peripheral nerve caused by constant mechanical irritation from an impinging anatomic structure. Entrapment may occur where a nerve passes through an osseofibrous tunnel or through a slit in fibrous tissue. One of the most commonly encountered peripheral entrapment neuropathies is the carpal tunnel syndrome (Fig. 7.6). In this condition entrapment occurs where the median nerve passes through the carpal tunnel in company with the flexor tendons

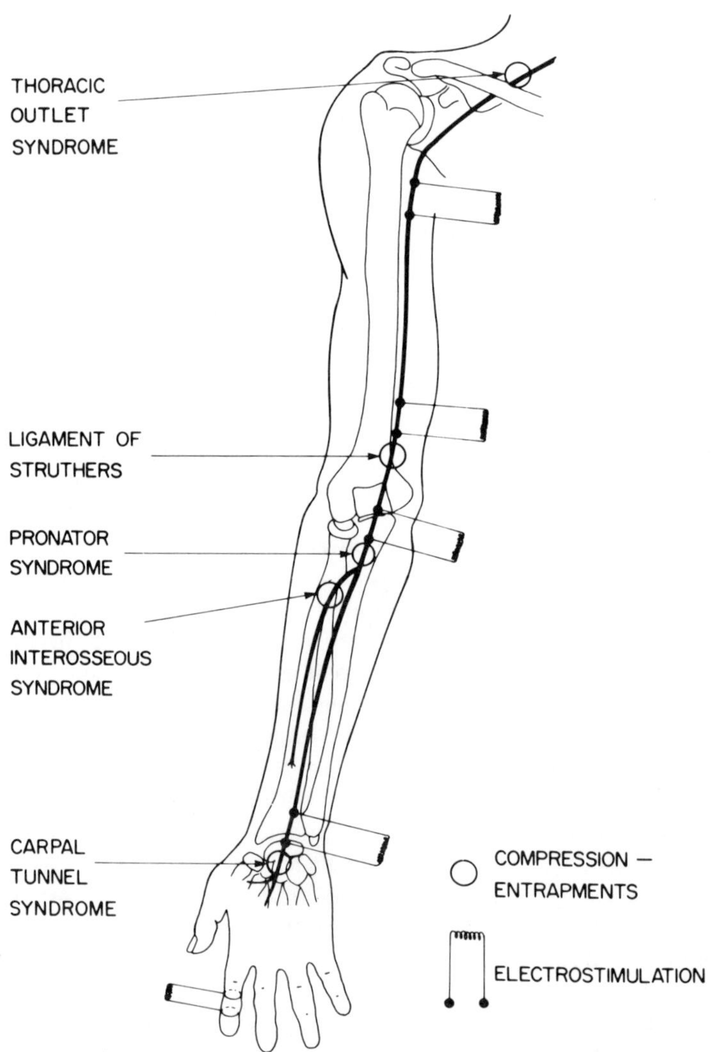

FIG.7.6. Diagram showing the median nerve, locations of compressive lesions and sites of electrostimulation useful in the demonstration of conduction defects. (From J. Goodgold: *Anatomical Correlates of Clinical Electromyography*, (p. 62. Williams & Wilkins, Baltimore, 1974.)

of the fingers. If, for example there is swelling of the tendons, harmful pressure can be exerted against the median nerve, because it takes considerable force to stretch the transverse carpal ligament which forms the roof of the tunnel.

The median nerve is a mixed nerve, carrying both motor and sensory impulses. Thus, in the carpal tunnel syndrome one would expect both motor and sensory functions to be impaired. Numbness and tingling of the fingers as well as weakness and atrophy of the thenar muscles are frequent symptoms. However, the signs of carpal tunnel syndrome not only may occur distal to the transverse carpal ligament, but retrograde distribution of pain even to the shoulder and neck may be present (35). The syndrome may occur from traumatic or nontraumatic sources. It may be a complication of a Colles' fracture, tenosynovitis, rheumatoid arthritis, or hypothyroidism; quite frequently it occurs without known cause. Characteristically, discomfort is worse at night than during the day, and the syndrome is often bilateral, although of different intensity or duration.

In most cases of the carpal tunnel syndrome, a prolonged distal latency is obtained to stimulation of the median nerve motor fibers at the wrist (36, 37). Depending on the severity of the compression, slowing of conduction may be associated with a prolonged duration of the evoked response, as well as a change in configuration to polyphasic and, of course, diminution in amplitude. The occurrence of repetitive firing after stimulation of the median nerve was noted as early as 1956 by Simpson (36). In a study of 300 patients, Thomas et al. (38) found abnormality of conduction in 67% of the symptomatic hands, which consisted of: (a) prolongation of distal latency to more than 4.7 msec in 60% of the hands; (b) failure to detect an action potential of thenar muscles in 4.4% of the hands; and (c) a difference in distal latency of more than 1 msec between the symptomatic and asymptomatic hand, even though both latencies were within normal limits in 13 hands. Distal latency ranged as high as 14.4 msec in some affected hands; the mean latency was 5.35 msec. A greater proportion of symptomatic hands showed abnormal sensory fiber conduction than motor fiber conduction. In sensory fiber examination, prolongation of latency of more than 3.5 msec was found in 35%, and no action potential was detected in 50% of the hands. Thus, 85% of the hands indicated sensory fiber abnormality. In addition, slow motor conduction in the median nerve between the wrist and elbow was found in a number of patients. When the conduction velocity was not below the normal range, it still often was significantly slower than in the unaffected arm.

Although it is evident that the most sensitive test of carpal tunnel disease is the sensory fiber conduction study, it is not an invariable abnormal finding. In a series of 55 patients reported from this laboratory (35), 95% did show abnormality, but three individuals had abnormal motor fiber latency without sensory fiber disturbance. To ensure completeness of examination, both studies should be performed.

The determination of the velocity of conduction both from digit to palm and from palm to wrist had made it possible to identify slowing in conduction along the median nerve in patients in whom conventionally recorded motor latencies are normal. Because the segment of the nerve from digit to palm may be little impaired, its exclusion enhances the degree of demonstrable abnormality. Thus, in six of eight patients with complaints suggestive of a carpal tunnel syndrome in whom motor latency was normal and sensory conduction to the wrist was normal, the maximum velocity from palm to wrist was significantly decreased (39).

In similar conduction velocity studies, Wiederholt (40) stated that sensory latency measurements do not accurately reflect conduction velocity because the exact site of stimulation is a function of stimulus intensity. He presented a method for determining sensory fiber conduction velocity through the carpal tunnel through which he found that the mean conduction velocity across the carpal tunnel in median nerve sensory fibers in healthy subjects was slower (54.43 m per sec) than that proximal to the tunnel (64.26 m per sec). Wiederholt considers the demonstration of abnormally slowed sensory fiber conduction a more sensitive method in evaluating patients with borderline latency measurements.

Downie (41) suggests that the sensitivity of the motor conduction examination may be increased by comparing the terminal latencies between the ulnar and median nerves. The difference in mean values was under 1.2 msec in controls, so that differences greater than 1.5 msec may support the diagnosis even though the median latency is within the normal range.

After examining 117 patients with carpal tunnel syndrome, Buchthal et al. (42) found that the ratio of findings in the median and ulnar nerve did not add information of diagnostic significance when findings were borderline. In 25% of the patients in whom motor conduction and electromyography were normal, the lesion was located from abnormalities in sensory conduction. They also found that motor conduction from elbow to wrist was slowed in two-thirds of the patients, although the slowing was not proportional to the increase in distal latency. Thus, proximal to the site of compression, motor fibers were affected differently from sensory fibers. A decrease in proximal motor velocity is no evidence against a carpal tunnel syndrome. Similarly, abnormalities in the potentials recorded from the ulnar nerve do not exclude a carpal tunnel syndrome, because 15% of the patients had clinical and electrophysiological signs of an ulnar nerve lesion as well. One or several electromyographic abnormalities, such as fibrillation potentials, positive sharp waves, polyphasic potentials, prolonged duration, and increased amplitude of motor unit potentials, were found in 90% of the abductor pollicis brevis muscles examined, including fasciculations in 18% of the patients examined.

The disappearance of pain or dysesthesia after surgical decompression is generally excellent; however, motor or sensory fiber conduction measurements have little value in prognosis (38). Approximately the same preoperative distribution of distal motor latencies was frequently found in those patients with complete recovery as in those who failed to obtain relief after surgery.

Electromyographic abnormality occurs with an incidence of about 40 to 45% (35, 38) and consists of the usual disturbances seen in neuropathy. The routine should include examination of median innervated forearm muscles so that the distribution of the lesion is confirmed.

The clinical features of carpal tunnel disease show a considerable resemblance to those encountered in the thoracic outlet syndrome, although careful examination and certainly electrodiagnostic study differentiate the two entities. In this laboratory, however, we have encountered several cases with concurrent lesions which necessitated specific therapy for each before clinical "cure." Crymble (43) reviewed 140 patients with brachial neuralgia and reported that 28 showed concurrent lesions, which he attributed to coincidence. It is the opinion of the authors that it is not a matter of coincidence but that the latent carpal tunnel disease manifests because of the superimposed distal lesion.

Case Report (J. M.). The patient is a 35-year-old white male outdoor workman. For the past few months he noticed Raynaud's phenomenon involving the fingers of both hands, first during severe cold weather and then on even slightly inclement changes. Physical examination was essentially negative except for evidence of obliteration of the brachial pulse on both sides in response to appropriate maneuvering and the precipitation of characteristic color changes of the digits on exposure to chilled water. Electrical studies showed delayed distal sensory and motor latency of both median nerves. EMG was normal. X-ray of the upper thorax showed no osseous abnormalities. After surgery was performed on both wrists, the patient had an uneventful postoperative course with considerable relief of pain and paresthesia. Upon return to work he noted that the vasospastic symptoms were happening about "half as much as before." In spite of the improvement in symptoms he was unable to carry out his work comfortably, so he returned several months later to the hospital for bilateral resection of the first rib. He has since been symptom-free, except for rare bouts of digital vasospasm involving only the right hand when the temperature is especially low.

Pronator Syndrome

Entrapment of the median nerve may also occur in the proximal forearm as the nerve passes through the two heads of the pronator teres and then dips under the sublimis bridge (Fig. 7.6). Three types of anatomic abnormalities called the pronator syndrome have been observed (44): (a) thickening of the lacertus fibrosis, (b) passage of the median nerve deep to both heads of the pronator teres, and (c) thickening of the flexor superficialis arch. According to Spinner and Spencer (44), patients usually have a 9- to 24-month history of nonlocalized forearm pain. The most consistent finding has been reproduction of pain in the proximal forearm on resistance to pronation of the forearm and flexion of the wrist. Numbness in some digits innervated by the median nerve has also been observed at times. Tenderness over the pronator teres was an invariable finding in seven patients with pronator syndrome (45). Intense nocturnal parasthetic discomfort is uncommon—which is not the case with the carpal tunnel syndrome.

In seven patients with a lesion localized to the trunk of the median nerve at the elbow, Buchthal et al. (42) found that three had abnormal sensory conduction (below to above elbow) and two had electromyographic abnormalities in the superficial and the deep flexor muscles of the forearm and in the abductor pollicis brevis muscle. In one patient the latency was prolonged to the deep flexor muscle, but electromyographic abnormalities were also found in the superficial flexor muscle. Another patient had prolonged motor latencies to both the deep and superficial flexor muscles, but electromyographic abnormalities only in the deep flexor muscles. As compared with entrapment at the wrist, the authors noted that compression at the elbow was located by electromyographic findings rather than by abnormalities in conduction. Abnormal conduction was observed in only four of the seven patients.

Anterior Interosseous Nerve Syndrome

Just distal to its passage through the pronator tunnel, the median nerve gives off the volar or anterior interosseous nerve, which supplies the flexor pollicis longus, the radial portion of the flexor digitorum profundus, and the pronator quadratus muscles. The anterior interosseous nerve is purely motor and frequently participates in anomalous distributions, e.g., innervation of all portions of the flexor digitorum profundus, cross-overs to the ulnar nerve, and others. This syndrome (also known as the Kiloh-Nevin syndrome after Kiloh and Nevin (46), who originally described it) may be a consequence of a forearm fracture or a supracondylar fracture of the humerus or compression by a fibrous band just below the origin of the branch. The hand may display a typical "pinch attitude" resulting from paralysis of the long flexor of the thumb and the flexor digitorum profundus to the index and long fingers (44).

Motor and sensory conduction in the main trunk of the median nerve are normal. Consistent with a lesion confined to the anterior interosseous nerve, electromyographic abnormalities are manifested in the deep finger flexors of the forearm and the pronator quadratus. Fibrillation potentials, positive sharp waves, and a reduced interference pattern during full effort are readily detected in these muscles (43, 47, 48).

Ligament of Struthers

Median nerve entrapment may also occur above the medial epicondyle (Fig. 7.6). An anomalous spur may be found 3 to 5 cm above the medial epicondyle in 1% of limbs (44). A fibrous-osseous tunnel is formed by the ligament of Struthers connecting the spur to the medial epicondyle. The median nerve and usually the brachial artery pass through this tunnel and consequently are subject to compression after trauma. The presence of this abnormality must be considered in the differentiation from more distal entrapments of the median nerve which it resembles, such as the pronator syndrome or the anterior interosseous nerve syndrome.

Thoracic Outlet Syndrome

Although the ulnar nerve is most frequently involved in this syndrome, compression of the median nerve can occur when the upper trunk or lateral cord of the brachial plexus is involved. Segmental conduction studies reveal low velocities which confirm the diagnosis (49).

Ulnar Nerve

Lesions at Wrist and Hand

In the area where the ulnar nerve enters the palm, it comes to lie in a shallow, oblique canal (canal of Guyon), the walls of which are the pisiform bone medially and the hook of the hamate laterally. The canal is covered by the volar carpal ligament and the palmaris brevis muscle. Near the pisiform bone the nerve divides into a deep muscular branch and superficial cutaneous branches. The deep branch, after innervating the abductor, flexor, and opponens digiti minimi, turns laterally to cross the palm at a deep plane, innervating the interossei, the medial two lumbrical muscles, the adductor pollicis, and the deep head of flexor pollicis brevis (Fig. 7.7).

Ulnar nerve lesions in the wrist and hand have been divided into three specific groups according to the symptoms and site of involvement (50, 51). According to the scheme of Shea and McClain (51), Type I syndrome represents motor weakness of all ulnar innervated muscles in the hand, as well as a sensory deficit to the palmar surfaces of the hypothenar eminence and of the ulnar two fingers, and can be caused by pressure on the nerve just proximal to the canal of Guyon or within the canal so that both superficial and deep branches are involved. Type II syndrome involves motor weakness of those muscles innervated by the deep branch, but normal sensation is present in the hand; it may occur with a lesion along the deep branch of the

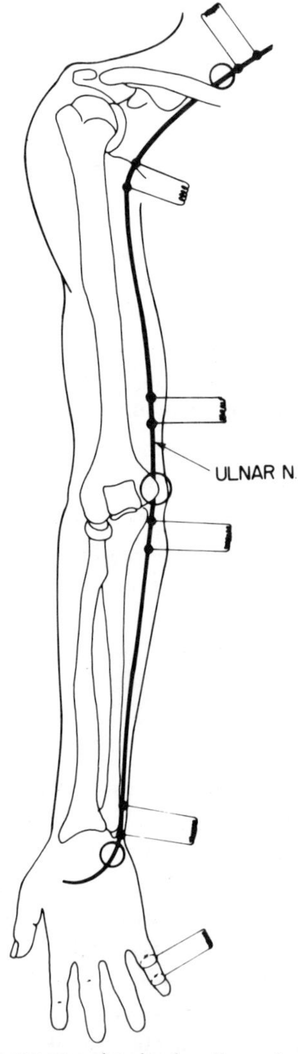

FIG. 7.7. Diagram of the ulnar nerve showing locations of compressive lesions and sites of electrostimulation useful in the demonstration of conduction defects. (From J. Goodgold: *Anatomical Correlates of Clinical Electromyography*, p. 70. Williams & Wilkins, Baltimore, 1974.)

ulnar nerve. Type III syndrome involves sensory deficits in the volar surface of the hypothenar eminence and in the fourth and little fingers due to pressure on the superficial branch. There is no muscle weakness or atrophy associated with the Type III syndrome.

Simpson (36) showed that a lesion involving the deep branch of the ulnar nerve may cause slowing of nerve conduction over the involved segment. Ebeling et al. (50) later confirmed this, observing profound increases in terminal latency of motor conduction to the affected muscles; they also noted a mild slowing of nerve conduction proximal to the local lesion. Their examinations were performed by placing concentric needle electrodes in the small muscles of the hand and stimulating the ulnar nerve trunk at the wrist, elbow, and axilla.

Bhala and Goodgold (52) describe a technique for measuring the conduction time in the deep branch of the ulnar nerve by stimulation of the ulnar nerve at the wrist and recording with surface electrodes over the abductor digiti minimi and the first dorsal interosseous muscles.

Shea and McClain (51) list 19 different causative lesions for compression of the ulnar nerve in the wrist and hand. In a review of the literature, they found the most frequent cause was ganglionic compression (28.7% of reported cases); next came occupational neuritis (23.5%), laceration (10.3%), ulnar artery disease (8.1%), and others. Most of the lesions (52%) involved the deep branch, Type II; 30% were Type I, and 18% were Type III. Occupation neuritis of the deep branch of the ulnar nerve may arise from prolonged pressure exerted on the hypothenar region; it is usually a unilateral condition characterized by weakness and wasting of the first dorsal interosseous muscle.

Lesions at the Elbow

The most common focus of ulnar nerve lesions is at the elbow, where the nerve is held in an osseous groove against the posterior aspect of the medial epicondyle of the humerus. At this point, the nerve is liable to direct trauma or, more commonly, to injury by being drawn tightly against the ulnar groove. Tightening of the nerve can be caused by a disturbance of the angular relationship at the elbow, such as a fracture, dislocation, or infection. The earliest symptom of motor involvement is usually weakness of adduction of the little finger, followed by weakness and wasting of the ulnar innervated intrinsic muscles of the hand (53). Sensation may be disturbed over the ulnar third of the palm and little finger and the medial aspect of the fourth finger. In the forearm, weakness is often found in the ulnar innervated portion of the flexor digitorum profundus and sometimes in the flexor carpi ulnaris, because the branch to this muscle varies in origination, arising slightly above the elbow or at the elbow level itself. Neuropathic findings may not be observed until years after an initiating trauma which is often forgotten. Under these circumstances, the abnormality has been called "tardy ulnar palsy." Surgical relief for a neuropathy at the elbow is usually not adequate unless the nerve is transplanted anteriorly, whereas a simple neurolysis may be sufficient for other entrapment areas (54).

Simpson (36), who first reported motor nerve conduction changes in a case of ulnar nerve lesion, found slow conduction through the involved region but relatively normal conduction above and below it. Gilliatt and Thomas (55) examined 14 patients with chronic lesions at the elbow and reported a substantial slowing of ulnar nerve conduction in the forearm and elbow region but only a very slight slowing in the upper arm. No sensory action potentials were detected from the wrist-to-above elbow segment or from the fifth finger-to-wrist segment; however, they were present at the axilla with stimulation above the elbow. It was the impression of the authors that conduction studies are likely to be helpful in localizing the level of an ulnar nerve lesion only when sufficient nerve damage has occurred to produce definite impairment of power or sensation in the hand.

Kaeser (56) also observed either none or very small sensory potentials at the wrist but was still able to localize 25 of 29 ulnar nerve lesions at the elbow by demonstrating slower motor conduction across the elbow.

In a study of 46 patients with lesions of one or both ulnar nerves, Payan (57) localized 48 of 50 lesions by combining results of the various electrophysiological examinations: (a) disproportionate slowing of sensory or motor conduction at elbow; (b) prolonged latency to the flexor carpi ulnaris; and (c) change in amplitude, duration, or shape of the sensory potential from below to above elbow. He found sensory fibers to be affected first in ulnar nerve lesions at the elbow.

A separate study by the same investigator (58) of 13 patients with ulnar lesions at the elbow, 11 of whom underwent anterior transposition of the nerve and two of whom were managed conservatively, indicated that the first sign of recovery in both sensory and motor fibers was an increase in conduction velocity across the elbow. Significant clinical improvement did not occur until the sensory action potential recorded at the wrist had increased in amplitude. Because the extent and rate of improvement of the patients managed conservatively equaled or exceeded the response in those who underwent transposition, Payan contends "that the operation is being performed more often than necessary: the course of the nerve need be altered only when it lies in adverse relation to its bed, and lesions caused by acute local trauma, avoidable occupational trauma, or a period of compression lack this essential criterion for surgical intervention."

Another ulnar nerve lesion at the elbow is due to a deficiency of the fascial roof over the epicondylar groove which results in complete dislocation of the nerve during flexion, or at least an abnormal hypermobility. The nerve in this way is exposed over the tip of the epicondyle to trauma, especially if it is somewhat tethered and not freely movable. In a study of 300 patients, 9 nerves were completely dislocated, 35 were incompletely dislocated, and 21 showed abnormal hypermobility (59). The lesion is frequently bilateral and often asymptomatic.

Thoracic Outlet Syndrome

Compression of the brachial plexus and the subclavian artery and vein, usually between the first rib and clavicle, results in the thoracic outlet syndrome. The signs and symptoms depend on whether the nerves or blood vessels or both are compressed at the thoracic outlet. In the majority of cases the ulnar nerve is involved, because it is formed by the lower trunk in the brachial plexus and lies directly on the first rib (Fig. 7.7). Pain and paresthesias, primarily in the ulnar distribution of the hand, are the most common symptoms. Caldwell et al. (60) found a nondermatonal sensory deficit roughly following an ulnar distribution in 48% of their patients with suspected thoracic outlet syndrome and weakness, usually involving the ulnar intrinsics and the wrist and finger extensors, in 20% of the patients.

Because measurement of ulnar nerve conduction velocity across the thoracic outlet is technically feasible and usually easily performed, it may be employed as an objective method for evaluation of patients with suspected thoracic outlet syndrome. Points of stimulation are over the supraclavicular fossa, the mid-upper arm, below the elbow, and the wrist. Recording electrodes are over the abductor digiti minimi muscle.

Caldwell et al. (60) obtained in normal subjects an average motor ulnar nerve conduction velocity across the thoracic outlet (neck to elbow) of 72.2 m per sec (range 68 to 75 m per sec). A similar measurement in patients clinically diagnosed as abnormal showed an average conduction velocity of 57.8 m per sec. A steel tape was used to measure the length of the proximal segment. Urschel et al. (49) reported an average ulnar nerve conduction velocity across the thoracic outlet in patients of 53 m per sec (range 32 to 65 m per sec).

Jebsen (61) used steel calipers to measure the neck-to-elbow segment in normal subjects and reported an average ulnar nerve conduction velocity of 61.3 m per sec (range 52 to 78 m per sec). London (62) completed a study in which the ulnar nerve conduction velocity across the thoracic outlet in 30 normal individuals was compared using caliper and steel tape measurements. With calipers, the length of the neck-to-elbow segment was 23.3 cm and the average velocity was 58.9 m per sec (range 50 to 67.7 m per sec); with steel tape, the length was 27.8 cm and the average velocity was 70.2 m per sec (range 58 to 82.4 m per sec). The 4.5-cm difference in apparent mean length of the ulnar nerve segment using the two types of measurement yields a difference of 11.3 m per sec in the calculated motor conduction velocity. This accounts for the different average normal values across the outlet. Applying Jebsen's results from studies in cadavers (61), London noted that caliper measurement more closely approximates the true nerve length than does steel tape measurement for this segment. He concludes, however, that meaningful results will be obtained if one consistently uses either measurement technique.

London (62) also investigated the possibility of using the opposite limb as a control. He found that the difference in the mean conduction velocity between the neck-to-elbow segment in the two arms of the same patient is greater than observed for the elbow-to-wrist segment. The explanation of this difference includes such factors as (a) temperature variation between the two limbs and (b) the variability of the depth of the skin-nerve interface. The depth is probably greater and more variable to Erb's point than at the other stimulation sites. A larger current is frequently required for supramaximal stimulation at Erb's point than at other sites. Thus, the effective point of stimulation might differ between the two limbs. London's recommendation was that the opposite limb may be used as a control if one is aware of the differences between the conduction velocities across this segment. If the velocity of each arm is within the established normal range but the two values differ by 9.0 m per sec (mean +2 SD), then the slower conducting ulnar nerve should be carefully studied serially.

These technicalities are exaggerated and compounded in stout subjects, especially those with short neck segments.

Radial Nerve

The radial nerve is involved in extensor-supinator movement of the upper extremity. From the axilla, the radial nerve passes down the arm, winding from the medial to the lateral side around the humerus in the spiral groove between the origins of the lateral and medial heads of the triceps muscle. Before entering the groove, it innervates the triceps and anconeus muscles. When the nerve reaches the lateral aspect of the humerus, it proceeds further forward by piercing the lateral intermuscular septum to occupy a position in front of the lateral condyle of the humerus between the brachialis and brachioradialis, innervating the brachioradialis and the extensor carpi radialis longus and frequently sending a twig to the brachialis. The radial trunk then bifurcates into a superficial branch which passes over the extensor carpi radialis brevis origin, down the forearm under the brachioradialis, and into a deep branch which passes through the fibrous edge of the extensor carpi radialis, through a slit in the supinator muscle to the posterior aspect of the forearm. In this region it is in contact with the interosseous membrane and is called the posterior interosseous nerve.

The deep branch is purely a motor nerve which innervates the muscles that dorsiflex the wrist and fingers. The superficial radial nerve innervates the skin over the radial side of the dorsum of the wrist and hand and then terminates in the dorsal digital nerves.

The radial nerve is subject to compression or injury in the spiral groove or in the proximal portion of the forearm immediately distal to the elbow (Fig. 7.8). In patients with fracture of the humerus, Trojaborg (63) found the site of injury of the radial nerve at the level of the spiral groove, with total interruption of motor function distal to this point. Sensation decreased in the dorsum of the hand and in one, two, or three radial fingers, with some involvement of a small area of the dorsal aspect of the forearm in one-half

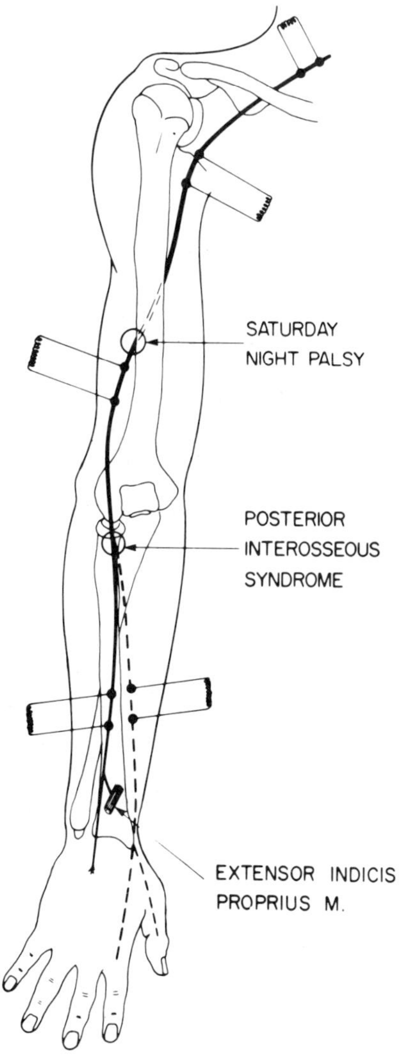

FIG. 7.8. Diagram of the radial nerve showing locations of compressive lesions and sites of electrostimulation useful in the demonstration of conduction defects. (From J. Goodgold: *Anatomical Correlates of Clinical Electromyography*, p. 72. Williams & Wilkins, Baltimore, 1974.)

of the patients. No response was detected in the brachioradialis and extensor muscles of wrist and fingers, and sensory potentials could not be discriminated with nerve stimulation. Trojaborg established that the rate of recovery of radial nerve motor and sensory fibers was equal, and estimated it to be about 1 mm per day.

"Saturday Night" Palsy

Prolonged compression of the radial nerve at the position of its penetration through the lateral intermuscular septum, which may occur during sleep, may result in the lesion commonly referred to as Saturday night palsy. This type of paralysis is usually classified as a neurapraxia or transient block. In a study of 29 patients with compression of the radial nerve during sleep, Trojaborg (63) found considerable slowing of conduction in both motor and sensory fibers across the site of the lesion. Normal conduction returned within 6 to 8 weeks. He suggests that the cause of the palsy is a local demyelination. Sunderland (64) proposed that the lesion occurs at the lateral border of the humerus, in the region where the radial nerve pierces the lateral intermuscular septum. This has been supported by other investigators (65).

Gassel and Diamantopoulos (65), and later Jebsen (66), measured motor conduction velocities for the proximal and distal segments of the same fibers of the radial nerve. They found that the distance between the sites of stimulation at Erb's point and above the elbow could be more reliably measured with obstetric calipers than with a surface tape measure; the true length of the proximal nerve segment averaged 0.54 cm longer than the caliper measurement (66).

Posterior Interosseous Nerve Syndrome

The posterior interosseous syndrome is a complex entity which involves a number of possible abnormalities.

1) As the radial nerve passes down toward the supinator, it passes the radiohumeral joint and is usually loosely tethered to the joint capsule. However, a firm, constricting band may be present which compresses the intact or bifurcated nerve trunk. Under these circumstances, the innervation to the brachioradialis and the extensor carpi radialis longus muscles remains intact.

2) A short distance distally, the nerve dips under the relatively sharp and tough edge of the extensor carpi radialis brevis, which may impinge on the nerve, especially during pronation.

3) The point at which the deep radial nerve enters the supinator muscle is not a simple slit but is an arch, called the arcade of Frohse, which may be fibrotendinous and compressive.

4) The posterior interosseous nerve may be compromised within the substance of the supinator mass itself by tumor or vascular anomaly. The resulting palsy is sometimes referred to as the "supinator channel syndrome" (67, 68).

Aside from demonstration of a segmental conduction defect, identification of the level of the lesion may be enhanced by the knowledge that the extensor carpi radialis longus is innervated above the bifurcation of the main trunk of the radial nerve and the supinator muscle begins to receive its innervation just before the deep branch penetrates its mass. After the posterior interosseous nerve leaves the supinator it innervates the superficial layer of extensor muscles (extensor digitorum communis, extensor carpi ulnaris, etc.) so that the brachioradialis, extensor carpi radialis, and supinator are spared in the "supinator syndrome," but the extensor digitorum and other distally innervated muscles are affected. The posterior interosseous nerve then descends on the superficial surfaces of the deep extensor muscles and gives branches into the surface of each of them; the last muscular branch goes to the extensor indicis proprius muscle.

An entrapment neuropathy involving the posterior interosseous nerve may occur from a single or repeated forceful supination, dorsiflexion, or radial deviation against resistance. In certain maneuvers, for example, with a hammer or tennis racket, the tough, thin, fibrous edges of the extensor carpi radialis brevis and the supinator slit may be drawn tight against the nerve, giving rise to a condition commonly called "tennis elbow" or lateral epicondylitis. The symptoms and signs of acute tennis elbow are pain and tenderness over the lateral epicondyle of the humerus and pain on passive stretching of the extensor muscles and on resisted extension of the fingers.

Sciatic Nerve

The sciatic nerve is formed in the posterior region of the pelvis and is derived from the $L_{4, 5}$, $S_{1, 2, 3}$ nerve roots. The nerve trunk leaves the pelvis through the greater sciatic notch and passes down the posterior thigh deep to the piriformis muscle to the region just above the popliteal space, where the two terminal branches form the tibial nerve medially and the peroneal laterally. There is a 10% incidence of anatomic variation in which the two portions of the sciatic nerve separate at the sciatic notch and the lateral division, the peroneal, frequently pierces the substance of the piriformis muscle to lie more posteriorly. In the usual arrangement, at the edge of the piriformis the nerve fascicles are already arranged to form the nerves to the hamstrings and part of the adductor magnus, the tibial nerve, common peroneal nerve, and the nerve to the short head of the biceps. A complete lesion of the sciatic results in a flail leg and foot.

A nerve lesion caused by direct trauma, except for that from penetrating missiles, is uncommon. In the region of the roots where the plexus and trunks form, space-occupying lesions (neoplasms, fetus during pregnancy) may cause a compressive neuropathy which wholly or maximally affects the peroneal portion. In the region of the buttock, the sciatic nerve may be compromised by fracture or dislocations involving the head of the femur, iatrogenic complications of surgery, and low, medially misplaced intramuscular injections in the buttock (69, 70). The postinjection paralysis may be immediate and associated with excruciating pain or may develop more slowly over a short interval of time. The injection mass need not be within the nerve but can be located adjacently. Surgical exploration has revealed relatively large intragluteal scars even in individuals uncomplicated by intramuscular injection. The problem is of greater magnitude and incidence in newborn and premature babies, even when injection is given in the upper and outer quadrant of the buttock. The only prophylactic measure is administration of parenteral therapy in the middle third of the lateral surface of the thigh (71). If injury is immediately perceived, then flooding the subgluteal area with 50 to 100 ml of normal saline may act to dilute the offending material.

Invariably, the common peroneal portion is maximally affected. When recovery does occur, any residue is more apt to involve this division of the sciatic nerve. Therapy should be quite conservative for 4 to 6 months to allow for spontaneous recovery; surgical intervention may involve neurolysis or resection and end-to-end anastomosis (72).

An unusual sciatic entrapment neuropathy was described (73) in which the entrapment was caused by a myofascial band between the biceps femoris and the adductor magnus. Nerve conduction measurements with needle stimulation of the sciatic nerve at the buttock were helpful in localizing a delay in conduction in the upper leg.

The piriformis syndrome represents a sciatic neuritis brought about by compression of the nerve between the bony edge of the notch and the piriformis muscle. Kopell and Thompson (54) have pointed out that an increase in lordosis with compensatory hip flexion tightens the nerve against the notch via pressure by the piriformis, which usually becomes hyperirritable.

Although it is difficult, at times, clinically to separate sciatica due to sciatic neuropathy from that produced by a lower lumbar compressive radiculopathy, the EMG evidence of a segmental distribution (i.e., involvement of glutei muscles and tensor fasciae latae) and conduction defects in the nerve serve to elucidate the problem.

At a more distal site, the sciatic (and/or its terminal branches) may be secondarily injured by fragment displacement after supracondylar fracture of the femur.

Posterior Tibial Nerve

Tarsal Tunnel Syndrome

The posterior tibial nerve is usually derived from the sciatic nerve just above the popliteal space and courses distally to innervate the posterior compartment muscles of the calf, the muscles and joints of the foot, and the skin of the heel and sole. The nerve may be compromised by lesions in the popliteal space (arterial aneurysm) or more distally at the ankle. The tarsal tunnel, located behind and inferior to the medial malleolus, has a bony floor and is roofed over by the laciniate ligament (flexor retinaculum). The tibial nerve passes through this fibroosseous passageway, and within it or immediately distal to it the nerve divides into three branches—the calcaneal, the lateral, and the medial plantar nerves. The calcaneal branch supplies the skin of the heel and a portion of the calcaneus, the medial plantar nerve innervates the skin and muscles of the medial aspect of the sole, and the lateral plantar is distributed to the lateral portion. The medial and lateral plantar nerves pass through individual openings, so that each is liable to an isolated entrapment neuropathy.

The tarsal tunnel syndrome, resulting from compression of all or part of the posterior tibial nerve, is not as readily recognized as its counterpart in the wrist, the carpal tunnel syndrome (Fig. 7.9). Its most common etiology involves spatial alteration as a consequence of fracture or dislocation of the region bones. Posttraumatic edema and tenosynovitis may be as important as the direct pressure of skeletal displacement. In some cases, no history of relevant antecedent trauma can be elicited.

The compression lesion may be partial or complete and may involve both

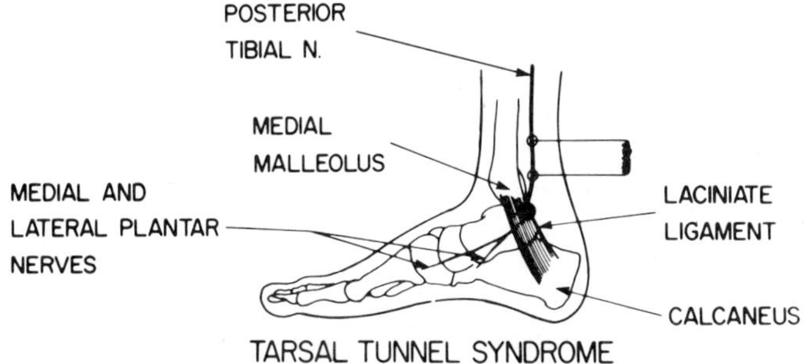

FIG. 7.9. At the proximal end of the tarsal tunnel, the entire trunk of the posterior tibial nerve may be compressed to produce weakness and sensory loss in the medial and lateral plantar distribution as well as in the distribution of the most proximal sensory branch, the calcanean, which supplies the medial surface of the heel. (From J. Goodgold: *Anatomical Correlates of Clinical Electromyography*, p. 138. Williams & Wilkins, Baltimore, 1974.)

motor and sensory fibers to a varying degree, so that signs and symptoms may include paralysis or paresis of the small muscles of the foot, numbness, burning pain, or paresthesia. Occasionally, a tender area is palpable at the margin of the medial malleolus, and percussion may trigger an acute attack of radiating pain. Frequently, pain is intensified at night.

In a report on two cases of tarsal tunnel syndrome, Goodgold et al. (74) found the latency from malleolus to the abductor hallucis was 9.5 msec on the affected side of one patient and that there was no response to stimulation for the abductor of the first toe in the other. Johnson and Ortiz (75) reported on six patients with tarsal tunnel syndrome (two had bilateral involvement) and found that the latencies in the medial plantar branch ranged from 6.0 to 7.6 msec and that those in the lateral plantar branch ranged from 7.0 to 9.0 msec. They concluded that a latency in excess of 6.1 msec for the medial plantar nerve and 6.7 msec for the lateral plantar nerve was indicative of tarsal tunnel syndrome. Similarly, Edwards et al. (76) recorded prolonged latencies (6.6, 6.5, and 8.0 msec) between ankle and abductor hallucis in three patients and abnormal electromyography only in the one with an 8.0-msec latency.

Femoral Nerve

The femoral nerve, the largest branch of the lumbar plexus, penetrates the psoas major muscle in the abdomen, courses downward through the muscle fibers, and emerges from the lower part of its lateral border to exit from the abdominal cavity under the inguinal ligament. Below the ligament, the nerve divides to supply innervation for the pectineus, sartorius, and quadriceps femoris muscles as well as sensory innervation to the skin over the anterior and lateral aspects of the thigh.

Femoral neuropathy may be caused by a variety of systemic factors, such as alcoholism and, particularly, diabetes mellitus, whereas compression and injury of the nerve may result from hemorrhage into the psoas muscle, adjacent pelvic fractures, or increased intraabdominal pressure during the birth process. Femoral neuropathy due to continuous pressure by retractor blades on the psoas muscle has been reported during the course of abdominal hysterectomy (77).

Gassel (78) determined femoral nerve conduction velocity by stimulating below the inguinal ligament and recording the response with needle electrodes in the rectus femoris muscle. Normal conduction in the femoral nerve was 70 m per sec. Prolongation of the latency and slow conduction velocity were observed in patients with neuritis of the femoral nerve but not in those with spinal muscular atrophy or primary muscle-wasting diseases, even in the case of severe muscle wasting. Chopra and Hurwitz (79) found a significant slowing of motor conduction velocity in diabetics with and without neuropathy.

In a study of 100 persons performed by Johnson et al. (80), latencies from above the inguinal ligament to the vastus medialis motor point ranged from 6.1 to 8.4 msec and those below the ligament ranged from 5.5 to 7.5 msec. The mean conduction velocity of the femoral nerve was 66.7 ± 7.4 m per sec. The technique devised by Johnson et al. was helpful in the diagnosis of femoral nerve compression by the inguinal ligament. Marked slowing in conduction was detected across the segment that passes under the inguinal ligament in a case of bilateral femoral nerve compression presumably due to a prolonged dorsal lithotomy position during surgery.

Peroneal Nerve

Peroneal Palsy

The common peroneal nerve, derived from the bifurcation of the sciatic nerve, travels down the popliteal fossa to the lateral aspect of the neck of the fibula and then passes through an opening in the origin of the peroneus longus muscle. At the fibular neck, it divides into three branches—the superficial, deep, and recurrent peroneal nerves. The deep peroneal nerve innervates the tibialis anterior, extensor digitorum longus, extensor hallucis longus, peroneus tertius, and extensor digitorum brevis. The superficial peroneal nerve supplies the peroneus longus and brevis and, with the deep branch, provides sensation to the skin over the distal lateral surface of the leg and dorsum of the foot. Peroneal nerve injury may cause pain in the lateral surface of the leg and foot as well as impaired dorsiflexion and reduced or lost eversion of the foot.

The common peroneal nerve is vulnerable to compression neuropathy, as it winds superficially over the fibular neck (Fig. 7.10). Damage may be caused by direct trauma, a tight plaster cast, or even sitting with legs crossed for prolonged periods. It appears also that patients with systemic disorders may be more susceptible to nerve compression. Gassel and Trojaborg (16), for example, reported peroneal nerve lesions in one patient with poliomyelitis and in another with spastic paraparesis.

In a study of compression palsy of the peroneal nerve, 9 of 10 cases showed conduction velocities of less than 45 m per sec (normal averaged 62.6 ± 3.4 m per sec) in the nerve fibers to proximal muscles (81). Often the velocity was reduced only over the nerve segment that was compressed, whereas the distal portion of the nerve to the extensor digitorum brevis was conducting normally. Also, the amplitude of the response of the anterior leg muscles in all cases of peroneal palsy was lower when stimulating above the fibular head than when stimulating below it. Redford (81) suggests that amplitude variations might be a better index of nerve dysfunction than velocity in the earliest stages of peroneal palsy.

Singh et al. (22) evaluated the diagnostic yield of electrophysiological

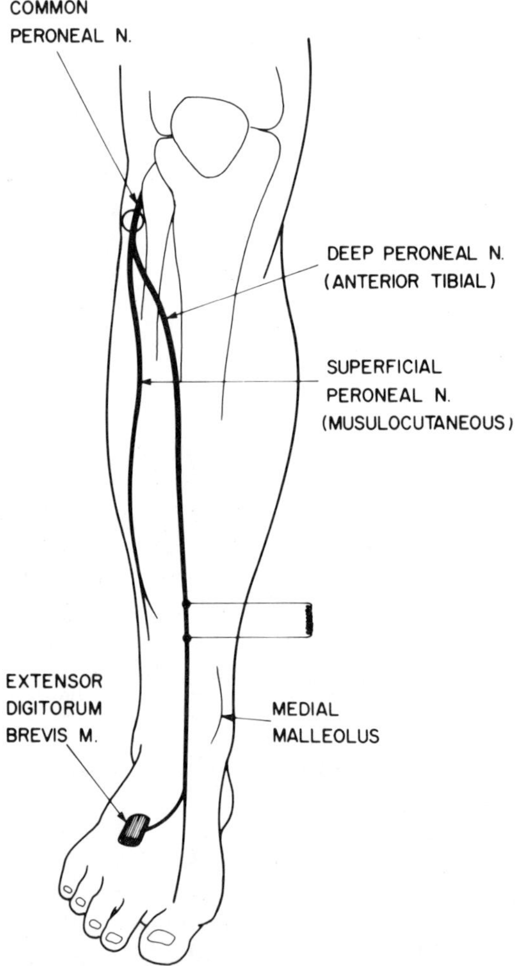

FIG. 7.10. Diagram of the peroneal nerve showing its superficial and deep branches. (From J. Goodgold: *Anatomical Correlates of Clinical Electromyography*, p. 140. Williams & Wilkins, Baltimore, 1974.)

procedures and criteria available to localize a lesion of the peroneal nerve in the region of the capitulum fibulae. Electromyography may fail to distinguish whether a peroneal palsy is due to involvement of a lumbar root or of the peripheral nerve. Weakness and wasting due to root compression may be limited to muscles innervated by the peripheral nerve, or affected muscles, other than those innervated by the peroneal nerve, may not show evidence of partial denervation. Conversely, although electromyographic examination may demonstrate widespread involvement of systemic neuropathy, it does not establish whether in addition there is local impairment of conduction after compression. To demonstrate slowing in conduction along the peroneal nerve segment across the capitulum fibulae, these authors found that it was important to confine measurements to this segment. Localized slowing may not be detected if a longer stretch of normal nerve is included. In fact, they found, in some patients with peroneal palsy and slowing along the nerve segment across the capitulum fibulae, sensory conduction in the normal range when measured from the superior retinaculum to the popliteal fossa. Conduction impairment from the superior retinaculum to the popliteal fossa or distal to it may or may not be due to a lesion localized to the region of the capitulum fibulae; it may be due to axonal neuropathy or more widespread demyelination.

Singh et al. found that slowing of sensory conduction velocity across the capitulum fibulae with normal conduction velocity distal to the capitulum fibulae gave the best diagnostic yield (localization of lesion in 64% of 74 consecutive patients). Slowing along the motor fibers (recorded in the extensor digitorum brevis muscle) across the capitulum fibulae gave only one-half of the diagnostic yield (localization of lesion in one-third of the patients). Differences in amplitude and in temporal dispersion of the sensory responses recorded in the popliteal fossa as compared with those recorded distal to the capitulum fibulae were of limited diagnostic value because of many false positive findings among patients whose peroneal palsy was not due to compression of the nerve at the capitulum fibulae. Stimulation of the superficial peroneal nerve for sensory conduction studies was performed with needle electrodes placed near the nerve at the superior extensor retinaculum, and the responses were recorded with one near-nerve needle electrode placed 1 to 2 cm distal to the capitulum fibulae and another at the popliteal fossa. The indifferent electrode was placed 3 to 4 cm transverse to the pickup electrode. Five hundred to 1000 sensory responses were electronically averaged. The maximum sensory conduction velocity was calculated from the latency to the first positive peak of the sensory potential. For motor conduction determination, near-nerve electrodes were placed in the popliteal fossa and distal to the capitulum fibulae. The following criteria were used to recognize slowing along the motor and sensory fibers: (a) the velocity across the capitulum fibulae was slowed to below the normal range, and the velocity along the segment distal to the capitulum fibulae was within the normal range; and (b) the conduction velocity across the capitulum fibulae was slower than that distal to it by more than 10 m per sec, although both values were within the normal range or the velocity was slightly slowed distal to the capitulum fibulae.

SOURCES OF ERROR

Determination of conduction velocity in motor and sensory fibers of peripheral nerves involves considerable sources of error. The discrepancies arise from problems in instrumentation, techniques of stimulation and recording, inaccuracies in mensuration, and misinterpretations.

Instrument faults are often quite inapparent and difficult to detect. When an error due to an improperly calibrated time base is uncovered (e.g., latency determinations, normal or abnormal, may be incorrectly slower), it reinforces the viewpoint that regularly scheduled checkout of all equipment is most desirable.

If a sweep which is blocked between shocks is triggered by the stimulus without a delay and is not synchronized with the time scale, an unstable triggering level may cause the first 2 msec to be so obscured as to introduce serious error in the latency measurements (82). The stimulus artifact should be delayed at least 1 msec beyond the start of the oscilloscope trace.

The most important variables of the stimulus which may give rise to errors relate to its intensity and the position of the electrodes on the patient.

When the stimulus is submaximal, the latency is usually incorrectly long. The fact that these apparently "lowest threshold" fibers are not the fastest conducting is probably related to the discrepancy between the precise position of the cathode and the "virtual cathode" which is actually affecting the nerve. The virtual cathode may be at an appreciable distance from the cathode position on the skin surface. Even when the cathode is perfectly placed, submaximal stimulus may only affect the few closest fascicles which do not happen to contain the fastest conducting fibers. To obtain an accurate measurement, it is necessary to ensure a supramaximal level of stimulus intensity by increasing the voltage about 25% above maximal or by determining threshold current and using 10 to 14 times this level during the determination. Simpson (82) has concluded that a 0.5-msec error is unavoidable in each latency measurement, making a 1.0-msec latency difference possible in repeated conduction velocity determinations.

A submaximal stimulus may also introduce serious error by evoking an "H" reflex. When the direct motor response is extremely small and the time sweep is slow, the configuration of the H wave coming at approximately 30 msec is undistinguishable in configuration from the direct "M" and is a potential source of difficulty to the unwary.

At supramaximal intensities, especially when the amplification is also high, the major areas of possible error relate to the spread of the stimulus to other nerves and the detection by the recording electrodes of volume-conducted potentials arising in other muscles.

The spread of the stimulus to other nerves is almost always encountered at the high intensities which are used when difficulty is encountered in evoking a response. When the median nerve, for example, is severely compressed in the carpal tunnel, the ulnar nerve is often stimulated by high intensity volume-conducted stimulation applied over the median nerve position. A similar spread may affect the median and ulnar nerves at the elbow region and, of course, in the brachium and axilla where they lie so much closer together. The common peroneal and tibial nerves in the popliteal area are also involved in similar patterns of unintentional stimulation.

The results of the spread of the stimulus to another nerve are readily appreciated when the muscles of both distributions are simultaneously monitored. The significance of spread to other nerves becomes more meaningful when it is noted that potentials are frequently recorded from muscles other than those whose nerve is being stimulated. Perhaps the most commonly recognized are the potentials recorded from the abductor pollicis brevis when the ulnar nerve is stimulated, and the volume-conducted potentials recorded from the extensor digitorum brevis when the small toe extensors are stimulated through the tibial nerve. Gassel (83) recorded potentials from the extensor digitorum brevis in 10 of 10 patients when the posterior tibial nerve was stimulated. It was noted that the volume-conducted potentials could not be distinguished from direct potentials by configuration, but characteristically they (a) appeared in both distributions when recorded, (b) required a higher threshold to stimulate, (c) persisted with the same configuration and amplitude when stimulation was carried out both proximally and distally, and (d), of greatest significance, if the muscle was infiltrated with 1% procaine, were unaffected, whereas the direct potentials were considerably attenuated. The type of recording electrode is significant because the volume pickup is greatest with surface discs and least with concentric bipolar electrodes in which the reference points to detect voltage differences are close together.

There are several other general features related to the evoked response which are noteworthy. (a) The stimulating electrode, of course, is the cathode. If both cathode and anode are placed over the nerve, and the polarity is switched so that the anode rather than the cathode is distal, an error of 0.5 msec in the latency measurement is possible. (b) The recording electrode should be placed over the belly of the muscle (end-plate zone) in order to avoid the theoretical error caused by the initial positive deflection not being detected. Simpson (82) calculated a possible error of 0.35 msec. (c) Recording with needle electrodes usually produces a sharper takeoff point of the response, but the recording is from a discrete area which may not be representative of innervation by the fastest conducting nerve fibers. (d) As the amplification is increased to higher gains with the stimulus at supramaximal, there is frequently noted an apparent decrease in the latency measurement. In Figure 7.11 such a recording is shown of superimposed tracings each at a different amplification. The difference in time measures approximately 0.4 msec. Therefore, the amplification used for recording at proximal and distal sites should not be changed. It has also been postulated (83) that at these high amplifications a potential with short latency may be recorded from the hand which is volume conducted from the forearm muscles. Perhaps the very high conduction velocities occasionally reported for humans may be erroneously calculated on the basis of these volume-conducted forearm flexor potentials. (e) Buchthal and Rosenfalck (9) and Simpson (82) have called attention to a small negative potential which precedes the muscle

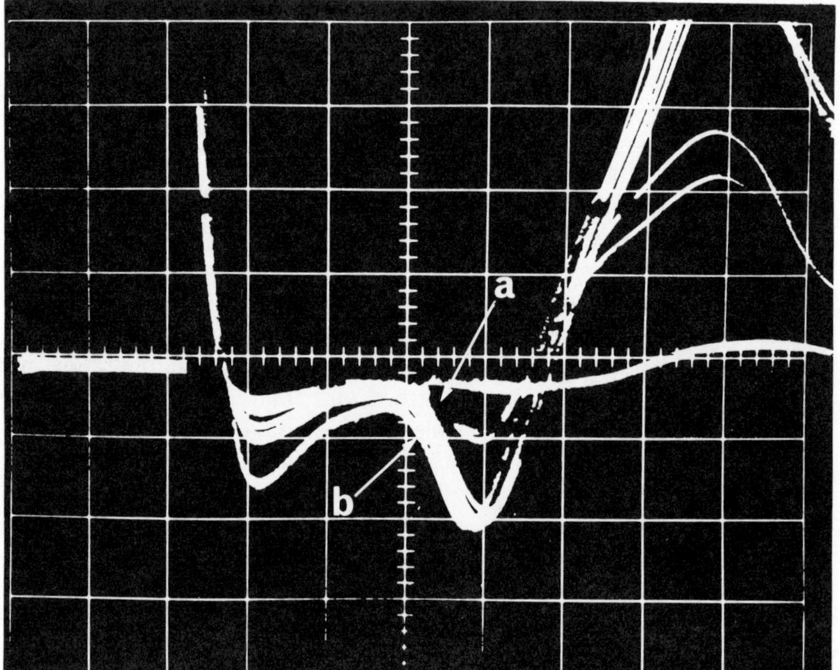

FIG. 7.11. Superimposed tracings of the same evoked response to supramaximal stimulation recorded at increasing levels of amplification. The *uppermost* response (*a*) is taken at the lowest amplification and the *bottom* response (*b*) at the highest amplification. The error in latency measurement between the two is equal to 0.4 msec. The horizontal calibration is equal to 1 msec per div.

action potential by about 1.0 msec (recorded at high gain) (Fig. 7.12). The activity is undoubtedly due to an intramuscular nerve action potential. Gutmann (84) has studied it in patients with severe loss of motor axons and concluded that although motor fibers may contribute, the major portion is derived from sensory axons conducting antidromically.

The measurement of the conduction distance is not an inconsequential source of error in spite of the fact that correlation between measurement on the surface of the extremity with tape and anatomic studies in cadavers appears to be good (85). The difficulty becomes more apparent when the course of the nerve is not direct (radial, ulnar); under these circumstances, obstetric calipers may be of considerable aid. In general an error of ± 0.5 cm is quite possible and becomes more significant as the distance is shortened. If the temporal error is ± 1.0 msec and the length measurement error is ± 0.5 cm, it is not unexpected to find a mean variation of 7.5 m per sec in conduction velocity in the same subject when examination is carried out on different days (86).

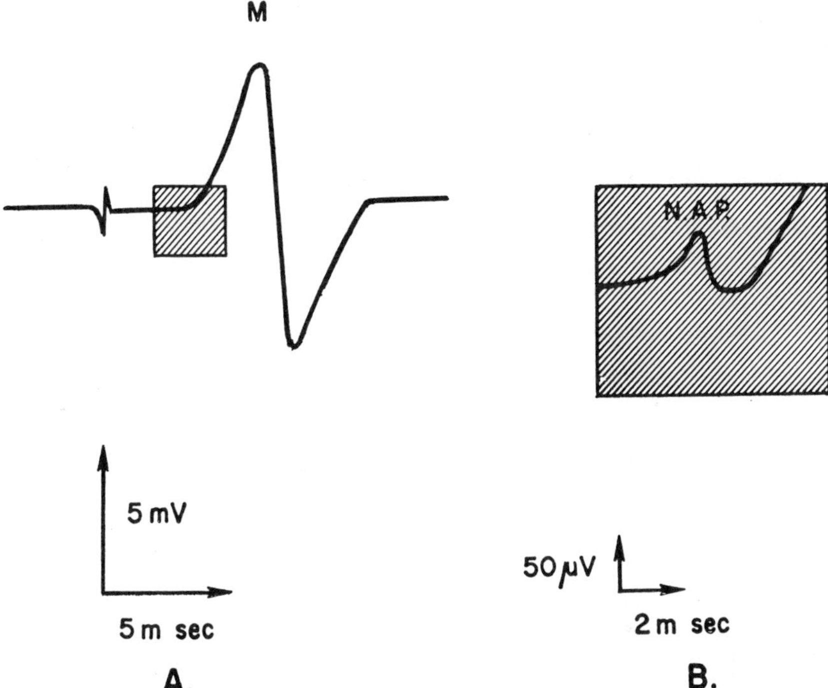

FIG. 7.12. Recording of muscle action potential (*M*) over the end-plate zone of the muscle. Higher amplification (*B*) reveals the presence of an intramuscular nerve action potential (*N.A.P.*)

The variation in the same subject (25 normal individuals) at the same time was calculated by recording simultaneously from three concentric needle electrodes (83). The greatest difference in a single individual ranged up to 10 m per sec, with an average greatest difference between the three electrodes of 3.5 m per sec. Finally, it seems quite obvious that the evoked responses to distal and proximal stimulation must have the same configuration if the measurement is to have any significance. Measurements made off the face of the scope are crude and inaccurate; the best method includes some type of permanent writeout which is easily visualized. Calipers are useful to set discrete points of measurement along the tracing. Measuring to the peak of the muscle action potential introduces some error because it is a complex waveform reflecting the diameter and velocity spectrum of its nerve fibers. The difference in dispersion when stimulating distally is sufficient to bring about some slight shift in the peak so as to introduce a small deviation.

The anomalous innervation of muscles of the extremities is by no means a recent discovery, although it is a potent source of misinterpretation of electrodiagnostic observations. Brooks (87) dissected the innervation to the flexor pollicis brevis in 30 cadavers; he found it totally innervated by the median in five cases and by the ulnar in five, and he found the "normal" dual variation in 19. In one case, all of the intrinsic muscles of the hand were innervated by the ulnar. Rowntree (88) reported that 20% of 226 patients with nerve lesions had anomalous innervation of the intrinsic muscles of the hand. About 20 to 25% of normal individuals show connecting strands between median and ulnar nerves in the forearm which coursed between the superficial and deep flexor muscle layers (Fig. 7.13). Recently

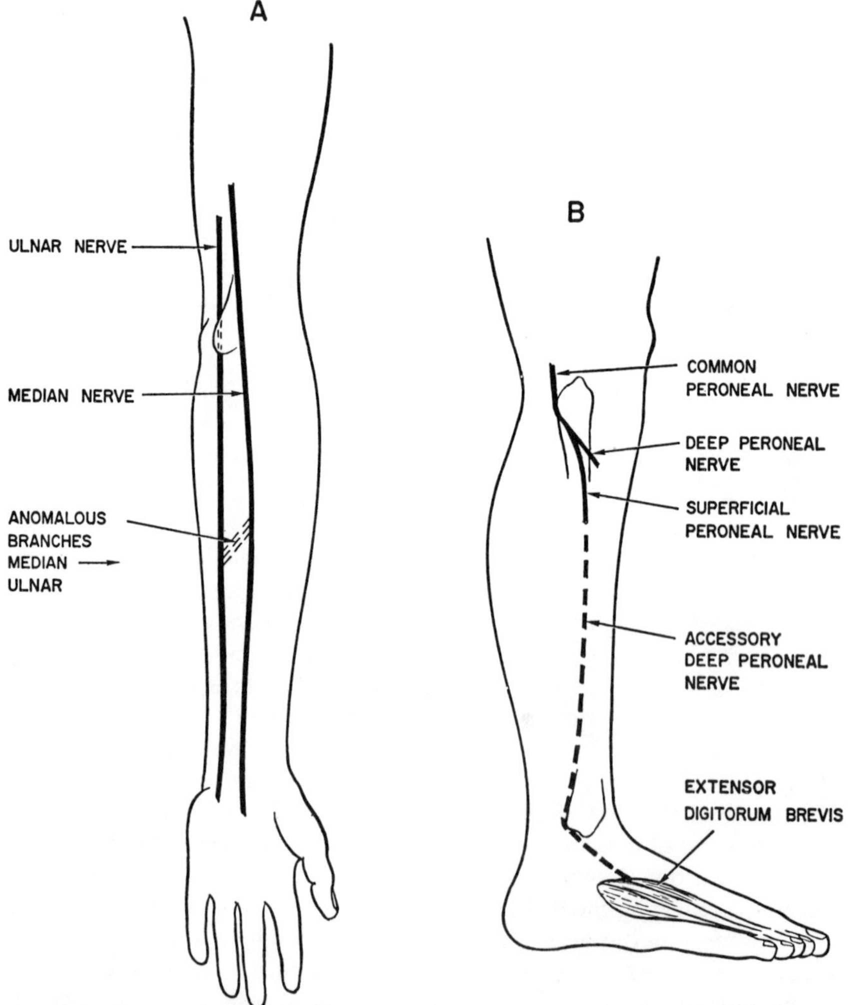

FIG. 7.13. *A*, diagram showing anomalous branching between median and ulnar nerves in the forearm; *B*, diagram showing accessory branch of the deep peroneal nerve arising from superficial peroneal and innervation of the extensor digitorum brevis.

a common anatomic variant of the innervation of the extensor digitorum brevis has been reviewed (89–91). Usually this muscle is innervated through the deep branch of the peroneal nerve, but in about 25 to 30% of normal individuals it derives an anomalous nerve supply through an accessory deep peroneal nerve which branches off the superficial peroneal.

Anomalous innervation is not difficult to detect if there is sufficient awareness of its possible existence supported by an accurate background of history and physical examination. For example, if a patient is examined 1 month after a severe trauma to the ulnar nerve at the elbow with irreplaceable destruction of a long segment of the nerve, the presence of motor units under voluntary control should evoke a strong reaction of suspicion. A muscle

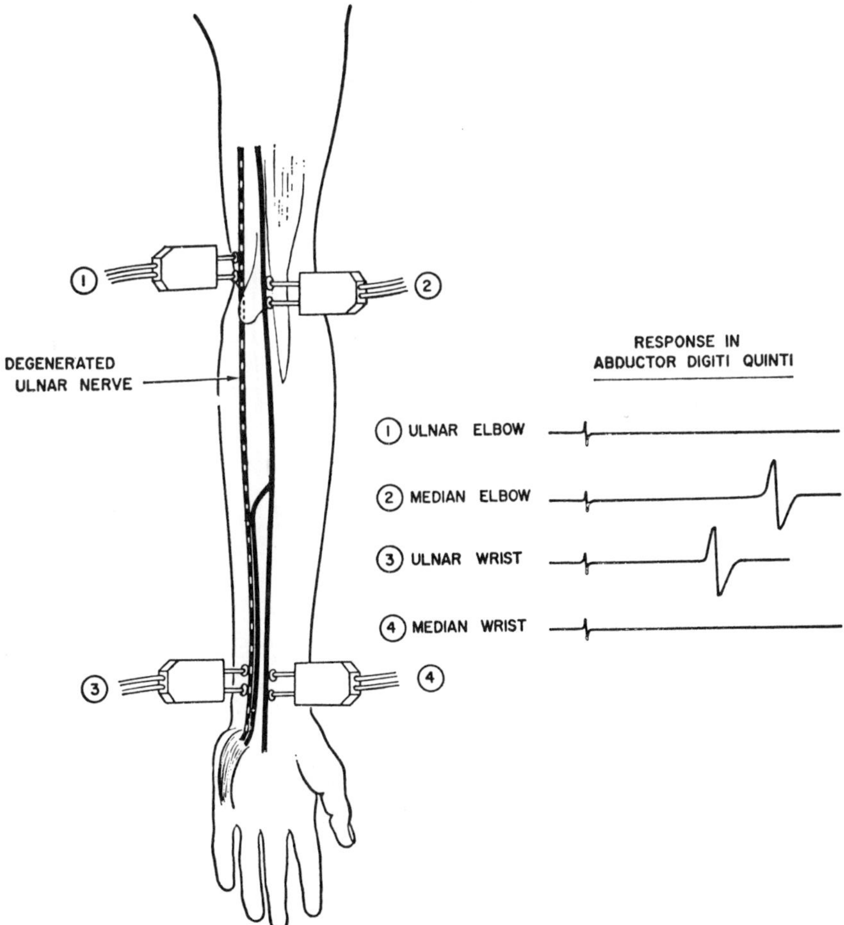

FIG. 7.14. Scheme for decision of anomalous cross-over median to ulnar nerve in forearm when a complete ulnar neuropathy exists (see text).

action potential response may be recorded from the abductor digiti quinti when the ulnar is stimulated at the wrist but not evoked when it is stimulated at the elbow. This is not miraculous reinnervation but is due to anomalous nerve supply. Specific identification of cross-over in the forearm may be established as follows: (a) demonstration of motor units under voluntary control in the abductor digiti quinti; (b) stimulation of the ulnar nerve at the elbow—no response; (c) stimulation of the median nerve at the elbow—evoked muscle action potential in abductor digiti quinti; (d) stimulation of

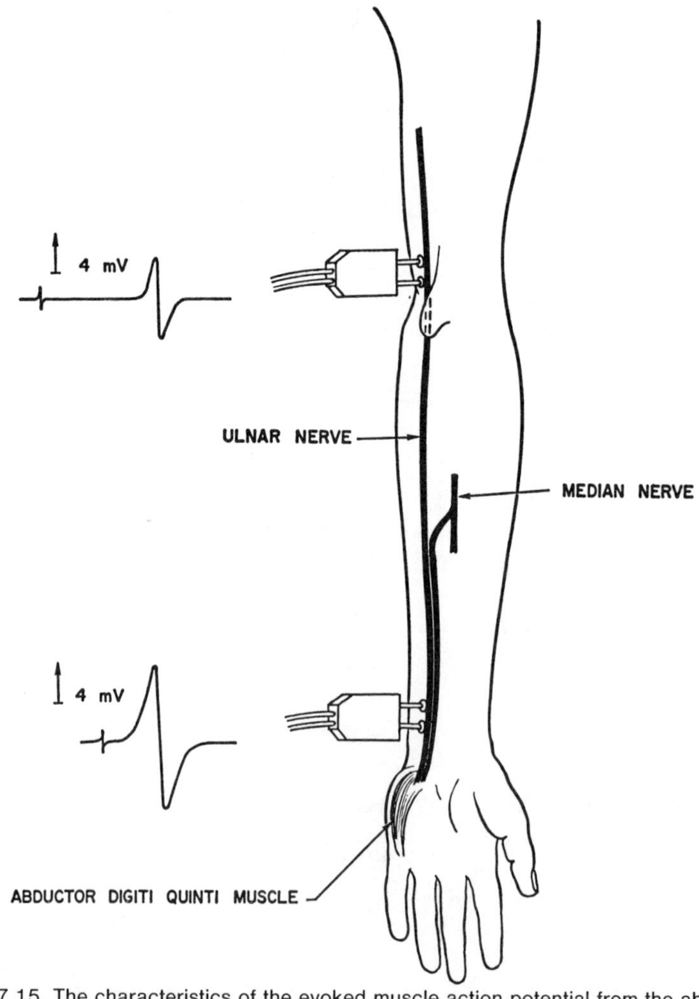

FIG. 7.15. The characteristics of the evoked muscle action potential from the abductor digiti quinti when the muscle has a dual innervation from the ulnar and a cross-over from the median nerve in the forearm. The amplitude of the response is greater when the nerve is stimulated distally.

ulnar nerve at wrist—evoked muscle action potential; and (e) stimulation of median nerve at wrist—no response in abductor digiti quniti (Fig. 7.14).

The entire hand may be innervated through the median in this manner, or there may be a dual innervation for the ulnar-innervated muscles as depicted in Figure 7.15. Dual innervation may be suspected in a normal individual if the amplitude of the evoked response to distal stimulation is significantly greater than that evoked proximally. With dual innervation, electromyographic examination may detect evidence of partial denervation.

The presence of an accessory deep peroneal nerve may give rise to an atypical deep peroneal neuropathy which is identified in a similar manner. If the anomalous innervation of the extensor digitorum brevis is total, then the electromyogram will not show the evidence of partial denervation that can be anticipated if the muscle derives part of its supply from the deep peroneal. Typically, a potential is evoked in the extensor by stimulation of the common peroneal nerve at the head of the fibula and the accessory deep peroneal nerve just behind the lateral malleolus, whereas stimulation of the deep peroneal at the dorsum of the ankle elicits no reaction. If this common anatomic variant is considered, erroneous conclusions regarding the completeness of deep peroneal lesions can be avoided.

The spread of the stimulus current to nearby nerves is also of some importance in evaluation of anomalous innervation. In the case of complete innervations of the intrinsic muscles by the ulnar in the hand while a complete and irreparable lesion of the median exists in the arm, high intensity stimulus over the median may spread to evoke an impulse in the ulnar. If the problem cannot be solved by some of the means already outlined, the answer will be clearly established by repeating the study after a 1% procaine block of the ulnar nerve at the wrist.

REFERENCES

1. von Helmholtz, H.: Messungen uber den zeitlichen Verlauf der Zuckung anamalischer Muskeln und die Fortpflanzungsgeschwindigkeit der Reizung in den Nerven. Joh. Muller's Arch. Anat. Physiol., 276–364. 1850.
2. Hodes, R., Larrabee, M. C., and German, W.: The human electromyogram in response to nerve stimulation and the conduction velocity of motor axons. Arch. Neurol. Psychiatry, *60:* 340–365, 1948.
3. Thomas, J. E., and Lambert, E. H.: Ulnar nerve conduction velocity of H reflex in infants and children. J. Appl. Physiol., *15:* 1–9, 1960.
4. Eaton, C. M., and Lambert, E. H.: Electromyography and electric stimulation of nerves in diseases of motor unit. J.A.M.A., *163:* 1117–1124, 1957.
5. Dawson, G. D., and Scott, J. W.: The recording of nerve action potentials through the skin in man. J. Neurol. Neurosurg. Psychiatry, *12:* 259–267, 1949.
6. Dawson, G. D.: The relative excitability and conduction velocity of sensory and motor nerve fibres in man. J. Physiol. (Lond.), *131:* 436–451, 1956.
7. Gilliatt, R. W., and Sears, T. A.: Sensory nerve action potentials in patients with peripheral nerve lesions. J. Neurol. Neurosurg. Psychiatry, *21:* 109–118, 1958.
8. Gilliatt, R. W., and Willison, R. G.: Peripheral nerve conduction in diabetic neuropathy. J. Neurol. Neurosurg. Psychiatry, *25:* 11–18, 1962.

9. Buchthal, F., and Rosenfalck, A.: Evoked action potentials and conduction velocity in human sensory nerves. Brain Res., *3:* 1–122, 1966.
10. Guld, C., Rosenfalck, A., and Willison, R. G.: Report of the committee on EMG instrumentation. Electroencephalogr. Clin. Neurophysiol., *28:* 399–413, 1970.
11. Peytz, F., Rasmussen, H., and Buchthal, F.: Conduction time and velocity in human recurrent laryngeal nerve. Dan. Med. Bull., *12:* 125–127, 1965.
12. Cherington, M.: Accessory nerve: Conduction studies. Arch. Neurol. (Chicago). *18:* 708–709, 1968.
13. Davis, J. N.: Phrenic nerve conduction in man. J. Neurol. Neurosurg. Psychiatry, *30:* 420–426, 1967.
14. Mavor, H., and Libman, I: Motor nerve conduction velocity measurement as a diagnostic tool. Neurology (Minneap.), *12:* 733–744, 1962.
15. Kraft, G. H.: Axillary, musculocutaneous and suprascapular nerve latency studies. Arch. Phys. Med. Rehabil., *53:* 383–387, 1972.
16. Gassel, M. M., and Trojaborg, W.: Clinical and electrophysiological study of the pattern of conduction times in the distribution of the sciatic nerve. J. Neurol. Neurosurg. Psychiatry, *27:* 351–357, 1964.
17. Shahani, B., Goodgold, J., and Spielholz, N. I.: Sensory nerve action potentials in the radial nerve. Arch. Phys. Med., *48:* 602–605, 1967.
18. Downie, A. W., and Scott, T. R.: An improved technique for radial nerve conduction studies. J. Neurol. Neurosurg. Psychiatry, *30:* 332–336, 1967.
19. DiBenedetto, M.: Sensory nerve conduction in lower extremities. Arch. Phys. Med., *51:* 253–258, 1970.
20. Lovelace, R. E., Myers, S. J., and Zablow,: Sensory conduction in peroneal and posterior tibial nerves using averaging techniques. J. Neurol. Neurosurg. Psychiatry, *36:* 942–950, 1973.
21. Behse, F., and Buchthal, F.: Normal sensory conduction in the nerves of the leg in man. J. Neurol. Neurosurg. Psychiatry, *34:* 404–414, 1971.
22. Singh, N. Behse, F., and Buchthal, F.: Electrophysiological study of peroneal palsy. J. Neurol. Neurosurg. Psychiatry, *37:* 1202–1213, 1974.
23. Sunderland, S.: *Nerve and Nerve Injuries*, pp. 277–280. Williams & Wilkins Co., Baltimore, 1968.
24. Trojaborg, W.: Motor nerve conduction velocities in normal subjects with particular reference to the conduction in proximal and distal segments of median and ulnar nerve. Electroencephalogr. Clin. Neurophysiol., *17:* 314–321, 1964.
25. Henriksen, J.D.: Conduction velocity of motor nerves in normal subjects and in patients with neuromuscular disorders. Thesis, University of Minnesota, 1956.
26. Johnson, E. W., and Olsen, K. J.: Clinical value of motor nerve conduction velocity determination. J.A.M.A., *172:* 2030–2035, 1960.
27. Baer, R. D., and Johnson, E. W.: Motor nerve conduction velocities in normal children. Arch. Phys. Med., *46:* 698–704, 1965.
28. Gamstorp, I.: Normal conduction velocity of ulnar, median and peroneal nerves in infancy, childhood and adolescence. Acta Pediatr. Scand., (*Suppl. 146*)*:* 68–76, 1963.
29. Thomas, J. E., and Lambert, E. H.: Ulnar nerve conduction velocity and H-reflex in infants and children. J. Appl. Physiol., *15:* 1–9, 1960.
30. Miglietta, O. E.: Sensory conduction of digital nerve fibers. Am. J. Phys. Med., *48:* 78–84, 1969.
31. Gilliatt, R. W., Melville, J. D., Velate, A. S., and Willison, R. G.: A study of normal nerve action potentials using an averaging technique (barrier grid storage tube). J. Neurol. Neurosurg. Psychiatry, *28:* 191–200, 1965.
32. Seddon, H. J.: Three types of nerve injury. Brain, *66:* 237–288, 1943.
33. Sunderland, S.: A Classification of peripheral nerve injuries producing loss of function. Brain, *74:* 491–516, 1951.
34. Wynn Parry, C. B.: Techniques of neuromuscular stimulation and their clinical application. In *Disorders of Voluntary Muscle,* edited by J. N. Walton, pp. 763–784. J & A Churchill, Ltd., London, 1969.
35. Kopell, H. P., and Goodgold, J.: Clinical and electrodiagnostic features of carpal tunnel syndrome: Arch. Phys. Med., *49:* 371–375, 1968.

36. Simpson, J. A.: Electrical signs in the diagnosis of carpal tunnel and related syndromes. J. Neurol. Neurosurg. Psychiatry, *19:* 275–280, 1956.
37. Thomas, P. K.: Motor nerve conduction in the carpal tunnel syndrome. Neurology (Minneap.), *10:* 1045–1050, 1960.
38. Thomas, J. E., Lambert, E. H., and Cseuz, K. A.: Electrodiagnostic aspects of the carpal tunnel syndrome. Arch. Neurol. (Chicago), *16:* 635–641, 1967.
39. Buchthal, F., and Rosenfalck, A.: Sensory conduction from digit and palm and from palm to wrist in the carpal tunnel syndrome. J. Neurol. Neurosurg. Psychiatry, *34:* 243–252, 1971.
40. Wiederholt, W. C.: Median nerve conduction velocity in sensory fibers through carpal tunnel. Arch. Phys. Med., *51:* 328–330, 1970.
41. Downie, A. J.: Studies in nerve conduction. In *Disorders of Voluntary Muscle*, edited by J. N. Walton, p. 800. J. & A. Churchill, Ltd., London, 1969.
42. Buchthal, F., Rosenfalck, A., and Trojaborg, W.: Electrophysiological findings in entrapment of the median nerve at wrist and elbow. J. Neurol. Neurosurg. Psychiatry, *37:* 340–360, 1974.
43. Crymble, B.: Brachial neuralgia and the carpal tunnel syndrome. Br. Med. J., *3:* 470–471, 1968.
44. Spinner, M., and Spencer, P. S.: Nerve compression lesions of the upper extremity. Clin. Orthop. Rel. Res., *104:* 46–67, 1974.
45. Morris, H. H., and Peters, B. H.: Pronator syndrome: Clinical and electrophysiological features in seven cases. J. Neurol. Neurosurg. Psychiatry, *39:* 461–464, 1976.
46. Kiloh, L. G., and Nevin, S.: Isolated neuritis of the anterior interosseous nerve. Br. Med. J., *1:* 850–851, 1952.
47. O'Brien, M. D., and Upton, A. R. M.: Anterior interosseous nerve syndrome. J. Neurol. Neurosurg. Psychiatry, *35:* 531–536, 1972.
48. Schmidt, H., and Eiken, O.: The anterior interosseous nerve syndrome: Case reports. Scand. J. Plast. Reconstr. Surg., *5:* 53–56, 1971.
49. Urschel, H. C., Razzuk, M. A., Wood, R. E., Parekh, M., and Paulson, D. L.: Objective diagnosis (ulnar nerve conduction velocity) and current therapy of the thoracic outlet syndrome. Ann. Thorac. Surg., *12:* 608–620, 1971.
50. Ebeling, P., Gilliatt, R. W., and Thomas, P. K.: A clinical and electrical study of ulnar nerve lesions in the hand. J. Neurol. Neurosurg. Psychiatry, *23:* 1–9, 1960.
51. Shea, J. D., and McClain, E. J.: Ulnar-nerve compression syndromes at and below the wrist. J. Bone Joint Surg. [Am.], *51:* 1095–1103, 1969.
52. Bhala, R. P., and Goodgold, J.: Motor conduction in the deep palmar branch of the ulnar nerve. Arch. Phys. Med., *49:* 460–466, 1968.
53. Preswick, G.: Peripheral entrapment neuropathies. Bull. Post-Grad. Comm. Med., Univ. of Sydney, *21:* 78–81, 1965.
54. Kopell, H. P., and Thompson, W. A. L.: *Peripheral Entrapment Neuropathies.* Williams & Wilkins Co., Baltimore, 1963.
55. Gilliatt, R. W., and Thomas, P. K.: Changes in nerve conduction with ulnar lesions at the elbow. J. Neurol. Neurosurg. Psychiatry, *23:* 312–320, 1960.
56. Kaeser, H. E.: Erregungsleitungssörungen bei Ulnarisparesen. Dtsch. Z. Nervenheilk., *185:* 231–243, 1963.
57. Payan, J.: Electrophysiological localization of ulnar nerve lesions. J. Neurol. Neurosurg. Psychiatry, *32:* 208–220, 1969.
58. Payan, J.: Anterior transposition of the ulnar nerve: An electrophysiological study. J. Neurol. Neurosurg. Psychiatry, *33:* 157–165, 1970.
59. Aschenhurst, E. M.: Anatomic defects in ulnar neuropathy. Can. Med. Assoc. J., *87:* 159–163, 1962.
60. Caldwell, J. W., Crane, C. R., and Krusen, U. L.: Nerve conduction studies: An aid in the diagnosis of the thoracic outlet syndrome. South. Med. J., *64:* 210–212, 1971.
61. Jebsen, R. H.: Motor conduction velocities in the median and ulnar nerves. Arch. Phys. Med. Rehabil. *48:* 185–194, 1967.
62. London, G. W.: Normal ulnar nerve conduction velocity across the thoracic outlet: Comparison of two measuring techniques. J. Neurol. Neurosurg. Psychiatry, *38:* 756–760, 1975.

63. Trojaborg, W.: Rate of recovery in motor and sensory fibres of the radial nerve: Clinical and electrophysiological aspects. J. Neurol. Neurosurg. Psychiatry, *33:* 625–638, 1970.
64. Sunderland, S.: Traumatic injuries of peripheral nerves. I. Simple compression of the radial nerve. Brain, *68:* 56–72, 1945.
65. Gassel, M. M., and Diamantopoulos, E.: Pattern of conduction times in the distribution of the radial nerve: A clinical and electrophysiological study. Neurology (Minneap.), *14:* 222–231, 1964.
66. Jebsen, R. H.: Motor conduction velocity in proximal and distal segments of the radial nerve. Arch. Phys. Med., *47:* 597–602, 1966.
67. Goldman, S., Honet, J. C., Sobel, R., and Goldstein, A. S.: Posterior interosseous nerve palsy in the absence of trauma. Arch. Neurol., *21:* 435–441, 1969.
68. Blom, S., Hele, P., and Parkman, L.: The supinator channel syndrome. Scand. J. Plast. Reconstr. Surg. *5:* 71–73, 1971.
69. Hanson, D. J.: Intramuscular injection injuries, G. P., *27:* 109–115, 1963.
70. Johnson, E. W., and Raptou, A. D.: A study of intragluteal injection. Arch. Phys. Med., *46:* 167–177, 1965.
71. Schneegans, E.: Sciatic nerve paralysis in newborn and premature babies. Ann. Pediatr. (Paris), *44:* 2425–2431, 1968.
72. Gilles, F. H., and Matson, D. D.: Sciatic nerve injury following misplaced gluteal injection. J. Pediatr., *76:* 247–254, 1970.
73. Banerjee, T., and Colin, D. H.: Sciatic entrapment neuropathy. J. Neurosurg., *45:* 216–217, 1976.
74. Goodgold, J., Kopell, H. P., and Spielholz, N. I.: The tarsal-tunnel syndrome. N. Engl. J. Med., *273:* 742–745, 1965.
75. Johnson, E. W., and Ortiz, P. R.: Electrodiagnosis of tarsal tunnel syndrome. Arch. Phys. Med., *47:* 776–780, 1966.
76. Edwards, W. G., Lincoln, C. R., Bassett, F. H., III, and Goldner, J. L.: The tarsal tunnel syndrome. J.A.M.A., *207:* 716–720, 1969.
77. Rosenblum, J., Schwartz, G. A., and Bindler, E.: Femoral neuropathy—a neurological complication of hysterectomy. J.A.M.A., *195:* 409–414, 1966.
78. Gassel, M. M.: A study of femoral nerve conduction time. Arch. Neurol. (Chicago). *9:* 607–614, 1963.
79. Chopra, J. S., and Hurwitz, L. J.: Femoral nerve conduction in diabetes and chronic occlusive vascular disease. J. Neurol., Neurosurg. Psychiatry, *31:* 28–33, 1968.
80. Johnson, E. W., Wood, P. K., and Powers, J. J.: Femoral nerve conduction studies. Arch. Phys. Med., *49:* 528–532, 1968.
81. Redford, J. B.: Nerve conduction in motor fibers to the anterior tibial muscle in peroneal palsy. Arch. Phys. Med., *45:* 500–504, 1964.
82. Simpson, J. A.: Fact and fallacy in measurement of conduction velocity in motor nerves. J. Neurol., Neurosurg. Psychiatry, *27:* 381–385, 1964.
83. Gassel, M. M.: Sources of error in motor nerve conduction studies. Neurology (Minneap.). *14:* 825–835, 1964.
84. Gutmann, L.: The intramuscular nerve action potential. J. Neurol. Neurosurg. Psychiatry, *32:* 193–196, 1969.
85. Carpendale, M. T. F.: Conduction time in the terminal portion of the motor fibers of the ulnar, median and peroneal nerves in healthy subjects and patients with neuropathy. Thesis, University of Minnesota, 1956.
86. Henriksen, J. D.: Conduction velocity of motor nerves in normal subjects and patients with neuromuscular diseases. Thesis, University of Minnesota, 1958.
87. Brooks, H. S. J.: Variations in nerve supply to the flexor brevis pollicis. Anat. Physiol., *20:* 641–644, 1886.
88. Rowntree, T.: Anomalous innervation of the hand muscles. J. Bone Joint Surg. [Br.], *31:* 505–510, 1949.
89. Lambert, E. H.: The accessory deep peroneal nerve: A common variation in innervation of extensor digitorum brevis. Neurology (Minneap.), *19:* 1169–1176, 1969.
90. Infante, E., and Kennedy, W. R.: Anomalous branch of the peroneal nerve detected by electromyography. Arch. Neurol. (Chicago), *22:* 162–165, 1970.

91. Gutmann, L.: Atypical deep peroneal neuropathy. J. Neurol. Neurosurg. Psychiatry, *33:* 453–456, 1970.
92. McQuillen, M. P., and Gorin, F. J.: Serial ulnar nerve conduction velocity measurements in normal subjects. J. Neurol. Neurosurg. Psychiatry, *32:* 144–148, 1969.
93. Lamontagne, A., and Buchthal, F.: Electrophysiological studies in diabetic neuropathy. J. Neurol. Neurosurg. Psychiatry, *33:* 442–452, 1970.
94. Trojaborg, W., and Sindrup, E. H.: Motor and sensory conduction in different segments of the radial nerve in normal subjects. J. Neurol. Neurosurg. Psychiatry, *32:* 354–359, 1969.
95. Jimenez, J., Easton, J. K. M., and Redford, J. B.: Conduction of the anterior and posterior tibial nerves. Arch. Phys. Med., *51:* 164–169, 1970.
96. Melvin, J. L., Harris, D. H., and Johnson, E. W.: Sensory and motor conduction velocities in the ulnar and median nerves. Arch. Phys. Med., *47:* 511–519, 1966.

chapter 8

Myopathy

Description of the electrophysiological characteristics of neuromuscular diseases for pedagogic purposes is a much more formidable task now than it was 15 or 20 years ago. Contributing to this state is the fact that of the 50 or so primary muscle diseases described as distinct entities by 1967, 15 were "discovered" in the prior 10-year period and eight since 1962 (1). In addition, the relatively new investigational methods of histochemistry and electron microscopy have shed new light on the fundamental nature of the pathology and pathophysiology of neuromuscular diseases so that unequivocable differentiation of primary neuropathic from myopathic disease is no longer quite that simple. At the same time, careful reevaluation of light microscopy observations of biopsied muscle at various intervals during the life history of a neuropathy has demonstrated that even a most sophisticated muscle pathologist cannot be absolute in diagnostic judgment in the later stages of the disease. What was formerly considered typically neuropathic in histological characteristics may appear typically myopathic; in many instances features of each type may be retained, so as to present a "mixed pattern." In a more advanced state of disease, no distinctive features may be identified; the pathological description is then identified as a graveyard variety—"end stage muscle."

The interpretation of the EMG must be carried out with cognizance that the electrophysiological observations play a counterpoint role to the lack of absolute specificity of histology and pathophysiology. Fibrillation potentials, for example, were not so long ago considered pathognomonic of lower motor neuron disease; however, critical reappraisal has forced the electromyographer to go beyond the "not never but hardly ever" phase inasmuch as these potentials were once described as never occurring in myopathy, then rarely seen, and now it is not unusual to review papers in which the presence of fibrillation in one-third to one-half of the individuals in a given series of patients with muscular dystrophy is reported. It is of more than passing interest that even the concept that muscular dystrophy itself is truly a primary muscle disease is under dispute. McComas and Sica (2) base their challenge of the conception of primary myogenic disease on their report that there is a significant loss of total numbers of motor units in the limb girdle and facioscapulohumeral types of muscular dystrophy. They interpret this observation as evidence of gross denervation and extend the thesis that chronic motor neuron dysfunction is the basic etiological factor. The myotonic and Duchenne types of muscular dystrophy are placed in the same category.

The fundamental studies on cross-innervations by Buller et al. (3) which demonstrated the nerve's profound influence on the metabolism of the muscle cell seem to lend further support to the idea that "myopathy" may really be an expression of neuronal dysfunction.

Parallel with these observations, it has become apparent that electromyography cannot be viewed as a sole determinant in identification of specific neuromuscular diseases. This is especially true in metabolic disease where ionic membrane disturbances occur, in cases involving specific enzymatic deficiencies, and in the congenital nonprogressive myopathies. The specific enzymatic deficiencies may be classified with this group as easily as with the metabolic disorders. The clinical signs of muscle disease may be quite obvious (e.g., atrophy and weakness), yet the EMG examination may yield little or no information. In McArdle's disease or nemaline myopathy, the EMG can be normal, yet a pathological diagnosis may be much more readily established by histochemical means.

Although not sine qua non, the EMG examination is of proven value in differential diagnosis because there are general characteristic patterns of electrophysiological change which can be correlated with neuropathic or myopathic disease. If the pathological characteristics are mixed, then the EMG may very well involve heterogeneous observations. In the congenital nonprogressive myopathic diseases, the electrical findings may be scant and nonspecific, but careful scrutiny may demonstrate the presence of subtle changes such as increased polyphasic activity, indicating that an observed muscle weakness truly reflects organic neuromuscular disease. Electromyographic examination can be carried out in multiple areas of a single muscle to determine universal or patchy distribution of the lesion or may be used to examine a large number of muscles. In this respect (examination of multiple sites or repeated examinations), muscle biopsy is seriously limited. In many clinics, EMG is used to guide the choice of specific muscles for histological study. In utilization of this approach caution must be exercised, because trauma incident to the needling procedure induces histopathological changes in the muscle which may persist for at least several weeks (4). In symmetrical diseases, the contralateral limb may be used for biopsy, or in restricted disease, the sites of EMG electrode puncture and examination may be widely marked on the skin with indelible ink.

It is interesting to note that localized histological changes characteristic of myopathy may be produced even by the minor trauma produced by massage or percussion with a reflex hammer. For the most part, the changes disappear within 2 weeks (5).

With this background, the significant electrophysiological observations useful in the classification of myopathy are presented.

CHARACTERISTIC ELECTRICAL CHANGES

Although certain electrophysiological observations serve generally to categorize the myopathies, there are no significant differences to distinguish one type from another. Perhaps the only exceptions, and then only as a group, are the true myotonias. Because the common electrophysiological features are not universally encountered in each individual disease, final diagnosis is enhanced by careful notation of as many of the electrophysiological clues as possible. What are the clues?

The characteristic features of the myopathies may be most often encountered in pseudohypertrophic muscular dystrophy. The most significant changes in turn relate to the configuration of the individual motor unit action potential (duration, amplitude, shape) and the process of recruitment of units in augmentation of the force of muscle contraction. Because the nerve supply is intact, conduction rates are normal.

Duration

The most consistent change of the motor unit action potential in myopathic disease is the considerable diminution in its duration (Fig. 8.1). The decrease in duration is due to the loss of muscle fibers in the individual motor unit.

The motor unit action potential is the result of the summation of action potentials from several muscle fibers of the unit, the contribution from each fiber depending on its distance from the electrode. Fibers situated at a distance from the recording electrode are recorded as the volume-conducted slow initial and terminal phases of the action potential and contribute to its duration. With a loss of muscle fibers in the individual motor units, the voltage amplitude is decreased and the contribution of distant fibers is undetectable, so the duration is diminished. The duration of the motor unit action potential in myopathy may decrease to 1 to 3 msec.

Configuration

The smooth triphasic action potentials are dependent on the integration of the electrical activity of the almost synchronously discharging individual muscle fibers of the motor unit. If, as in muscular dystrophy, there occurs a

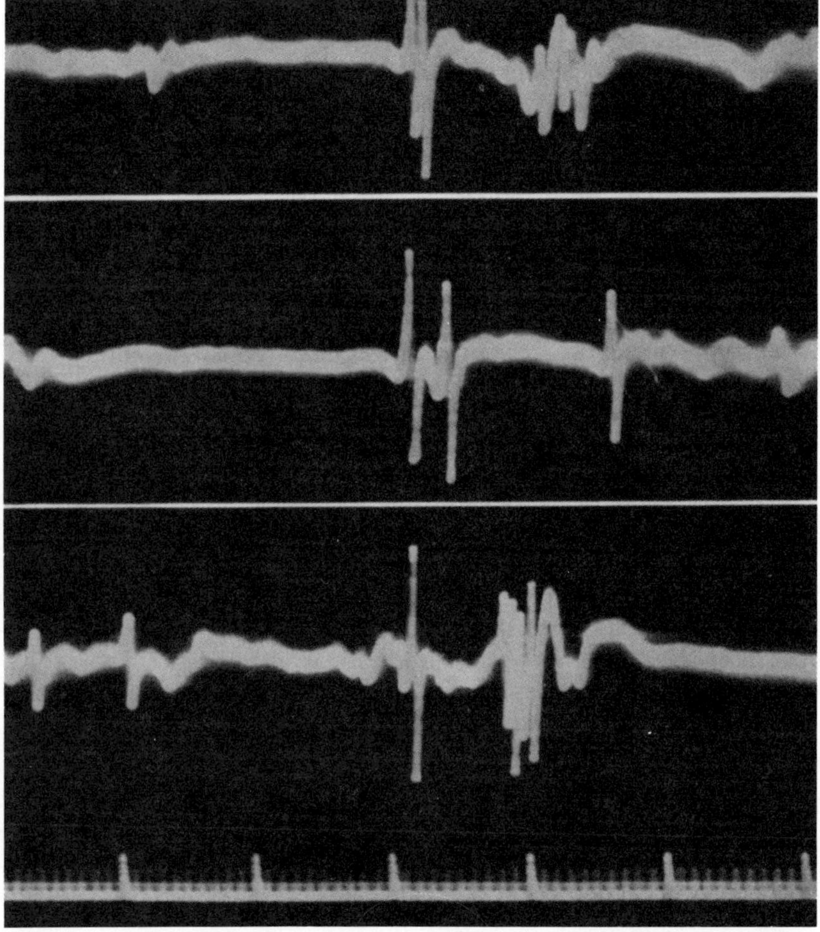

FIG. 8.1. Recording from patient with hypertrophic muscular dystrophy showing short duration motor unit action potentials and short duration polyphasic potentials. Time scale = 1 msec per div.

patchy destruction of fibers, the slight asynchrony becomes much more apparent and results in a "splintering" of the action potential. In this way a polyphasic action potential is generated. In myopathy, it is characteristic that the total duration of the polyphasic unit does not exceed that of a normal motor unit (it is usually considerably shorter), and the spike components of the polyphasic motor unit potential are all sharp (Fig. 8.2). The peak-to-peak amplitude of the unit is frequently diminished as well.

Augmentation of muscle contraction is mainly accomplished by increasing the number of motor units discharging and the firing rate of the individual units. If the motor unit output is viewed on the oscilloscope at maximal effort, individual motor unit potentials cannot be recognized and the base line cannot be visualized. In chronic motor neuron disease, on the other hand, in which motor neurons are destroyed, maximal voluntary effort results in limited recruitment, so that single motor unit potentials separated by considerable lengths of flat base line are easily recorded. These two extremes are, respectively, called "full interference pattern" in the normal patient and "discrete activity" in neuronal disease. An intermediate state of reduced interference pattern is somewhat more nebulous and subjected to individual interpretation (or misinterpretation!).

In myopathy, the neuron is presumably intact. Because of the loss of viable muscle fibers, a comparable range of movement of a limb or intensity of muscle contraction requires a greater firing rate and recruitment of motor units. Such a necessary level of recruitment is apparent by the presence of a full interference pattern at a phase of activity far lower than in the normal. It follows then that a full interference pattern at less than maximal, or at small or moderate effort, is characteristic in myopathy. The short duration potential and the short duration, sharply spiked polyphasics which occur in such profusion at maximal effort in myopathy are associated with a sharp, high pitched sound which is easily recognized with even minimal experience.

Insertional Activity

Increased insertional activity is a nonspecific finding observed in a host of neuropathic and myopathic diseases. It is, however, significant of abnormality and may be observed early in myopathic disease. Normal insertional activity consists of a brief (few hundred milliseconds) deflection of the base

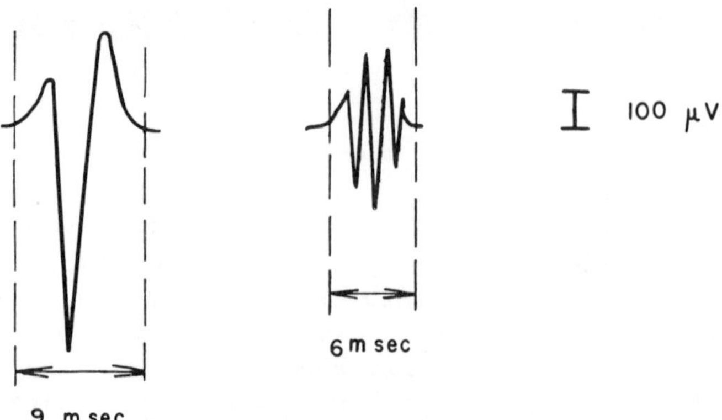

FIG. 8.2. *Left* figure is representative of a triphasic normal motor unit action potential. The figure on the *right* shows the typical short duration, low amplitude polyphasic potential seen in muscular dystrophy. Positive deflection is upward.

line. Abnormal activity appears as trains of sharp, spiky potentials, usually of low amplitude. Positive sharp potentials are not infrequently present.

Fibrillation potentials are more likely to be encountered during examination of the patient with muscular dystrophy (usually in a moderately advanced stage) than in any of the other myopathies, exclusive of polymyositis. Their presence is a reflection of a state of decreased membrane stability rather than of an anatomic denervation. For the same reason, positive sharp waves are also detected in some of these patients, perhaps from partially damaged (i.e., degenerated) muscle fibers.

Myotonic-like Discharges

High frequency, bizarre discharges which resemble the trains of potentials seen in myotonia are not unusually found during electrophysiological study of myopathic muscle. True electromyographic myotonia is identified by a fluctuation of both amplitude and frequency, whereas the repetitive discharges encountered here exhibit only the amplitude variation. This type of trains of potentials is not solely seen in myopathy but occurs in a great number of neuromuscular diseases, including the peripheral neuropathies. These trains are, therefore, also not pathognomonic of myopathy but are a distinctly abnormal phenomenon.

Amplitude of the Motor Unit Action Potential

The peak-to-peak amplitude of motor unit action potentials recorded while exploring a single normal muscle is one of the most variable parameters. Buchthal and Rosenfalck (6) consider only deviations of 40% or more from average normal voltage levels as significant; in actual practice, only changes toward both extremes of the normal range are really of value. For example, to label a motor unit as "hypertrophied" is hazardous unless the voltage level is at least 5 mV.

It is true that the amplitude of a motor unit action potential is a function of the number of its component muscle fibers, but in reality the peak-to-peak amplitude is mainly due to the few fibers which subtend the recording electrode—the voltages caused by fibers even at a distance of 1 mm are remarkably attenuated. The amplitude of the individual motor unit potential in diffuse myopathy is classically diminished. Sometimes the reduction is more apparent with recording of the interference pattern at maximal effort. In the other myopathies, such as facioscapulohumeral dystrophy, the amplitude may be reduced, normal, or even far greater than the average (Fig. 8.3).

MUSCULAR DYSTROPHY

If we permit a classical case of progressive muscular dystrophy of the Duchenne type to serve as a model in the description of the electrophysio-

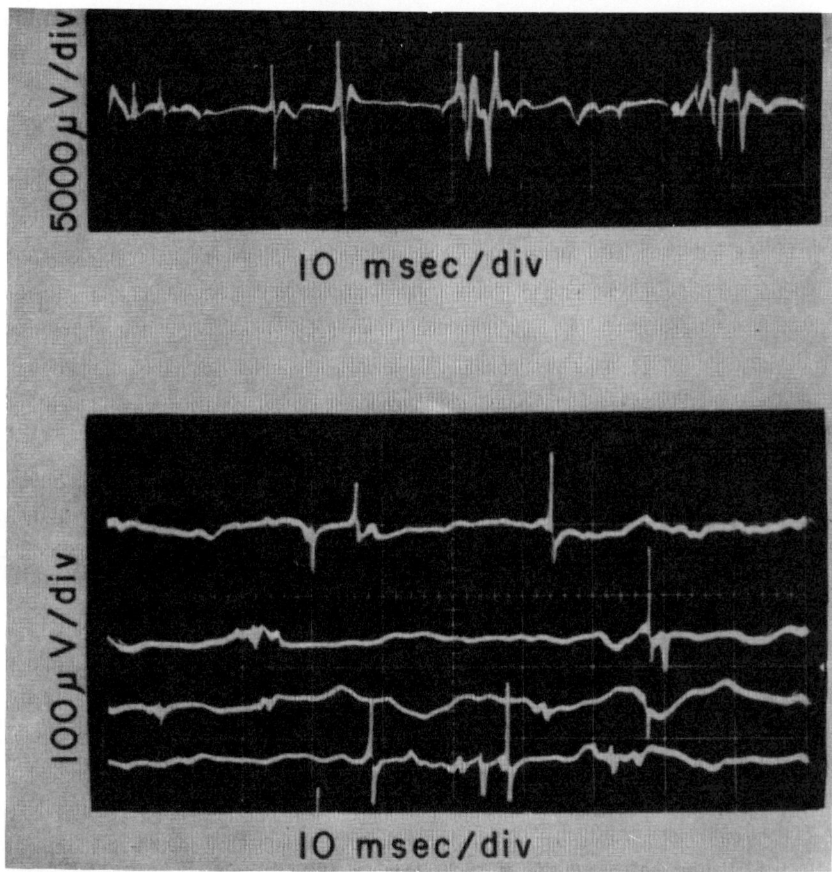

FIG. 8.3. *Top*, short duration motor unit potential in patient with facioscapulohumeral muscular dystrophy showing "hypertrophied" motor unit, amplitude over 10 mV; *bottom*, adjacent area of same muscle (deltoid), showing units with maximal peak-to-peak voltage of 175 μV.

logical observations in myopathy, then a review of the findings during an examination could reveal the following: (a) full interference pattern at moderate and maximal volitional effort (with a peak-to-peak voltage of the pattern significantly reduced); (b) prolonged insertional activity; (c) reduction in the average duration of the motor unit potential, measuring 1 to 3 msec (relative to patient's age and particular muscles studied); (d) increased incidence of polyphasic motor unit potentials with short duration spike components (total duration of unit equal to or less than normal); (e) spontaneous discharges: fibrillations, positive sharp potentials; (f) bizarre high frequency discharges; (g) normal nerve conduction velocity; (h) contraction of the motor unit territory (multielectrode studies).

The changes are not found in all muscles; they are usually observed best in the presence of atrophy and/or weakness. In the individual muscle, the involvement is spotty so that in some areas no abnormalities may be recorded, whereas in other locations there is complete electrical silence. Fibrous tissue produces resistance to insertion of the needle electrode so that a gritty sensation is frequently experienced when the probe is advanced into the muscle.

It is most advisable to select a muscle which is clinically involved but not so advanced in pathology that almost total fibrous and fat tissue replacement has occurred. Manual muscle testing may be used as a guide in selection of muscles, choosing those which test at about an antigravity level.

In facioscapulohumeral and limb girdle muscular dystrophy, the findings may be essentially the same. Frequently, however, they are quite different. For example, in facioscapulohumeral muscular dystrophy the interference pattern may be "discrete" type with giant motor units. Perhaps the most consistent EMG positive findings linking all of the myopathies are increased polyphasia and individual short duration motor unit potentials. The occurrence of the other stigmata is variable but frequent enough so that they can be correlated with clinical signs and symptoms to support a diagnosis of muscular dystrophy.

In the late distal muscular dystrophy originally described by Gowers and later in greater detail by Welander, the EMG again presents a variation in findings ranging from typically myopathic to very questionable. The distal distribution is, of course, a distinguishing feature; the normal conduction velocity, which can be determined by evoking responses from musculature which is not completely atrophied, and the intact perception of vibration help in differential diagnosis from Charcot-Marie-Tooth disease.

There is some question whether a juvenile form of hereditary distal myopathy exists. McGee and DeJong (7) have reported myopathic EMG and biopsy findings in a family with onset before age 2, and bilateral foot drop as the earliest paretic symptom. Cessation of progression after the age of 18 appears to be characteristic.

It has become apparent that the disorder, formerly considered an isolated myopathy of the quadriceps muscle, is not a distinct entity but usually represents cases which start mainly in the quadriceps or appear as incomplete, aborted cases of muscular dystrophy of the limb girdle or late onset types. As a matter of fact it would be more concise if the isolated atrophy (unilateral or bilateral) of a quadriceps muscle were viewed under the heading of "quadriceps syndrome." Such nomenclature would indicate that the lesion could be due to myopathy or, equally, to neuropathy (e.g., isolated femoral neuropathy or part of a polyneuropathy). To differentiate, electromyographic examination of more than the quadriceps muscle should be done to include other muscles of the same limb, the contralateral limb, and, in many cases, the upper extremities as well. Under these circumstances, findings of diffuse myopathy or polymyositis, for example, would be encountered and identified. In the same way, conduction velocities of nerves of the upper and lower extremities, including the femoral nerve itself, would be revealing of primary neuropathic disease. Thage (8) reviewed 46 individuals presenting with the quadriceps syndrome and noted the incidence of femoral neuropathy in 15, limb girdle muscular dystrophy in five, and polymyositis in five others.

The muscular dystrophies alluded to thus far are so classified because they develop primarily in the muscle fiber as a degenerative process and are genetically determined. They are, of course, included in the broader classification of myopathy which also encompasses inflammatory, metabolic, toxic, and endocrine etiologies which cannot be attributed to the central nervous system or a peripheral nerve dysfunction. The information derived from electromyographic examination in the endocrine and metabolic myopathies is best described as supportive study, with few exceptions. The paucity of observations reflects the frequent reversibility of the pathological alterations.

PERIODIC PARALYSIS

Normal neuromuscular function is dependent on the level and distribution of K^+ in the fluid compartments of the body. For example, a complaint of weakness is not unusual if corticosteroid therapy results in excessive loss of K^+ in the urine. Periodic paresis or paralysis is characteristically seen in the hypokalemia of primary hyperaldosteronism.

Hypokalemic Periodic Paralysis

Familial periodic paralysis is a hereditary variety of disease in which episodic flaccid paresis or paralysis is the cardinal symptom. The inheritance is autosomal dominant. The attacks are associated with low plasma K^+ levels (i.e., 2 to 3 mEq per liter). If an EMG is performed during the period of flaccid paralysis, there is complete electrical silence. Electrical stimulation of the muscles or their motor nerves evokes no response. If the EMG is performed before the height of paralysis, a few isolated motor unit potentials of shortened duration may be recruited on maximal effort (9).

During paresis: discrete activity pattern; short duration potentials. During paralysis: EMG—complete electrical silence; electrical stimulation—no response (nerve or muscle).

A permanent variety of myopathic weakness has also been described in hypokalemic periodic paralysis. EMG findings in two cases were described by Dyken et al. (10) as typically myopathic, whereas an older paper by Olivarius and Christensen (11) reported EMG and muscle biopsy findings typical of neurogenic origin in one patient, and in another, EMG and biopsy results were at the opposite pole—typically myopathic. Complete elucidation awaits additional and more elaborate studies, such as histochemistry, enzymes, etc.

Adynamia Episodica Hereditaria

Adynamia episodica hereditaria, or hyperkalemic periodic paralysis, as the name implies, involves a second form of episodic paresis associated with an alteration of plasma K^+ concentration, in this instance an increased level. It is also autosomal dominant.

Electromyographic examination between attacks reveals no abnormalities. During paresis, the findings are distinctly different from the hypokalemic form.

EMG

Spontaneous activity (at rest): increased insertional activity, fibrillation potentials, myotonic discharges. During voluntary effort: fewer total number motor unit potentials, diminished mean duration of motor unit potential (i.e., 70 to 80% of normal).

Because of the occurrence of myotonia induced or enhanced by exposure to cold, on the one hand, and the episodic paresis which may be seen in paramyotonia, on the other hand, Drager et al. (12) have postulated that the two disorders are really a single disease. The electrical myotonia is not a prominent finding in adynamia; as a matter of fact, it was not reported at all in the early publications.

A hereditary form of normokalemic periodic paralysis has also been clinically and biochemically described.

ENDOCRINE DISEASES

Although the complaint of weakness may be a prominent symptom in disorders of the endocrine glands, specific histological identification of a myopathy has been accomplished in only a few. The electromyographic findings in Addison's disease, Cushing's syndrome, or thyrotoxic myopathy offer no features which differentiate these disorders from each other or the other myopathies. The EMG changes may vary so as to include one or all of the features discussed in the review of pseudohypertrophic muscular dystrophy. There are, however, some helpful facts. In thyrotoxic myopathy, for example, initially the involvement is of proximal muscles, and the prominent abnormal EMG finding of shortened duration action potentials has been observed to disappear after an interval of successful therapy.

The myopathy may appear gradually in a chronic form or as an acute event associated with a fulminating hyperthyroidism. The most common localized myopathy involves the extraocular muscles; in its most severe form it is identified as exophthalmic ophthalmoplegia. There is a rare association of hyperthyroidism and myasthenia gravis, so that electrophysiological features of the latter may be a superimposed feature. The same relationship, to a lesser degree, pertains to the association of thyroid disease and hypokalemic periodic paralysis. The myopathy of Cushing's syndrome has been mimicked in an animal model by administration of large doses of corticosteroids. In humans under therapy with steroids, the α-fluoro compounds are the most likely to produce myopathic proximal musculature side effects.

The proximal muscles of acromegalics frequently show a patchy myopathic involvement which may be the basis of the common complaint of weakness. EMG examinations may reveal a significant shortening of the average mean action potential duration (13).

Weakness is a very common complaint in hypothyroid disease (14). Usually the muscles show normal or increased bulk rather than atrophy. Slow contraction and, especially, relaxation are commonly present and are often clinically identified by testing the deep tendon reflexes and by evoking the "mounding" phenomenon by percussion of the muscle. The prolonged phase of relaxation of a reflex muscle contraction is the basis of the Lambert photomotographic examination (15).

The complex of muscle weakness and enlargement associated with slowness of movement and muscle aching, stiffness, and cramping has been identified as the Hoffmann syndrome. This is seen in adults with myxedema.

The EMG reports on hypothyroid myopathy associated with a clinical picture of proximal weakness have varied from normal to "typical" of myopathy.

Occasionally, rare cases of myxedema are associated with a true myotonia identified by clinical and electrical signs, but the usual high frequency discharges reported on hypothyroid patients with clinical signs of myopathy most probably should be classed as bizarre high frequency discharges or myotonic-like discharges. They are provoked by movement of the needle electrode; the sustained repetitive discharges and the waxing and waning of true myotonia have not been observed to follow voluntary muscle contraction.

A report by Frame et al. (16) concerns the occurrence of myopathy in primary hyperparathyroidism. The electromyograms revealed increased numbers of small polyphasic potentials. In one patient a biopsy was performed and showed spotty areas of muscle fiber degeneration with a cellular infiltration indicative of a myositis. A previous paper on parathyroid myopathy by Bischoff and Esslen (17) reported similar electrical changes interpreted as a slight degree of myopathy. In the three patients reported in the study by Frame et al., the EMG returned to normal after surgical removal of parathyroid tumors. The muscle weakness seen in many cases of hyperparathyroidism may be related to a renal deficiency with associated electrical imbalance, to osteitis fibrosa cystica, where the muscle weakness may be associated with severe pain, and finally to the direct effects of hypercalcemia on the nervous system.

METABOLIC MYOPATHY

McArdle's Disease

This is a glycogenosis in which there is a deficiency of muscle phosphorylase. The clinical symptoms of pain, weakness, and cramps during exercise are most characteristic. Biochemical study reveals that the normal increase of blood lactic and pyruvic acid after a period of ischemic exercise does not occur and that myohemoglobinuria may be detected in some patients. Between attacks, the routine electromyographic examination is negative. If an EMG examination is performed when cramping has occurred after exercise, there is electrical silence, a finding typical of contracture.

Dyken et al. (18) have suggested an electromyographic screening test in McArdle's disease which is based on the observation that repetitive stimulation of the median nerve with supramaximal stimulation at a rate of 18 stimuli per sec produces a rapid decrement in the amplitude of the evoked muscle action potential. The EMG change is associated with severe muscle cramping of the thenar eminence muscles. These observations were recorded in a study of a single patient and were performed with the use of bipolar concentric needle electrodes inserted into the muscle. A reliable test of this variety would be of immeasurable value in the identification of mild phosphorylase and perhaps phosphofructokinase deficiency. Caution must be used, however, in interpretation of repetitive stimulation studies, because small displacements of the tip of the recording electrode, which do occur in strong muscle contractions, may be responsible for severe attenuation of the amplitude of the responses.

Phosphofructokinase Deficiency

As described in man by Tarui et al. (19) in 1965, this is another type of muscle glycogenosis. It involves a deficient conversion of fructose-6-phosphate to fructose-1,6-diphosphate. In the absence of the enzyme, glycogen cannot be broken down to lactic acid. For practical purposes, the clinical features are identical with those of muscle phosphorylase deficiency.

Pompe's Disease

As described in several reports (20–22), this is the most severe form of glycogenosis with severe cardiac, skeletal muscle, and nervous system involvement. Death usually ensues within the first 1 or 2 years of life. The deficient enzyme is identified as acid maltase or lysosomal α-1,4-glucosidase.

Cardiomegaly and hypotonia are the outstanding clinical symptoms. The electrodiagnostic findings may be summarized as follows:

Abnormal spontaneous activity: (a) increased insertion activity, (b) diffuse presence of bizarre high frequency discharges resembling true myotonia, and (c) diffuse fibrillation and positive sharp potentials.

Voluntary effort: because the patients are infants, "voluntary effort" is observed at incomplete rest or in response to a mild noxious stimulus. Most significant is the shortened duration of the potentials and the low amplitude, short duration polyphasics which are most frequently encountered during small weak contractions.

Conduction velocity has invariably been reported as normal.

Hirschhorn et al. (23) have reported a technique which may prove significant in detecting carriers of this inherited disease. Multiple enzyme analysis is performed after stimulation of lymphocytes with phytohemaglutinin. The deficiency of α-1,4-glucosidase appears to be clearly demonstrable.

The clinical presentation of the more benign forms of acid maltase deficiency is indistinguishable from that of a relatively mild limb girdle dystrophy or chronic polymyositis. In some cases, there may be slowly progressive weakness of pelvic and pectoral girdle muscles with some involvement of the sternocleidomastoid and trunk muscles, whereas in others, only the iliopsoas, glutei, and adductors may be weakened and later the pectoral, sternomastoids, and facial muscles. Tendon reflexes are decreased, and serum levels of muscle enzymes are raised to 2 to 3 times normal. Electromyographic examination reveals increased insertion activity, low amplitude, short duration motor unit potentials, increased frequency of polyphasic potentials, and myotonic-like bizarre high frequency discharges (24, 25).

ALCOHOLIC MYOPATHY

The syndrome of alcoholic myopathy with muscle pain, tenderness, and swelling associated with fever, abnormal enzyme levels, and myoglobinuria is now a well recognized clinical entity. The chronic syndrome of proximal muscle weakness has been more recently described and supported by biopsy and EMG studies (26, 27). The electromyographic findings parallel the chronic myopathic changes observed in microscopic examinations.

PARASITIC MYOPATHY

Trichinosis

Infestation with *Trichinella spiralis* induces a severe myositis with electromyographic characterizations quite similar to those encountered in polymyositis. Waylonis and Johnson (28) reported early findings (fourth day) consisting of marked spontaneous activity with fibrillations and long trains of positive sharp waves. One week later the electromyogram showed the diffuse presence of spontaneous activity, but in addition there was a marked diminution in the amplitude and duration of the motor unit action potentials. Follow-up electromyographic examinations of the four patients reported in this series revealed a reversion to normal 2 to 3 months after the onset.

Toxoplasma gondii

This also invades the skeletal muscles and causes a diffuse focal myositis. Buchthal and Rosenfalck (6) reported that in six of 12 patients with diagnostic serological findings, EMG revealed some evidence of myopathy. The observations included reduced voltage and duration of motor unit potentials, increased polyphasic potentials, and abnormal spontaneous activity.

POLYMYOSITIS

The diseases which fall into the classification of polymyositis present weakness as the cardinal clinical symptom (29, 30). The distinguishing common pathological feature is nonsuppurative inflammatory changes in skeletal muscles. Approximately 50% of the cases are associated with skin lesion and are identified as dermatomyositis, whereas most of the others are associated with collagenosis or malignancy. Tenderness and pain of the involved muscles are usually present but not invariably so (i.e., in about 50% of the patients). In the past, polymyositis was often mistakenly dismissed from consideration in differential diagnosis if this sign and/or symptom was not elicited. Polymyositis is the most frequently occurring primary myopathy in adults and is second in overall incidence to the muscular dystrophies.

The important electrophysiological findings may be presented as follows:

1) There is abnormal spontaneous activity—prolonged insertional activity which blends into the abnormalities found in the resting muscle (fibrillation potentials and trains of positive, sharp potentials).

2) Bizarre high frequency potentials are seen which resemble myotonic discharges.

3) There is a myopathic pattern—i.e., short duration motor unit action potentials, short duration polyphasic potentials, etc.

4) In some patients a certain degree of neuromuscular block may be demonstrated by the responses to repetitive electrical stimulation. In some instances the pattern of fatigue is typical of myasthenia gravis, whereas in others the early incrementation is more characteristic of the myasthenic syndrome (31).

The abnormal spontaneous activity is not present in all patients with polymyositis; EMG changes consistent with myopathic lesions are more uniformly encountered.

It is characteristic that motor and sensory fiber conduction velocity determinations are normal in polymyositis. This fact is of value in the occasional unusually difficult diagnostic problem when polymyositis and polyneuritis must be differentiated.

COLLAGEN GROUP

Scleroderma, lupus erythematosus, and rheumatoid affections of joint and soft tissue are included with polymyositis in the group identified as collagen diseases. Electrophysiological abnormalities are present only in a proportion of these patients, with the variation in specific EMG changes no different from those described for all of the myopathies. In the patients with scleroderma, the electromyographic abnormalities are most prominent in muscle subjacent to sclerodermatous patches of the skin (32).

In a study of 110 patients with collagen diseases, Vilppula (33) found that the mean duration of motor unit potentials was decreased in 84% of the cases and that this was most frequently observed in proximal muscles. The decreased duration as well as the increased incidence of polyphasic potentials was most pronounced in adult polymyositis. The electromyographic pattern during maximal effort was normal except for a 50% diminution in amplitude in one-half of the patients. According to the author, the electromyographic findings are not specific for any one of the collagen diseases, but the degree of abnormalities may help to distinguish between the different types of collagen disease. For example, severe electromyographic abnormalities including spontaneous activity and a high incidence of polyphasic potentials are more likely to occur in polymyositis and dermatomyositis than in the other forms of collagen disease. Electromyographic changes that are pronounced, but with fewer polyphasic potentials and often without spontaneous activity, may be indicative of systemic lupus erythematosus or polymyalgia rheumatica.

SARCOIDOSIS (34, 35)

Although sarcoid granulomata occur in over 50% of muscle biopsies performed on patients with this systemic disease, muscular weakness of any functional significance is rather infrequent. Occasionally a progressive picture resembling muscular dystrophy does occur. EMG studies may reveal the typical gamut of decreased action potential duration, decreased amplitude, polyphasic potential, etc.

CONGENITAL MYOPATHIES

There is an increasing number of inherited myopathies which are generally nonprogressive clinically and noninflammatory in histopathological character. The classification may include muscular glycogenosis, megaconial and pleoconial myopathies, congenital muscular dystrophy, central core disease, nemaline myopathy, and myotubular myopathy. These are the diseases in which the electrophysiological examination may and frequently does contribute nothing to establishment of a diagnosis. Although the answers lie within the realm of histochemical and electron microscopic investigation, the clinical neurophysiologist must include these diseases within the index of suspicion when considering patients who have presented with weakness. Most frequently the problem is concerned with the evaluation of infantile hypotonia.

Central Core Disease (36)

In central core disease, hypotonia and weakness are prominent, in body distribution similar to that of hypertrophic muscular dystrophy. The muscle biopsy shows large fibers with abnormal central areas devoid of enzymatic activity.

Nemaline Myopathy (37, 38)

Special histochemical staining reveals characteristic inclusions in the muscle fibers referred to as myogranules, nemaline, or rods. For the most part, the patients are infants, although a late onset (age 40 to 44) rod myopathy has been reported (39). The essential histopathological changes involve progressive enlargement of the Z bands of the skeletal muscle fiber. The exact chemical nature of the rods which are formed is unknown. In most of the cases reported, the EMG has been described as "typically" myopathic, with shortened duration of individual motor unit potentials as the most recurrent finding.

Abnormalities of the Mitochondria

The abnormal enlargement and increased number of mitochondria as seen in electron microscopic studies are respectively referred to as megaconial and pleoconial changes. Both have been identified with diffuse muscular weakness and growth retardation. The affected fibers also show a marked decrease or total lack of myofibrils. The exact pathogenesis of the myopathy is unknown. Hulsmann et al. (40), however, have reviewed the relationship of an abnormal "loosely coupled" state of oxidative phosphorylation of the muscle mitochondria to generalized myopathy. Luft et al. (41) reported this type of abnormal electron microscopic finding in a patient with severe weakness and myopathy associated with a hypermetabolic state (basal metabolic = +140 to +210%).

Myotubular Myopathy

The abnormal cells seen in myotubular or centronuclear myopathy resemble the myotubes seen in fetus muscle (42). In some cases a distinct Type I fiber atrophy is a predominant feature (43). The weakness is symmetrical, with ptosis, facial muscle involvement, and ocular palsy as common clinical features.

Arthrogryposis multiplex congenita falls within the inherited disease category but is now accepted as a physical syndrome with either a myogenic or neurogenic etiology. Children with this disease are born with severe contractures caused by extensive joint, muscle, and ligament pathology. When the etiology is myogenic the EMG presents a corresponding pattern. In the rare case of congenital muscular dystrophy substantiated histologically, the initial clinical picture may be that of arthrogryposis multiplex congenita (44, 45).

MALIGNANCY AND MYOPATHY

In spite of the fact that muscle wasting and weakness are familiar symptoms in neoplastic disease, the occurrence of a true myopathy is infrequent. If all lesions are thrown together into the "carcinomatous neuromyopathies" (46, 47), then the incidence of these remote effects of malignant neoplasia is 7%. The implication of the nomenclature that neuropathy and myopathy occur simultaneously is quite exaggerated. Shy and Silverstein (48) reported that only five of 27 cases of myopathy showed concomitant electrophysiological evidence of neuropathy; one of 82 patients electrophysiologically studied by Moody (49) revealed evidence of combined lesion.

If only electrophysiological criteria of myopathy are considered, Shy (50) has described a late onset muscular dystrophy in which 70% of the males manifest a malignancy within 3 years of onset of the muscle disorder.

EMG Findings

In general, the frequency of occurrence of the EMG picture typically seen in myopathy is low. In 55 patients with carcinoma of the lung, Trojaborg et al. (51) found only one individual with a myopathic pattern. In those patients in whom the malignancy is associated with dermatomyositis, the electrophysiological findings occur as described previously. The "myasthenic syndrome" with its characteristic electrophysiological features is a fascinating example of carcinomatous myopathy, but it too is relatively rare. The incidence in patients with all types of carcinoma of the lung is only 1%. If the pulmonary lesion is a small cell carcinoma, then the incidence is higher, at 6%.

NEOPLASM AND MYOPATHY

There are several general EMG patterns seen in neoplastic disease which are indistinguishable from the descriptions of the specific disorders presented in this text: generalized myopathy, dermatomyositis/polymyositis, and myasthenic syndrome.

MYOTONIA

Myotonia is a disorder characterized by an impaired ability to relax a previously contracted muscle and is the common denominator of three inherited diseases: myotonia congenita, myotonia dystrophica, and paramyotonia (52).

Myotonia Congenita (Thomsen's Disease)

This is a genetically determined (usually autosomal dominant) disease characterized by muscle "stiffness" which is aggravated by cold temperature and relieved by exercise. The muscles are usually hypertrophied, giving the young patient the body configuration of a tiny Hercules. The disease is compatible with normal longevity. The myotonic phenomenon may be evoked by volitional effort, so that there is difficulty in opening the clenched fist or opening the eyelids after they are closed tightly. The myotonia may also be evoked mechanically, by striking the thenar eminence sharply with a percussion hammer, or electrically, by direct stimulation of the muscle or its motor nerve. The electrophysiological characteristics of myotonia congenita do not show any essential differential features from the other myotonias except that there are no "myopathic" (dystrophic) EMG changes. The myotonia seems to be more severe and involves all of the skeletal muscles, distal and proximal, although the lower extremities may be preferentially involved. A differential feature from myotonia dystrophica is the increase of creatine tolerance in myotonia congenita as compared to the characteristic diminution in the dystrophic variety. The clinical and electrical signs of myotonia are relieved by exercise, as is the usual case in the inherited myotonias. (Occasionally the term myotonia paradoxica is seen, usually in reference to paramyotonia; it denotes an aggravation, rather than relief, of the phenomenon by exercise.)

Myotonia Dystrophica

This is most often identified as Steinert's disease. It is also inherited as an autosomal dominant and is characterized by myotonia, muscle weakness and atrophy, cataracts, and multiple system involvement, including the endocrines. Although the disease usually starts in the second or third decade, early onset myotonic dystrophy does occur (53). The effect on the facial muscles, which produces a typical myopathic facies, the nasal speech, due to pharyngeal and laryngeal involvement, and the atrophy of the sternocleidomastoid muscles are some clinical features which are very helpful diagnostic clues. The distal axial muscles are usually most affected.

Paramyotonia Congenita (Eulenberg's Disease)

The tendency for myotonia to appear after exposure to cold is a major symptom in paramyotonia with a predilection for involvement of the facial muscles and tongue. The severe episodic paresis which occurs and relates this disorder to adynamia episodica hereditaria has already been reviewed. There are no dystrophic features in paramyotonia.

Electrophysiological Features of Myotonia

The myotonic response has several characteristics which are important in its identification and its differentiation from myotonic-like responses. In true myotonia, the response involves high frequency repetitive discharges which show a recurrent variation of the frequency and amplitude (54) (Fig. 8.4). The waxing and waning in amplitude and frequency are responsible for the associated divebomber-like sound. The myotonic response may be evoked by voluntary movement, mechanically, by percussion or needle movement, and in response to electrical stimulation.

The activity which occurs in myotonic muscle after a voluntary contraction is most impressive with regard to the long persistence of the waving and waning repetitive discharges. The motor unit action potentials are usually seen in fine fibrillation potentials or, just as often, take the form of positive sharp waves. In some instances they have normal configurations. There is no relationship between the degree of atrophy and the presence of myotonic discharges, so that the wasted intrinsic muscles of the hands of the patient with myotonia dystrophica may not show the expected reaction. Even when the myotonic discharges are present, repeated efforts at demonstration will often be followed by a short interval when they disappear, returning after a brief period of rest. During the time when the myotonic response is not excited by voluntary movement, it still may be evoked mechanically by displacement of the electrode. If multiple electrodes are placed in the muscle at intervals of several centimeters, it can be demonstrated that the myotonia is not uniformly present in all muscle fiber bundles because only one of multiple electrode sites may show myotonic activity. Local blockage of the motor nerve or curarization does not abolish the myotonia. In some mild cases the myotonic response may be provoked by exposure to lowered temperature, e.g., 15°C for 30 to 40 min.

Myotonic muscles which are at apparent rest are the seat of some activity, which is not a product of mechanical irritation by the needle electrode, because it has been recorded with surface electrodes (55). Buchthal and Rosenfalck (6) have reported the presence of random showers of spontaneous potential which are indistinguishable from fibrillation except for the fact that they are enhanced by provocatively lowering the temperature of the limb.

The myotonic response may be evoked electrically only if the stimulation

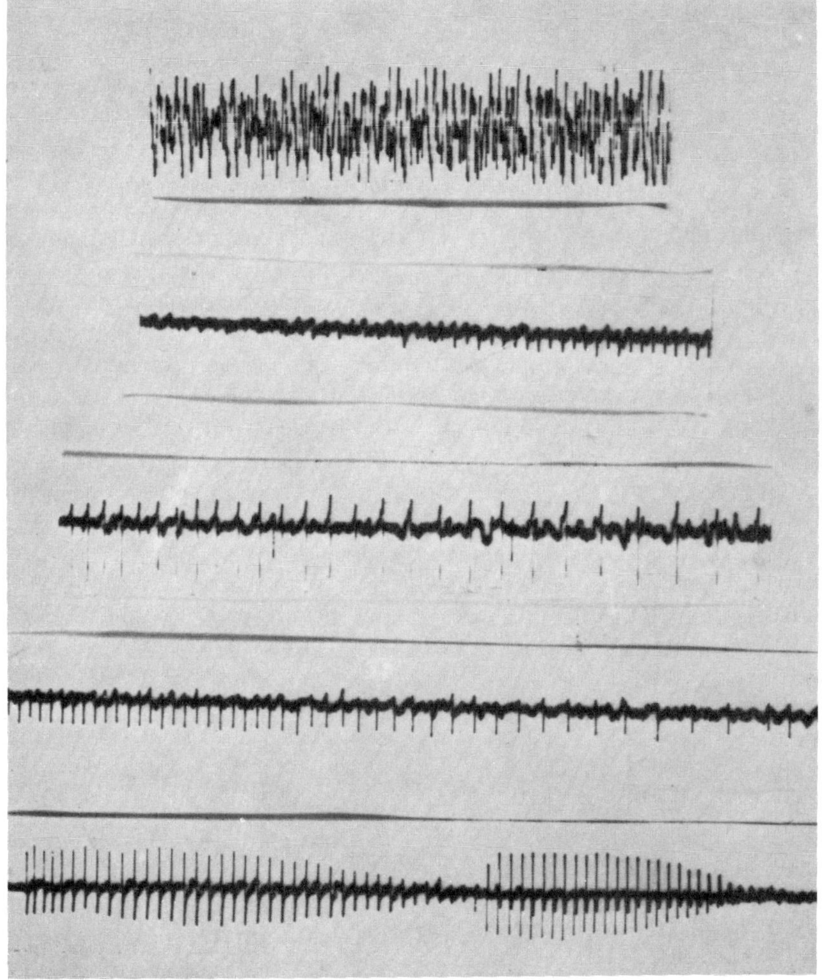

FIG. 8.4. Myotonic discharge. These tracings represent portions of a continuous record, starting with voluntary effort (*top*) and progressing into the myotonic response during relaxation of the effort. The variation in amplitude and frequency is apparent.

is repetitive (at least 2 to 20 repetitions per sec). A single excitation does not evoke a discharge (56). After repetitive stimulation, a rest period is required before typical discharging trains can be again evoked. Percussion elicits a localized myotonic response because the sharp blow acts in a manner comparable to a brief train of repetitive electrical stimuli.

Pharmacologically, myotonia is lessened or abolished by quinine, calcium, and procainamide, whereas potassium and acetylcholine are excitatory to it.

It is interesting that Foster Kennedy, a leading neurologist of this century, said of the "symptomatic cure" of myotonia congenita by quinine, "that is a fact, a fact so striking and so definite that it is comparable, perhaps, with the giving of insulin to a diabetic" (57). The passage of time has brought the realization that the cure of both is only an apparent one. Also within the context of therapeutics is the reported iatrogenic complication of a syndrome resembling systemic lupus erythematosus during the course of treatment with procainamide (58). The effect, however, appears to be transient and subsides when the drug administration is stopped.

Aside from the generally accepted premise that the myotonic response is a local event in the muscle, the observation that a powerful involuntary spasm occurs in muscles remote from the prime mover (involuntary spasm of forearm extensors and flexors when the hand is clenched) led to the view that a second, centrally determined event was also operative. These disabling generalized afterspasms were considered reflexly originated, afferent proprioceptive discharges induced by the myotonic contraction in the prime movers (59). Landau (55) considered the afterspasm to be a physiological response of the nature of a lengthening reaction in muscles stretched by sustained myotonic contraction in antagonists.

In myotonia dystrophica, the muscular dystrophy is manifested in varying degrees within the full spectrum of the EMG pattern identified as typical of myopathy.

Although the "dystrophic" changes in myotonia dystrophica are not limited to the muscles but are expressed in involvement of lens, gonads, skin, skeleton, etc., there has recently been described another familial group in which nonprogressive myopathy is associated with myotonia: dwarfism, skeletal deformities different from those described in myotonic dystrophy, and abnormalities of the face and orbital region. Aberfeld et al. (60) have unified the cases reported as dysotosis enchondrales metaepiphysaria of the Catel-Hempel type (61) and the Schwartz-Jampel syndrome (62) of congenital blepharophimosis associated with myopathy under the more appropriate and inclusive nomenclature of "chondrodystrophic myotonia." The EMG characteristics encompass true myotonic responses increased by cold and decreased by repetitive activity.

"CONTINUOUS MUSCLE FIBER ACTIVITY" SYNDROME

Isaacs in 1961 and 1967 (63, 64) described three patients with symptoms and postural disturbances resulting from involuntary continuous muscle activity which could not be classified as myotonia or stiff man syndrome. The specific features of this entity served to separate it from other known forms of neuromuscular disease, and it was called "a syndrome of continuous muscle fiber activity." It has since been described in other case reports (65, 66). The disorder affects males and females of any age, with complaints of muscle stiffness and difficulty with voluntary movement. On clinical examination, the sensory nervous system is completely normal but the involuntary contractions and fasciculations are particularly noticeable in the facial muscles and eyelids. The extraocular muscles do not seem to be affected and swallowing remains normal, although chewing may be affected. The abnormal activity persists during sleep (67).

According to Isaacs, the key to diagnosis is the electromyographic examination. Electromyography reveals a persistent, rapid dysrythmic discharge at rest consisting of a mixture of motor unit activity and low amplitude, short duration potentials which was considered to indicate both single fibers and motor units with varying degrees of fiber depletion. A period of electrical silence of 10 to 20 sec follows strenuous activity. In less involved muscles, occasional repetitive bursts of motor unit activity were seen, with corresponding coarse undulating movements in the muscle. Nerve conduction in both motor and sensory fibers was found to be at the lower limits of normal, and the terminal latencies may be prolonged (64, 65). The muscular stiffness and spontaneous electromyographic discharges were abolished by curare but persisted during spinal anesthesia and after peripheral nerve block. Unlike the activity of myotonia, that of this syndrome is not induced by percussion.

Considerable variation in muscle fiber size, numerous aggregates of nuclei, and significant grouping of fiber types were the major histological and histochemical findings in biopsy specimens. Motor nerve terminal and endplates showed evidence of excessive terminal branching (67).

Symptomatic relief was obtained with administration of diphenylhydantoin (63), an agent which facilitates the active extrusion of intraneuronal sodium. Follow-up of two patients by Isaacs after 12 years revealed almost complete remission of the syndrome, accompanied by improvement in the muscle histology and lack of spontaneous myoelectric discharges at rest.

The site of pathology is considered to be mainly in the motor nerve terminal, with involvement of the distal motor axon to a lesser degree. The etiology is unknown, although the possible causative effect of 2,4-D (dichlorophenoxyacetic acid) poisoning has been considered in one case (65).

STIFF MAN SYNDROME

The stiff man syndrome bears a certain resemblance to the continuous muscle fiber activity syndrome, because electromyography reveals a constant activity at rest which subsides during sleep. Clinically the stiff man syndrome is characterized by chronic board-like stiffness involving the proximal limb muscles and especially the abdominal and back muscles. The facial muscles are usually spared. Superimposed on the stiffness is a severe and painful spasm excited by fright or any mild external stimulation. In general there is a paucity of neurological symptoms, and pathological examination has revealed little of a definitive nature. The patient characteristically moves about with the appearance of a tin soldier; the body is hyperextended and flexion of the trunk is carried out with great difficulty. There are no fasciculations.

The electromyogram shows a constant discharge of motor unit potentials which are normal in configuration. The clinical stiffness and the electromyographic findings are inhibited by neuromuscular blocking agents, peripheral nerve block, and general anesthesia. The exact physiological mechanism is unknown, but it is suspected that it concerns an insufficiency of inhibitor interneuron activity. This concept is considerably enhanced by the observation that diazepam exerts a remarkable clinical effect in reducing activity and clinical symptoms (68, 69).

REFERENCES

1. Pearson, C. M.: Skeletal muscle: Basic and clinical aspects and illustrative new diseases. Ann. Intern. Med., *67:* 614–650, 1967.
2. McComas, A. J., and Sica, R. E. P.: Muscular dystrophy: Myopathy or neuropathy. Lancet, *1:* 119, 1970.
3. Buller, A. J., Eccles, J. C., and Eccles, R. M.: Interactions between motoneurones and muscles in respect of the characteristic speeds of their responses. J. Physiol. (Lond.), *150:* 417–439, 1960.
4. Engel, W. K.: Focal myopathic changes produced by electromyographic and hypodermic needles. Arch. Neurol. (Chicago), *16:* 509–511, 1967.
5. Hathaway, P., Dahl, D., and Engel, W. K.: Myopathic changes produced by local trauma. Arch. Neurol. (Chicago), *21:* 355–357, 1969.
6. Buchthal, F., and Rosenfalck, P.: Electrophysiologic aspects of myopathy with particular reference to progressive muscular dystrophy. In *Muscular Dystrophy in Man and Animals,* edited by G. H. Bourne and M. N. S. Calorz, ch. VI, pp. 193–262. Karger Publishing Co., New York, 1963.
7. McGee, K. R., and DeJong, R. M.: Hereditary distal myopathy with onset in infancy. Arch. Neurol. (Chicago), *13:* 387–390, 1965.
8. Thage, O.: The quadriceps syndrome. Acta Neurol. Scand., *41:* 245–249, 1964.
9. Shy, G. M., Wanko, T., Rowley, P. T., and Engel, A. G.: Studies in familial periodic paralysis. Exp. Neurol., *3:* 53–121, 1961.
10. Dyken, M. L., Zeman, W., and Rusche, T.: Hypokalemic periodic paralysis. Neurology (Minneap.), *19:* 691–699, 1969.
11. Olivarius, B., and Christensen, E.: Histopathological muscular changes in familial periodic paralysis. Acta Neurol. Scand., *41:* 1–18, 1965.
12. Drager, G. A., Hammill, J. G., and Shy, G. M.: Paramyotonia congenita. Arch. Neurol. Psychiatry, *80:* 1–9, 1958.
13. Mastaglia, F. L., Bazwick, D. D., and Hall, R.: Myopathy in acromegalics. Lancet, *2:* 907–909, 1970.
14. Grob, D.: Myopathies and their relation to thyroid disease. New York J. Med., *63:* 218–228, 1963.
15. Lambert, E. H., Underdahl, L. O., Beckett, S., and Mederos, L. O.: A study of the ankle jerk in myxedema. J. Clin. Endocrinol., *11:* 1186–1205, 1951.
16. Frame, B., Heinze, E. G., Jr., Block, M. A., and Manson, G. A.: Myopathy in primary hyperparathyroidism. Ann. Intern. Med., *68:* 1022–1027, 1968.
17. Bischoff, A., and Esslen, E.: Myopathy with primary hyperparathyroidism. Neurology (Minneap.), *15:* 64–68, 1965.
18. Dyken, M. C., Smith, O. M., and Peake, R. C.: An electromyographic diagnostic screening test in McArdle's disease and a case report. Neurology (Minneap.), *17:* 45–50, 1967.
19. Tarui, S., Okuno, G., Okuka, Y., Tanaka, T., Suda, M., and Nishikawa, H.: Phosphofructokinase deficiency in skeletal muscle: A new type of glycogenosis. Biochem. Biophys. Res. Commun., *19:* 517–523, 1965.

20. Bordiuk, J. M., Legato, M. J., Lovelace, R. E., and Blumenthal, S.: Pompe's disease. Arch. Neurol. (Chicago), *23:* 113–119, 1970.
21. Hogan, G. R., Gutmann, L., Schmidt, R., and Gilbert, E.: Pompe's disease. Neurology (Minneap.), *19:* 894–900, 1969.
22. Swaiman, K. F., Kennedy, W. R., and Sauls, H. S.: Late infantile acid maltase deficiency. Arch. Neurol. (Chicago), *18:* 642–648, 1968.
23. Hirschhorn, K., Nadler, H., Waithe, W. I., Brown, I. B., and Hirschhorn, R.: Pompe's disease, detection of heterozygotes by lymphocyte stimulation. Science, *166:* 1632–1633, 1969.
24. Hudgson, P., Gardner-Medwin, D., Warsfold, M., Pennington, R. J. T., and Walton, J. N.: Adult myopathy from glycogen storage disease due to acid maltase deficiency. Brain, *91:* 435–460, 1968.
25. Engel, A. G.: Acid maltase deficiency in adult life: Morphology and biochemical data in 3 cases of a syndrome simulating other myopathies. In *Proceedings of the International Congress of Muscle Disease*, edited by J. N. Walton, N. Conal, and G. Scarlato, series 199, pp. 236–245. Excerpta Medica, Amsterdam, 1969.
26. Perkoff, G. T., Dioso, M. M., Bleisch, V., and Klinkerfuss, G.: A spectrum of myopathy associated with alcoholism. I. Clinical and laboratory features. Ann. Intern. Med., *67:* 481–492, 1967.
27. Ekbom, K., Hed, R., Kirstein, L., and Astrom, K. E.: Muscular affections in chronic alcoholism. Arch. Neurol. (Chicago), *10:* 449–458, 1964.
28. Waylonis, G. W., and Johnson, E. W.: The EMG in acute trichinosis—Report of 4 cases. Arch. Phys. Med., *45:* 177–183, 1964.
29. Vignos, P. J., Bowling, G. F., and Watkins, M. P.: Polymyositis. Arch. Intern. Med., *114:* 263–277, 1964.
30. Richardson, A. T.: Clinical and EMG aspects of polymyositis. Proc. R. Soc. Med., *49:* 111–114, 1956.
31. Simpson, J., and Lenman, A. E.: The effect of frequency of stimulation in neuromuscular disease. Electroencephalogr. Clin. Neurophysiol., *11:* 604–605, 1959.
32. Hausmanowa-Petrusewicz, H. P., and Kozminska, A.: Electromyographic findings in scleroderma. Arch. Neurol. (Chicago), *4:* 281–287, 1961.
33. Vilppula, A.: Quantitative electromyographic findings in some collagen diseases. Scand. J. Rehabil. Med., Suppl. 3: 69–72, 1974.
34. Crompton, M. R., and MacDermot, V.: Sarcoidosis associated with progressive muscular wasting and weakness. Brain, *84:* 62–74, 1961.
35. Kim, C., and Lee, M.: Muscular dystrophy and sarcoidosis. New York J. Med., *70:* 2354–2358, 1970.
36. Shy, G. M., and McGee, K. R.: A new congenital non-progressive myopathy. Brain, *79:* 610–621, 1956.
37. Shy, G. M., Engel, W. K., Somers, J. E., and Wanko, T.: Nemaline myopathy—A new congenital myopathy. Brain, *86:* 793–810, 1963.
38. Hefferman, L. P., Newcastle, M. B., and Humphrey, J. G.: The spectrum of rod myopathies. Arch. Neurol. (Chicago), *18:* 529–542, 1968.
39. Engel, W. K., and Resnick, J. S.: Late-onset rod myopathy: A newly recognized, acquired, and progressive disease. Neurology (Minneap.), *16:* 308–309, 1966.
40. Hulsmann, W. C., Bethlem, J., Meijer, A. E. F. H., Fleury, P., and Schellens, J. P. M.: Myopathy with abnormal structure and function of muscle mitochondria. J. Neurol. Neurosurg. Psychiatry, *30:* 519–525, 1967.
41. Luft, R., Ikkos, D., Palmieri, G., Ernster, L., and Afzelius, B.: A case of severe hypermetabolism of nonthyroid origin with a defect in the maintenance of mitochondrial respiratory control: A correlated clinical, biochemical and morphological study. J. Clin. Invest., *41:* 1776–1804, 1962.
42. Spiro, A. M., Shy, G. M., and Gonatas, N. K.: Myotubular myopathy. Arch. Neurol. (Chicago), *41:* 1–4, 1966.
43. Bethlem, J., Van Wijngaarden, G. K., Mumenthaler, M., and Meijer, A. E. F. H.: Centronuclear myopathy with type I fiber atrophy and "myotubes." Arch. Neurol. (Chicago), *23:* 70–73, 1970.
44. Gubbay, S. S., Walton, J. N., and Pearce, G. W.: Clinical and pathological study of a case of congenital muscular dystrophy. J. Neurol. Neurosurg. Psychiatry, *29:* 500–508, 1966.

45. Banker, B. Q., Victor, M., and Adams, R. D.: Arthrogryposis multiplex due to congenital muscular dystrophy. Brain, *80:* 319–334, 1957.
46. Brain, R., and Adams, R. D.: A guide to the classification and investigation of neurological disorders associated with neoplasms. In *Remote Effects of Cancer on the Nervous System*, edited by W. R. Brain and F. H. Norris, Jr., pp. 216–221. Grune and Stratton, New York, 1965.
47. Brain, R., and Henson, R. A.: Neurological syndromes associated with carcinoma: The carcinomatous neuromyopathies. Lancet, *2:* 971–974, 1958.
48. Shy, G. M., and Silverstein, I.: A study of the effects upon the motor unit by remote malignancy. Brain, *8:* 515–528, 1965.
49. Moody, J. F.: Electrophysiological investigations into neurological complications of carcinoma. Brain, *88:* 1023–1035, 1965.
50. Shy, G. M.: The late onset myopathy: A clinicopathologic study of 131 patients. World Neurol., *3:* 149–158, 1962.
51. Trojaborg, W., Frantzen, E., and Andersen, I.: Peripheral neuropathy and myopathy associated with carcinoma of the lung. Brain, *92:* 71–82, 1969.
52. Caughey, J. E., and Myrianthepoulos, M. C.: *Dystrophica Myotonica and Related Disorders.* Charles C Thomas, Springfield, Ill., 1963.
53. Watters, G. V., and Williams, T. W.: Early onset myotonic dystrophy. Arch. Neurol. (Chicago), *17:* 137–152, 1967.
54. Report on Subcommittee of the Pavia Committee on Terminology on Electromyography. Bull. Am. Assoc. Electromyogr. Electrodiag., *14:* 34–36, 1967.
55. Landau, W. M.: The essential mechanism in myotonia: An electromyographic study. Neurology (Minneap.), *2:* 362–388, 1952.
56. Denny-Brown, D., and Foley, J. M.: Evidence of a chemical mediator in myotonia. Trans. Assoc. Am. Physicians, *62:* 187–191, 1949.
57. Kennedy, F., discussant in Russel, C. K., Odom, G., and McEachern, D.: Physiological and chemical studies of neuromuscular disorders. Trans. Am. Neurol. Soc., *64:* 120–124, 1938.
58. Prockop, L.: Myotonia, procaine amide, and lupus-like syndrome. Arch. Neurol. (Chicago), *14:* 326–330, 1966.
59. Denny-Brown, D., and Nevin, S.: The phenomenon of myotonia. Brain, *64:* 1–18, 1941.
60. Aberfeld, D. C., Nomba, T., Vye, M. V., and Grob, D.: Chondrodystrophic myotonia: Report of 2 cases. Arch. Neurol. (Chicago), *22:* 455–462, 1970.
61. Catel, W.: *Differential diagnostische Symptomatologie des Kindesalters*, p. 48. Georg Thieme, Stuttgart, 1951.
62. Schwartz, O., and Jampel, R. S.: Congenital blepharophimosis associated with a unique generalized myopathy. Arch. Ophthalmol. (Chicago), *68:* 52–57, 1962.
63. Isaacs, H.: A syndrome of continuous muscle-fiber activity. J. Neurol. Neurosurg. Psychiatry, *24:* 319–325, 1961.
64. Isaacs, H.: Continuous muscle fibre activity in an Indian male with additional evidence of terminal motor fibre abnormality. J. Neurol. Neurosurg. Psychiatry, *30:* 126–133, 1967.
65. Wallis, W. E., Van Poznak, A., and Plum, F.: Generalized muscular stiffness, fasciculations and myokymia of peripheral nerve origin. Arch. Neurol., *22:* 430–439, 1970.
66. Welch, L. K., Appenzeller, O., and Bicknell, J. M.: Peripheral neuropathy with myokymia, sustained muscular contraction, and continuous motor unit activity. Neurology, *22:* 161–169, 1972.
67. Isaacs, H., and Frere, G.: Syndrome of continuous muscle fibre activity: Histochemical, nerve terminal and end-plate study of two cases. South Afr. Med. J., *10:* 1601–1607, 1974.
68. Gordon, E. E., Januszko, D. M., and Kaufman, L.: A critical survey of stiff-man syndrome. Am. J. Med., *42:* 582–599, 1967.
69. Olafson, R. A., Mulder, W. W., and Howard, F. M.: "Stiff-man" syndrome: A review of the literature, report on three additional cases and discussion of pathophysiology and therapy. Mayo Clinic Proc., *39:* 131–144, 1964.

chapter 9

Myasthenia Gravis and Other Disorders of the Neuromuscular Junction

Myasthenia gravis is a chronic disease of voluntary muscle characterized by (a) onset of abnormal weakness after repetitive or sustained contractions, (b) recovery of power after a short interval of rest, and (c) in most cases, temporary repair of the defect by administration of anticholinesterases such as Tensilon (Roche) or prostigmine.

The disease was first described by Willis in 1672 (1). Two centuries later, the clinical features were thoroughly documented following contributions by Erb (2), who differentiated the disorder from other neurological syndromes, and Goldflam (3). Also at this time, Jolly (4) provided the first evidence that the disorder was in the peripheral nervous system. He observed a rapid deterioration in the size of the muscle response after faradic current stimulation and then recovery of the response after rest. Jolly also discovered that faradic current could not easily stimulate a myasthenic muscle fatigued by a series of volitional contractions. Although his experimental arrangements were very crude, e.g., maximal stimulation could not be achieved with the stimulator, his results have been confirmed with modern equipment. Jolly suggested naming the disorder "myasthenia gravis pseudoparalytica," its present appellation (5).

The important signs and symptoms are reviewed in capsular form in Table 9.1. From the practical viewpoint of the electrophysiological tests which are employed, there are several clinical features worthy of emphasis: (a) The muscle weakness is not constant but varies from day to day as well as within

TABLE 9.1. Symptom Review of Myasthenia Gravis

Parameter	Finding
Painless muscle weakness	Variably transient or persistent from day to day or within the 24-hr period; recovery with rest
Distribution of muscles affected	
Extraocular	Diplopia, ptosis
Cervical muscles	Drooping head
Shoulder girdle	
Hip girdle	
Facial	"Bell's palsy snarl"
Mastication	Jaw drop
Deglutition	Dysphagia
	Dysphonia
Respiratory muscles	Dyspnea, respiratory failure
Deep tendon reflexes	Normal
Precipitating factors	Infections, especially upper respiratory; cold; emotional distress; menstruation; pregnancy
Significantly associated with	Thymus tumor, thyroid disease, pernicious anemia
Sex predominance, female:male	2:1
Age	Variable, average 20+ years; neonatal period

a single day. (b) There is not universal affection of the voluntary muscle but a distinct preferential distribution (1). Extraocular muscles probably rank first, followed by cervical muscles, and then the shoulder girdle musculature. It is not unusual for the defect to involve only the eye muscles and apparently spare all others. A routine examination of solely the intrinsic hand muscles, therefore, may fail to reveal a potent abnormality. (c) The extraocular muscle involvement is usually associated with paresis of the levator palpebrae and orbicularis oculi, so that ptosis and inability to close the eyes tightly are common symptoms. (d) In 10 to 20% of the patients, late permanent weakness and atrophy (especially of the extraocular, triceps, and quadriceps muscles), which is due to myasthenic myopathy, occur.

Significant advances in research during the past few years have promoted our understanding of the nature and origin of myasthenia gravis; in fact, it is now considered the foremost example of an autoimmune disease in humans. Before discussing the pathophysiology, the basic events involved in neuromuscular transmission will be reviewed.

PHYSIOLOGY OF THE END-PLATE

The neuromuscular junction, shown in diagrammatic form in Fig. 9.1, includes the presynaptic nerve terminal, the synaptic cleft, and the postsynaptic region on the muscle fiber. The gap between the presynaptic and postsynaptic sides, known as the synaptic cleft, averages around 10 to 50 nm and is discernible only under the electron microscope. Numerous spherical membranous structures, the *synaptic vesicles*, are also seen with the electron microscope in the presynaptic terminal that are about 50 nm in diameter. The synaptic vesicles contain acetylcholine (ACh), the neurotransmitter substance, which is released into the synaptic cleft when a propagating nerve impulse arrives at the terminal. Thus, the neuromuscular junction acts as an electrochemical transducer; electrical activity is first transduced into a chemical signal and then, at the subneural part of the muscle cell membrane, back again into electrical energy.

ACh is synthesized in the motor nerve terminal cytoplasm from choline and actyl-coenzyme A, derived from the mitochondria, by the enzyme choline acetylase. Following release, ACh acts on the subsynaptic receptors for a short time when it is hydrolyzed by the enzyme, acetylcholinesterase, into two inactive components, choline and acetic acid. Approximately 50% of the choline released in the reaction is returned into the nerve terminal, presumably by the circulation.

As stated, ACh is not distributed uniformly within the nerve terminal but is concentrated in vesicles and released into the cleft at specific sites along the terminal membrane by a process of exocytosis (6). The specific release sites are situated directly opposite the regions of highest concentration of ACh receptors on the postsynaptic membrane (7) (see Fig. 9.1).

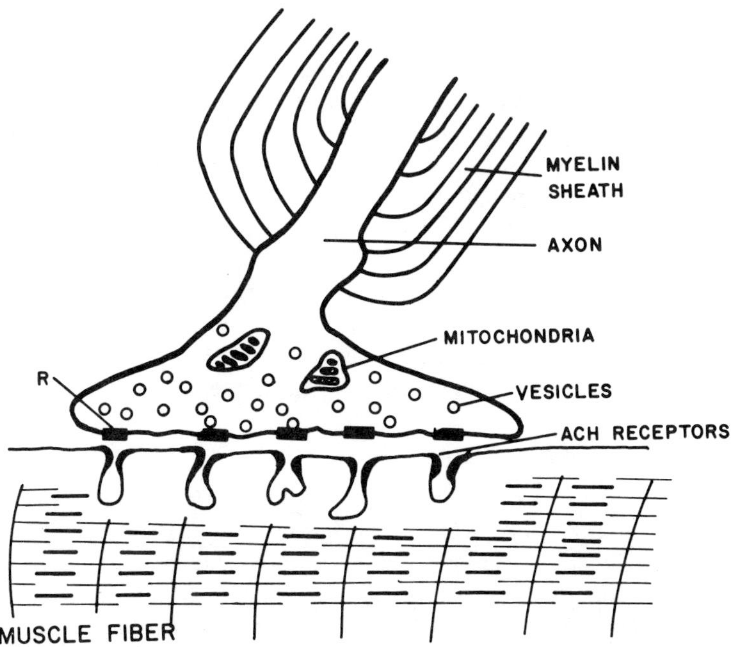

FIG. 9.1. A diagrammatic drawing of the neuromuscular junction showing the presynaptic nerve terminal, the synaptic cleft, and the postsynaptic region on the muscle fiber.

Quantal Release of ACh

The contents of the vesicles are released in two ways: (a) spontaneously and (b) following a nerve terminal action potential. The spontaneous release of ACh occurs randomly and results in small depolarizations at the postsynaptic membrane, called *miniature end-plate potentials* (MEPP), which do not reach threshold nor initiate action potentials. Normal MEPP are approximately 1 mV in amplitude and appear only once per sec on the average. ACh is not released in a continuous stream, one molecule at a time, but in discrete packets, where each packet is called a *quantum* and includes all the ACh associated with a vesicle, ranging from 5000 to 10,000 molecules.

When an electrical nerve impulse propagates into the motor nerve terminal, a greater amount of ACh is released into the synaptic cleft, approximately 100 to 200 quanta. This ACh can interact with ACh receptors on the postsynaptic side to enhance the permeability of the muscle membrane to cations, such as sodium, potassium, and calcium, producing a large membrane depolarization, the *end-plate potential* (EPP). If the EPP is equal to or greater than threshold, an action potential is triggered which propagates along the muscle membrane.

ACh not attached to receptors is removed by either the action of acetylcholinesterase, which rapidly hydrolyzes the ACh, or by diffusional spread away from the synapse. The entire action from release to generation of the muscle action potential requires only a few milliseconds.

In normally innervated skeletal muscle, only the region directly underneath the nerve terminal has the receptor protein specific for ACh. The density may reach 30,000 receptors per μm^2 at the junction and then falls off precipitously a short distance away. The end-plate potential may be either suprathreshold or subthreshold in amplitude, depending on the number of quanta that combine with the receptors. Only a small fraction of the total ACh released interacts with only a few of the available receptors, which normally is more than sufficient to generate an end-plate potential far above threshold. The excess amount of released ACh represents a *safety margin* for neuromuscular transmission. Stated another way: normally, the end-plate potential is much bigger than is nècessary for triggering the action potential.

Storage Sites of ACh

A useful model to explain some of the responses observed following nerve stimulation describes three sites of vesicle storage in the nerve terminal (Fig. 9.2). The main storage pool contains most of the quanta, estimated at 300,000; however, only a small fraction is available for immediate release by a nerve impulse. Quanta released from this pool and "mobilized" for release at the membrane are considered another storage compartment. Finally, the quanta adjacent to the membrane comprise the immediately available store of ACh, estimated at 1000 quanta.

During a repetitive stimulation, it is the size of immediately available store and the rate at which ACh is replenished from the main pool into that store which determines the amount of ACh liberated by each nerve impulse. Thus, the rapid fall in amplitude of the end-plate potential during a high frequency nerve stimulation is attributed to the decrease in the number of quanta released by each impulse which, in turn, is due to partial reduction of available quanta.

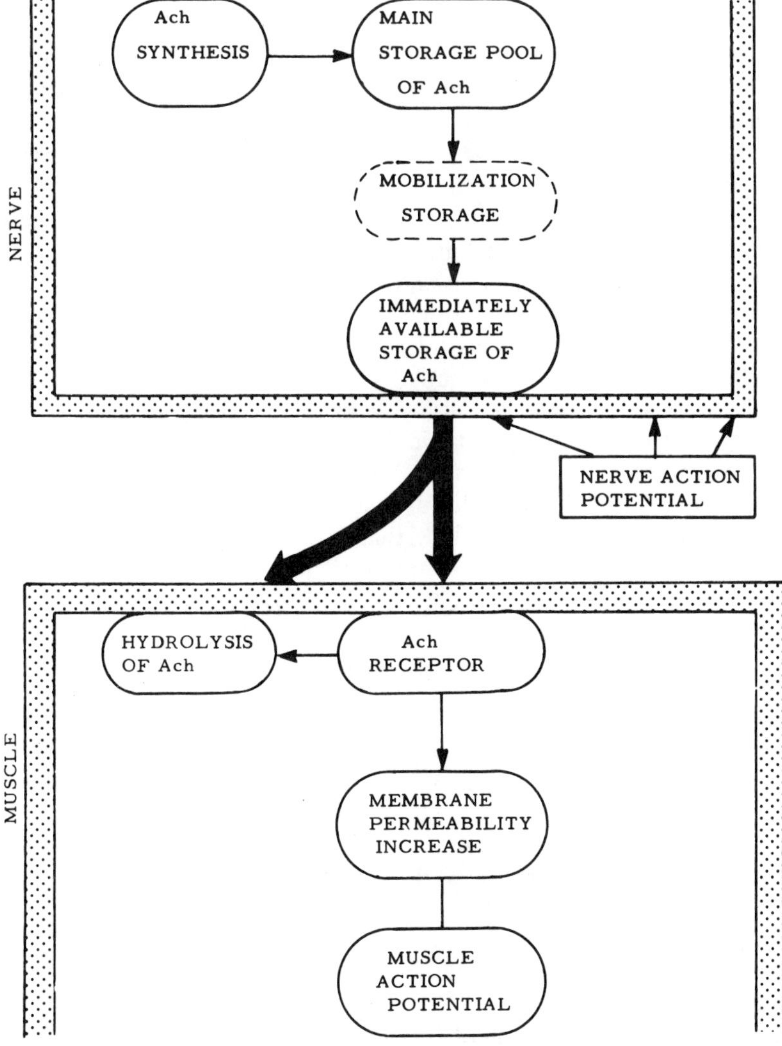

FIG. 9.2. A drawing of the model used to show the main steps in neuromuscular transmission.

The Role of Calcium in Transmitter Release

The presence of calcium ions in the extracellular fluid is absolutely necessary for the normal release of quanta by a nerve action potential. Calcium must be present before depolarization of the nerve terminal membrane, despite the fact that it does not act until after depolarization. Following depolarization of the nerve terminal membrane, calcium ions enter into the ending from the extracellular fluid and, through an as yet unknown process, stimulate the release of ACh. Since ACh is released when the vesicles fuse with the terminal membrane, it has been suggested that calcium is necessary to empty the vesicles into the synaptic cleft. Recent studies have suggested that some of calcium's effects may be modulated by a calcium-dependent regulator protein called *calmodulin.* Calmodulin appears to be a calcium receptor protein with a specific and strong binding affinity for calcium and unique among the calcium-binding proteins for its widespread distribution and multiplicity of functions. In the nerve terminal, recent experimental results suggest that calcium stimulation of neurotransmitter release and protein phosphorylation requires calmodulin (8).

The whole process of calcium entry and outward diffusion takes 100 to 200 msec. Repetitive nerve stimulation at frequencies of 5 Hz or greater (intervals of 200 msec or less) will lead to facilitation of ACh release due to the presence of extra calcium. Similarly, the augmented response of normal muscle to a single nerve impulse following a period of high frequency stimulation (posttetanic potentiation) has been explained by the raised intraterminal calcium concentration.

The effect of botulinum toxin as well as Mg^{2+} on the nerve ending is similar to that of removing Ca^{2+}, that is, they are both neuromuscular blocking agents. Botulinum toxin and Mg^{2+} prevent the influx of Ca^{2+} and thereby inhibit the release of ACh.

SITE OF DEFECT

Although the peripheral nature of the disease was known since the 1890's, the locus of the lesion was not established until 1934 when Mary Walker (9) reported that physostigmine, an inhibitor of cholinesterase, alleviated the weakness of myasthenic muscle. Coincidentally, Dale and Feldberg (10) confirmed the role of acetylcholine in neuromuscular transmission.

Mary Walker's report provided the first evidence that the neuromuscular junction was the site of the defect and is considered a milestone in the study of myasthenia gravis. From that time onward, clinical as well as laboratory studies concentrated on finding the transmission defect at the neuromuscular junction.

In 1964, Elmquist and his colleagues reported the results of experiments that were crucial in focusing the site of the defect at the presynaptic terminal.

From intercostal muscles biopsied from myasthenia gravis patients, they found that the amplitude of MEPP was decreased but that the frequency was normal (11). They interpreted the results as indicating a reduced ACh content of each vesicle, i.e., "small quanta." This was supported by demonstrating normal end-plate sensitivity in myasthenic muscles: iontopheretically applied ACh produced normal end-plate depolarization.

Grob (12) disagreed with the Elmquist et al. findings regarding end-plate sensitivity. Grob observed that the spontaneous end-plate activity in myasthenic patients had the same amplitude and frequency as in normal subjects, but that it was more difficult to locate the discharges in the myasthenic muscle. In addition, Grob found that the end-plate zone of myasthenic patients was less responsive than that of normal subjects to the excitatory action of ACh. Even though these studies reported a postsynaptic rather than a presynaptic disorder, myasthenia gravis was generally considered to be a presynaptic disease coupled with an abnormal immune system.

The early implication of the immune system in myasthenia gravis was based on circumstantial evidence (see review by Simpson (13)). The hypothesis formulated by Simpson (14) in 1960 that myasthenia gravis was caused by antibodies to ACh receptors that impaired neuromuscular transmission has now, more than 20 years later, been confirmed. The high incidence of thymic abnormalities and the association of myasthenia gravis with a number of diseases immunological in nature formed the basis of the concept. Smithers (15) and Nastuk et al. (16) also independently proposed about 1960 that an immunological disorder was associated with myasthenia gravis.

The breakthrough in our understanding came in 1973. Availability of neurotoxins from certain snake venoms which bind specificially to the activities of ACh receptors finally enabled the exact site of the abnormality to be localized. The toxin most commonly used is α-bungarotoxin from the Formosan many-banded krait which binds specifically and irreversibly to the active sites of the postsynaptic receptors and blocks the action of ACh both in vivo and in vitro. Since it can be labeled with radioactive iodine, the number of ACh receptor sites can be determined from the amount of bound radioactive isotope. Using this technique, Fambrough et al. (17) calculated the number of receptor sites per neuromuscular junction in muscles taken from 10 patients with myasthenia gravis and compared it with the number in muscles obtained from normal individuals. A marked reduction was observed in receptor sites of the patients with myasthenia gravis, averaging 80% less than the controls. This implicated a defect of the ACh receptors.

Coincidentally with the receptor studies, an experimental model of myasthenia gravis was discovered, almost accidentally, by Patrick and Lindstrom (18) which provided the most direct evidence that the autoimmune response was directed against ACh receptors. Attempting to identify ACh receptors with antibodies from myasthenia gravis patients, they found that injection of purified ACh receptors (derived from the electric organs of electric eels) in complete Freund's adjuvant into rabbits caused the development of antibodies which cross-reacted with the muscle receptors. The animals developed a condition analogous to myasthenia gravis, and the disease was designated experimental autoimmune myasthenia gravis (EAMG). EAMG has been induced in all species tested by immunization with ACh receptors purified from fish electric organs, such as rabbits, rats, mice, guinea pigs, goats, monkeys, and frogs. It has been most thoroughly studied in rats. It is interesting to note that as little as 1 μg of purified ACh receptor in complete Freund's adjuvant produces antibody and loss of ACh receptor (19). Although chronic EAMG closely resembles the human form of myasthenia gravis, there are differences which have not been explained as yet. For example, the nature of the initiating event in the human disease is unknown, and the active phase in the animal model does not occur in humans.

Subsequently, a search was begun for a sensitive anti-ACh receptor antibody assay. Initial procedures depended upon the inhibition of α-bungarotoxin binding to ACh receptor extracted from denervated rat muscle. Almon et al. (20), with this assay, demonstrated the presence of serum immunoglobulins directed against the ACh receptors in one-third of 15 patients with myasthenia gravis. Of the various procedures, the one developed by Patrick and Lindstrom (18) employing the immunoprecipitation of α-bungarotoxin-labelled ACh receptors has been established to be the most sensitive and reliable. In a group of myasthenia gravis patients, 85% positive results have been obtained (21). Lindstrom et al. (22) published the first detailed assay of the anti-Ach receptor antibodies in normal individuals and myasthenia gravis patients.

The measurement of anti-ACh receptor antibodies is a useful test for myasthenia gravis, but its efficacy is reduced by some problems still unsolved. Antireceptor antibody values vary widely from patient to patient, and also there is no particular correlation with the severity of the disease (21, 22). More than 10% of the patients with generalized myasthenia gravis have no detectable antibody by present assay methods, and in ocular myasthenia the proportion is up to 25%. These problems, as well as the etiology of the disease itself, are currently under investigation in many laboratories. One proposal for the possible triggering factor is a viral infection (23).

EVOKED MUSCLE ACTION POTENTIALS

The most useful electrophysiological test that will demonstrate a defect of neuromuscular transmission in most cases is the recording of evoked muscle action potentials. Jolly published in 1895 (5) the results of the first neurophysiological investigation of myasthenia gravis. He reported a continuous decrease in the mechanical response of the muscle during submaximal faradic stimulation of the nerve, recovery of the response followed a period of rest. The muscle response was also diminished when faradic stimulation was applied after voluntary muscle exercise. The Jolly test occasionally is used to refer to a test of the muscle mechanical response with repetitive nerve stimulation, but use of this term is discouraged.

The electrophysiological test for the diagnosis of myasthenia gravis as we know it today had its beginnings with the study of Harvey and Masland (24). Using supramaximal stimulation to ensure activation of all fibers of the nerve, they observed in myasthenic muscle a progressive decline in action potential amplitude with trains of stimuli of 3 to 50 Hz. The same stimulation applied to normal subjects caused no change in the electrical response. Prostigmine reversed the reduction in amplitude observed in the myasthenic patients. This procedure, modified somewhat over the years, has become the most widely used to detect the presence of myasthenia.

Procedure

The examination of muscle action potentials evoked by single stimulation does not greatly differ from the procedure used in conduction velocity determinations, but the technical difficulties become apparent when repetitive stimulation is used. There is little doubt that movement and slippage of the contiguous surfaces of recording electrodes and the skin are the greater source of error. Slight displacement results in considerable change of the amplitude of the recorded potential; the attenuation is frequently not regular, because the contrast may vary from moment to moment. Movement of the stimulating electrode with respect to the underlying nerve defeats the strict requirement for maintenance of supramaximal intensity of stimulation. Hand-held stimulating electrodes, therefore, notoriously involve erroneous results because they are easily dislodged by motion during muscular contraction.

It is absolutely necessarly that the limb be firmly restrained and that if surface electrodes are used they are carefully affixed to the skin. With regard to recording electrodes, the best and most reproducible results have been obtained with short subcutaneous needle electrodes (25).

It is important to use supramaximal intensity of stimulation because all of the axons must be activated if variation of the amplitude of the evoked potentials is to be avoided. Supramaximal stimulation may be absolutely ensured by increasing the intensity required for maximal response by 25%. In a more concise method, the stimulus current flow is monitored and a stimulus strength 10 to 14 times the threshold current is used.

The preliminary requirements for repetitive stimulation studies, then, are: (a) immobilization of the limb, (b) fixation of stimulation electrodes, (c) fixation of recording discs or preferential use of short subcutaneous electrodes, and (d) supramaximal stimulation, e.g., 10 to 14 times threshold current.

With modern stimulators and isolation techniques, the size of the shock artifact is usually of no consequence. In some cases where its size is excessively large, attenuation of this relatively high voltage source is desirable and can often be attained by simply placing the stimulating electrodes at a more proximal site, e.g., stimulation of ulnar or median nerve at elbow level instead of at the wrist when recording from the hand. It is helpful, too, to place the ground electrode in the path between stimulating and recording electrodes.

Since myasthenia gravis usually shows a proximal distribution, the diagnostic yield is significantly lower for distal than for proximal muscles. In a study of 80 myasthenia patients, a decrementing response was obtained in 82% with the deltoid muscle, 50% with abductor digiti minimi muscle, 62.5% with orbicularis oculi muscle, and 52% in wrist flexors (26). The likelihood of demonstrating a positive response rose to 95% with examination of all these muscles. Thus, proximal muscles as well as distal muscles should be tested. Stålberg (27) has stated that in his experience when the distal muscles were abnormal then the proximal muscles were similarly involved at the same time.

A typical examination may begin with stimulation of the ulnar nerve at the wrist and recording from the hypothenar muscle; then proceeding to median nerve stimulation also at the wrist and recording from the thenar muscle. The biceps muscle may be checked with stimulation of the musculocutaneous nerve at the axilla, and the deltoid muscle response similarly recorded by stimulation at the supraclavicular. In the lower limbs, the anterior tibial and quadriceps may be examined by stimulation of the peroneal nerve at the knee and the femoral nerve at the inguinal region, respectively.

One should be aware that in the less accessible nerves, such as the musculocutaneous at the axilla, the muscle contraction can displace the stimulating electrode and cause spurious decrementation of the responses.

For diagnostic accuracy, the recorded abnormal responses should be reproducible and demonstrable in two different muscles.

Low frequency (1 to 3 Hz) stimulation of the motor nerve has been found to be the most reliable. The usual procedure involves stimulating the motor nerve with a brief train of six supramaximal pulses at 3 per sec and measuring the amplitude of the fifth electrical response with respect to that of the first in the same train. The authors of this procedure (28–30) consider it to be the most sensitive and consistent method for estimating the amount of neuromuscular block.

The reasons for choosing a stimulation rate of 3 per sec were carefully delineated: (a) It is high enough to elicit a maximum decrease of successive responses, and nothing is gained by stimulating at a higher frequency. (b) It is low enough to avoid interference from conduction block in the presynaptic nerve arborization or from postactivation facilitation of neuromuscular transmission. At 3 per sec it is fairly certain that the action potentials invade the terminal arborization and that the decremental responses recorded from the muscle are related to neurochemical failure at the junction. (c) It is much less painful, when the stimulating electrodes are placed properly, than is stimulation at higher rates. (d) In mildly affected myasthenic muscles tested at 10 to 50 per sec, facilitation obscures the early decrement, which is more developed at 3 per sec. In such muscles the decrement of the fifth response is less at the higher rates than at 3 per sec, whereas in a severely involved muscle neuromuscular block can be demonstrated by stimulating at any rate between 0.5 and 50 per sec. (e) It does not produce long term changes in the level of block if repeated at an interval of at least 30 or 60 sec.

In practice, the decrement at 3 per sec is determined first in the rested muscle and then in the same muscle after it has been exercised (either by stimulating the nerve at 3 per sec for 4 min or through a volitional maximum contraction for about 20 sec). In the rested condition, the amplitude of the successive responses decreases up to the fifth response and then remains fairly fixed. Normal subjects can occasionally show a decrease of as much as 8% of the fifth response with respect to the first. Therefore, the decrement of the fifth response at 3 per sec must exceed 10% to be considered indicative of neuromuscular block in a possible myasthenic muscle. The decrement may not be significant in some cases, but only after exercise will an increased decrement of the fifth response be distinguished (postactivation exhaustion).

Evaluation of the evoked muscle responses is usually performed by measuring the amplitude of the negative phase of the compound action potential. However, the amplitude is a function of the synchrony of firing of the muscle fibers and may vary at times, e.g., in "*pseudofacilitation*" the increase in amplitude is due to improved synchronization of firing and not recruitment. To circumvent this problem some investigators have taken to also measuring the area enclosed by the compound action potential because the area is proportional to the number of active muscle fibers (30). Stålberg (27) employs a computer to determine both the amplitude and the area and found that the change in area is usually close to the change in amplitude.

In the routine examination for myasthenia gravis, high frequency repetitive stimulation (over 10 Hz) is generally unnecessary. It is uncomfortable to the patient and can produce considerable movement artifact.

Responses to Single Stimulus

When the ulnar nerve is stimulated, the amplitude of the negative spike of the evoked muscle action potential recorded from normal hypothenar muscles is related to the type and precise placement of the recording electrodes. With surface recording the average value may be 11.4 ± 0.29 mV with a range of 5.6 to 20.8 mV (31). With the use of subcutaneous recording electrodes, the values may be 20% higher. In patients with myasthenia gravis the amplitude of the rested muscle response to a single maximal shock does not frequently fall outside the normal range, although statistically the mean values appear to be somewhat lower (25, 31, 32). The precise measurement of the amplitude of the single evoked muscle action potential, therefore, probably renders no practical diagnostic help in myasthenia gravis. By comparison, the first potential in patients with myasthenic syndrome secondary to pulmonary neoplasm is consistently of low amplitude.

Responses to Repetitive Stimuli

The amplitude of a normal muscle action potential does not change appreciably when the rate of stimulation is slow or moderate (i.e., 1 to 10 per sec). At a frequency of 10 per sec, the amplitude is usually maintained for several minutes; at 10 to 30 per sec it is maintained for ½ to 1 min. At these frequencies fatigue is usually insignificant or manifests as a small gradual decrement in amplitude. At a frequency of 50 per sec applied for longer than a 30-sec interval, the decrement may equal 50%. The decrease in amplitude is due to the fact that successive stimuli occur during the muscle's refractory period (33).

There are individual variations in the response of normal subjects, but it is unusual for fatigue to occur at a frequency less than 25 per sec.

At a stimulation frequency of 3 Hz in normal adults, the amplitude of the fifth response with respect to the first may be decreased by 8% or less. In patients with severe or moderate myasthenia gravis, the ratio of the fifth to first response is usually distinctly abnormal, that is, the decrement is larger than 10%. The first response in the series is normal in amplitude (or may be lower than normal), followed by a gradual decrease starting with the second and continuing to about the fifth, at which time the amplitude may gradually increase slightly. In mild cases of myasthenia, the electrical as well as the mechanical responses to stimulation may not deviate from normal.

The decrement indicates that the safety factor at the neuromuscular junction has been reduced. In the normal neuromuscular junction, the high safety factor permits action potentials to be generated even with some reduction of the EPP amplitude; however, myasthenia gravis has a reduced safety factor, that is, the EPP amplitude may be too low to stimulate the muscle. The decrementation in responses is observed with repetitive stimulation because a progressively increasing number of end-plates do not reach threshold.

It is noteworthy to mention here that any disorder with a decreased safety factor (which may be due to different mechanisms) may demonstrate a decrementation: curarized normal muscle, botulism, or myasthenic syndrome, such as Eaton-Lambert. Considering that this type of response is not exclusive to myasthenia gravis, and that at times it may be insignificant, further specialized testing is required.

The response following a period of maximum contraction is considerably different in normal and myasthenic muscles. After normal muscles have been exercised by a maximum voluntary contraction for 15 to 20 sec or by nerve stimulation at 3 Hz for about 4 min, a 3-Hz stimulation applied afterwards shows that the amplitude remains essentially unchanged (Fig. 9.3).

In myasthenic muscle, 3-Hz test trains applied immediately after the exercise reveal a short period of moderate facilitation, followed by a rapid decrease in amplitude that reaches a minimum (or maximum decrement) in 2 to 4 min postexercise. The amplitude subsequently recovers slowly to the original level (Fig. 9.3). In the Eaton-Lambert syndrome the facilitation component is particularly pronounced; whereas, in intoxication with organophosphorus compounds (34) or overtreatment with cholinesterase inhibitors (35), there is only an immediate decrementation of the response following exercise. Stålberg (27) points out that the amplitude of the response at the peak of the facilitation is an indication of the total number of motor endplates that can be activated and thus has a practical value.

The decrement in response following exercise is called *postactivation exhaustion* and is the most characteristic feature of myasthenia gravis. It was first described by Desmedt (36). In this procedure, it is important that the test trains of 3-Hz stimulation be applied intermittently, for example, at intervals of at least 30 sec. Also the patient should be rested before the test (for at least 30 min), tested before and after exercise, and suitably deprived of anticholinesterase drugs.

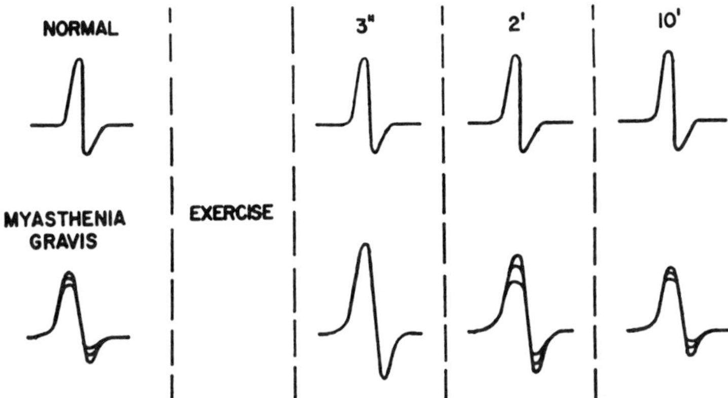

FIG. 9.3. Eaton-Lambert test comparing normal response with that in mild to moderate myasthenia gravis. The moderate increment immediately after exercise and the increased defect in transmission after 2 min are easily discernible in the myasthenic recording.

In some mild cases of myasthenia, postactivation exhaustion is clearly observable even though the decrement following 3-Hz test trains may be insignificant. However, even this phenomenon is not invariably present, so the test is not an absolute method of screening.

In the Eaton-Lambert test, the response to 3-Hz supramaximal stimulation is recorded before and at fixed intevals—3 sec, 2 min, 10 min—after a brief period of exercise (Fig. 9.3).

Another technique involves the response to pairs of stimuli which is considerably different in normal and myasthenic muscles (29, 32, 37). The first or "conditioning" stimulus is separated from the second or "test" stimulus by varying intervals. In normal muscle, the electrical response to the second stimulus remains constant for intervals longer than 20 msec. In clinically weak myasthenic muscles, the response of the second stimulus shows a dip in the interval vs. time recovery curve. The minimum occurs for intervals between 0.1 and 0.7 sec, but it is reduced by anticholinesterase drugs.

Effects of Temperature

Intramuscular temperature is an important parameter in neuromuscular transmission (14, 27). A decrease in temperature of a myasthenic muscle by only a few degrees from the normal 37°C may markedly reduce the recorded decrement (Fig. 9.4). Conversely, raising the temperature of a cooled muscle increases the decrement; for example, a change of 26°C to 35°C produces an increase in decrement from 0% to 29% (Fig. 9.4*B*). It is thus essential to measure the muscle temperature and maintain it close to 37°C. A thermistor needle probe inserted through the skin into the muscle is the most reliable procedure.

Intramuscular temperature in the hand may drop 30°C within 30 min in a warm room, whereas proximal muscles may show a decrease of only 2°C (27). A heat lamp may be conveniently used to raise the temperature of distal musculature. When the intramuscular temperature cannot be measured, the skin temperature should be 34°C or higher (29).

The Mechanical Response

Studies of the mechanical responses of myasthenic muscles have been few, lagging behind the many reported for electrical activity. Techniques have been developed to determine the mechanical responses of human muscles in situ (25, 29, 38). Slomic et al. (25) demonstrated that in moderate and severe myasthenia the decrement in force with 3-Hz stimulation was greater in myasthenic patients than in normal individuals (Fig. 9.5). With higher rates of stimulation, the decrement in force was less likely to be seen. The

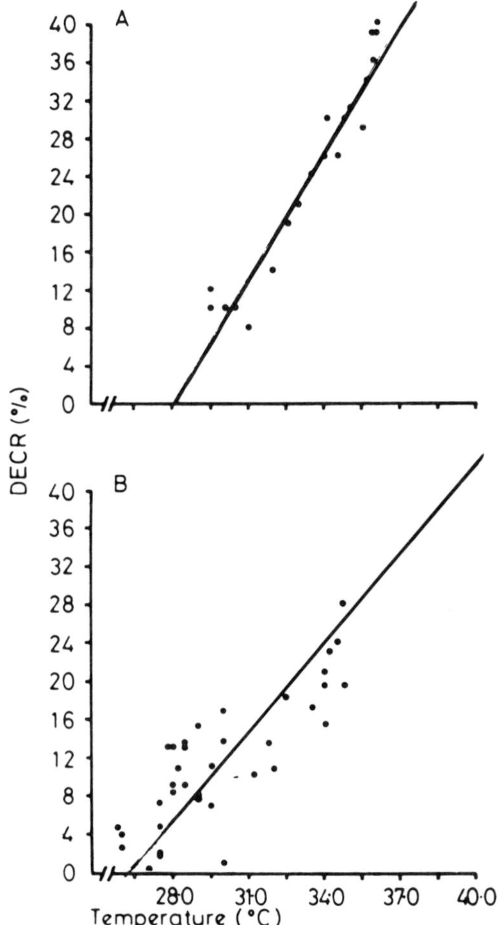

FIG. 9.4. Effect of temperature on the decrement (first/fourth response) in two patients with myasthenia gravis. *A*, from deltoid muscle; *B*, from abductor digiti minimi muscle. The temperature is slowly changed with a heating lamp and icebags and is measured with an intramuscular thermocouple. (From E. Stålberg: Clinical electrophysiology in myasthenia gravis. J. Neurol. Neurosurg. Psychiatry, *43:* 626, 1980.)

maximum tetanic force for the myasthenic patients was 50 to 70% of that observed in normals.

Observations regarding the staircase phenomenon in myasthenia gravis are of considerable interest. If the force of a twitch response to slow rates of stimulation is recorded in a normal subject, it can be demonstrated that the force of the successive twitches gradually increases. At a rate of stimulation of 2 per sec for 1.5 min, the increase is 42 ± 5% above the first twitch. In approximately 50% of normal subjects an initial decrement of about 16% may be seen within the first 10 sec. The initial decrement in force is called the *negative staircase*; the gradual increase is identified as the *positive staircase* (Fig. 9.6).

In patients with myasthenia gravis the positive staircase was absent or

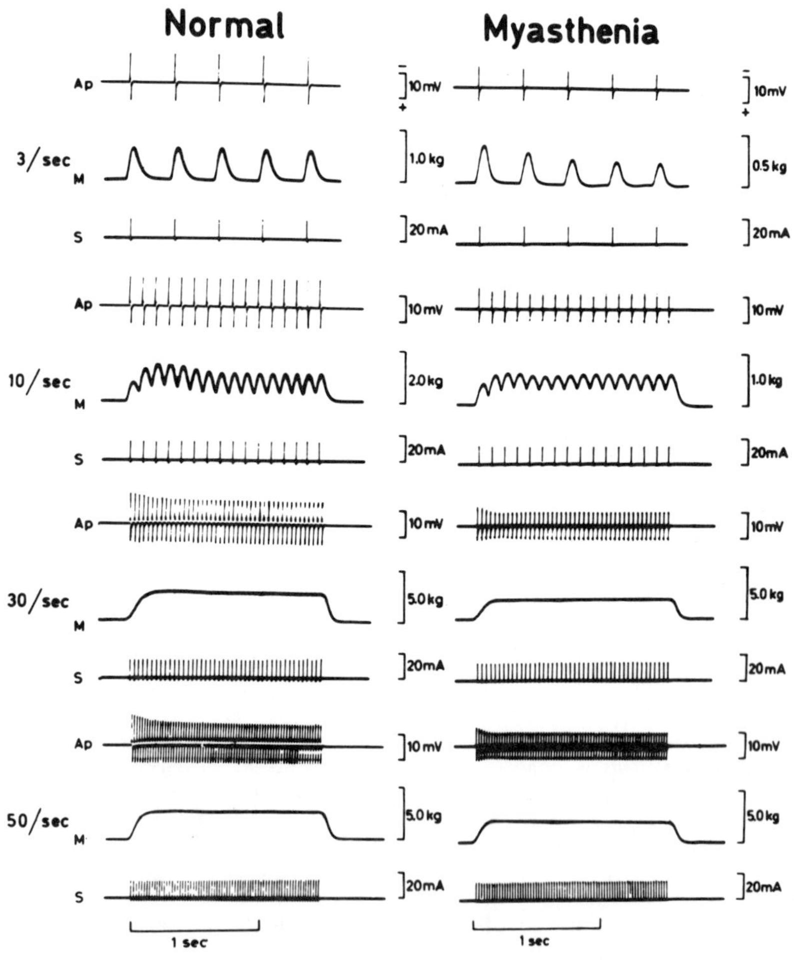

FIG. 9.5. Action potentials (*Ap*), mechanical responses (*M*), and stimulus current (*S*) in trains, 1.5 sec in duration evoked by stimuli given at a rate of 3, 10, 30, and 50 per sec. Normal subject, male, 19 years old. Patient, severe myasthenia gravis, female, 19 years old. The intramuscular temperature was 34 to 35°C. (From A. Slomic, A. Rosenfalck, and F. Buchthal: Electrical and mechanical responses of normal and myasthenic muscle. Brain Res., *10:* 41, 1968.)

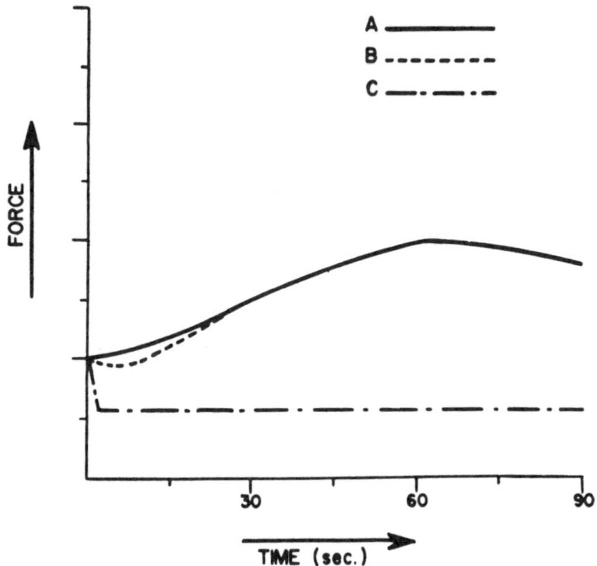

FIG. 9.6. Comparison of staircase phenomenon in normal individual and a severe myasthenic patient. *A*, normal positive staircase; *B*, normal negative staircase; *C*, Severe myasthenia gravis showing sharp decrement of force and absence of positive staircase.

reduced in 91% of the patients, including seven of eight whose muscles showed no clinical weakness (25). In severe myasthenics the force of the twitch may decrease 20 to 40% from the initial response. Tensilon injection may increase the amplitude of the evoked muscle action potential and the twitch force but does not reverse the absence of the positive staircase.

Reinhold et al. (39) demonstrated a similar dissociation of the mechanical and electrical responses. He partially curarized a fully conscious normal human subject with intravenous *d*-tubocurarine and measured the force of the adductor pollicis when the ulnar nerve was stimulated at 2 per sec. Initially both muscle action potential and mechanical responses showed parallel decrement. After the fifth stimulus, the electrical response increased and then remained constant at about 70% of the control value recorded before the experiment, whereas the twitch force did not level off but increased steadily.

Desmedt et al. (40) reported that the staircase phenomenon was present in their myasthenic patients. This result contradicts that of Slomic et al. (25), who found the staircase to be absent or reduced. This controversy has not been resolved, and, obviously, further study is required. An abnormal staircase phenomenon in myasthenia gravis would indicate that the contractile mechanism may be involved.

ELECTROMYOGRAPHY

The examination of muscles which are not clinically affected is usually futile and yields no useful information. In muscles observed to be abnormal, the most characteristic EMG finding is made during weak voluntary effort and consists of an irregular variation in the amplitude of the single recurring muscle action potential (Fig. 9.7). With somewhat stronger efforts, whole motor units may fail. The amplitude of the first motor unit potential appears to be at a maximum and is followed by a series of three to 10 decreasing potentials. A recovery of amplitude then occurs and persists for a finite interval dependent on the degree of involvement. In general, there is an overall pattern of progressive failure with continued effort. The oscillation of amplitudes and the decrement are not pathognomonic of myasthenia gravis but may be encountered in other diseases in which a degree of changing block of neuromuscular transmission may occur. The phenomenon, for example, may be observed in some diseases of the anterior horn cell, such as poliomyelitis and chronic motor neuron disease (41, 42).

There are no other consistently significant EMG abnormalities in myasthenia gravis except for the occasional observation of a typically myopathic pattern (short duration motor units and increased short duration polyphasic potentials) in approximately 10 to 20% of patients with long-standing disease. This finding is consistent with the designation of myasthenic myopathy (43, 44). Pinelli et al. (45) demonstrated that thymectomy performed in myasthenic patients apparently increases the signs of myasthenic myopathy. After thymectomy, the average duration of motor unit action potentials was diminished (7.1 ± 2.1 msec) compared with the values before thymectomy (9.2 ± 2.3 msec). The percentage of polyphasic motor potentials was also increased from 14 to 322. No fibrillation potentials were observed.

ADDITIONAL METHODS OF TESTING

Single Fiber Electromyography

Single fiber electromyography is another method which has been used to study neuromuscular transmission in myasthenia gravis (46–48). Stålberg et

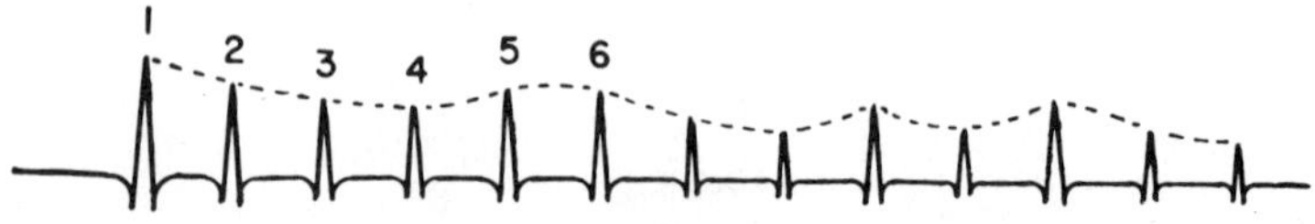

FIG. 9.7. Recording of voluntary motor unit action potentials in myasthenia gravis during a weak contraction. The peaks of the negative spikes are joined by a *stippled line* to emphasize the characteristic variation in amplitude. Unit *1* is of normal amplitude, *2*, *3*, and *4* show a decrement, and *5* and *6* have recovered due to facilitation.

al. (47) applied this approach to 32 patients with myasthenia gravis with symptoms ranging from 5 months to 23 years in duration. Most of the tests were performed on the extensor digitorum communis muscle, but some were made on biceps brachii and tibialis anterior and a few on frontalis and quadriceps muscles. At least 20 jitter recordings were attempted in each patient; however, it sometimes was difficult to obtain jitter recordings in severely affected muscles because two muscle fibers from the same unit rarely occurred together. Jitter, it will be recalled, is the variability at consecutive discharges in the time interval between action potentials from two muscle fibers from the same motor unit.

In all myasthenic muscles increased jitter was observed, as well as occasional blocking of single fiber action potentials (Fig. 9.8). In more severely involved patients, jitter increased to a greater extent and impulse blocking occurred more often. In fact, when the neuromuscular transmission defect was very pronounced, impulse blockings appeared after only a few discharges and at times were long lasting. Jitter, as well as the frequency of impulse blockings, was increased during prolonged activity. In addition, the size of the jitter and the degree of blocking was augmented at higher discharge rates.

Stålberg et al. (47) found that end-plates in a particular muscle were affected unequally by the disease. Some end-plates showed a very high jitter with frequent blockings, whereas others had jitter within the normal range. They also observed a considerable variation in the response to Tensilon even on end-plates in the same muscle. Tensilon (2 mg) was injected intravenously during 15 sec, and after 45 sec another 8 mg were injected if there was no adverse reaction to the first dose. The size of the jitter increased, decreased, or was unaffected. Blom and Ringqvist (48) also obtained equivocal results with Tensilon.

Explanation of these experimental results may be derived from experiments of Elmqvist et al. (49), who measured end-plate potentials in preparations of isolated human intercostal muscle obtained from patients with myasthenia gravis. The variability in size of end-plate potentials which they observed resulted in considerable variability in the latency between the stimulus and the initiated action potentials. It is probable that this variation in amplitude of the end-plate potentials is the cause of the increased jitter in myasthenia gravis (49). Similarly, the decline in end-plate potential recorded during continuous stimulation (49) could explain the increase in blockings and jitter during continuous muscular activity. Stålberg et al. (47) consider the increase of the degree of blocking during continuous activity as myasthenic "fatigue" in the individual motor end-plate.

Blom and Ringqvist (48) point out that increased jitter can also occur in neuromuscular diseases in which nerve sprouting exists or during reinnervation after a nerve injury. Pronounced electrolyte disturbances and some

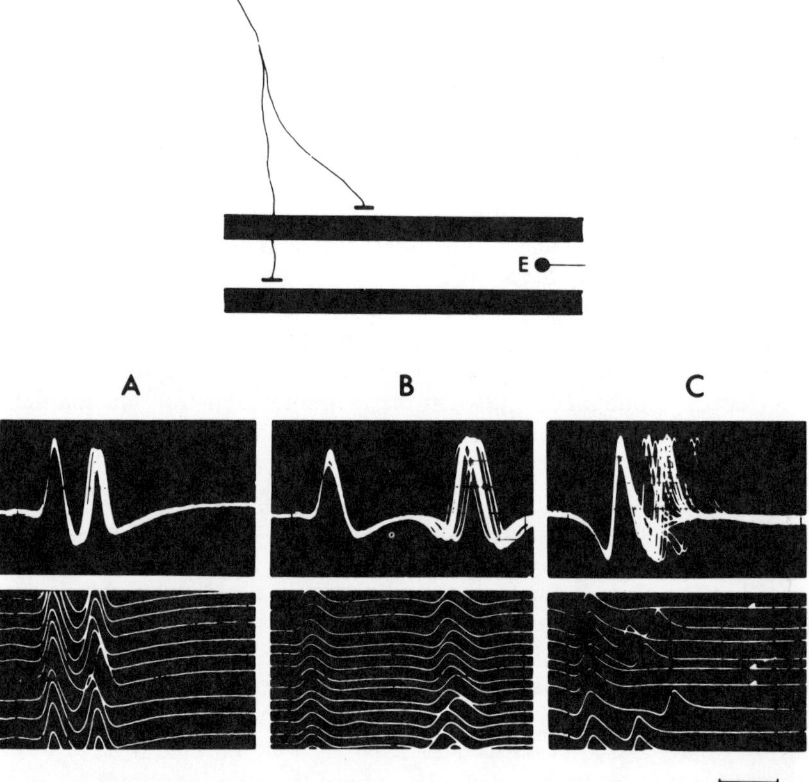

FIG. 9.8. Electrode *E* is recording activity from two muscle fibers belonging to the same motor unit. *A* represents a recording from a normal muscle, *B* and *C* from a myasthenic muscle. The oscilloscope sweep is triggered by the first action potential, and interval variability between the potentials is seen as a variable position of the second potential. In the *upper row*, 10 to 15 action potentials are superimposed. In the *lower row*, the oscilloscope sweep is moved downward. In *A*, there is normal jitter; in *B* there is increased jitter but no impulse blockings; in *C* there is increased jitter and occasional blockings (*arrows*). Calibration: 500 μsec. (From E. Ståberg: *Single Fiber Electromyography*, p. 8. Disa Elektronik, Skovlunde, Denmark, 1974.)

myopathies, particularly polymyositis, may also show increased jitter. It should be stressed, as Stålberg does (27), that increased jitter and partial impulse blockings are not pathognomonic for myasthenia gravis but indicate disturbed neuromuscular transmission or at times an abnormal impulse propagation in the terminal nerves. Thus, it is necessary to perform conventional electromyographic and nerve conduction studies along with the measurement of jitter.

The single fiber recording technique was extended to include testing a muscle during repetitive submaximal stimulation of the nerve to that muscle (50). With 2-Hz stimulation, impulse blockings and facilitation were found in patients with myasthenia gravis, even those with only the ocular form of myasthenia and without surface decrement in the abductor digiti minimi muscle. Minimally involved motor end-plates, as well as those with pronounced neuromuscular disturbance, may be detected.

An excellent detailed discussion of single fiber electromyography can be found in the book by Stålberg and Trontelj (51).

Ischemia

The sensitivity of the test for detection of subclinical involvement (e.g., when no decrement or exhaustion is observed in the regular test) can be increased by checking the postactivation exhaustion after exercise with and without ischemia of the limb. For example, stimulation of the ulnar nerve at 3 per sec for 4 min with an inflated cuff around the upper arm produces a marked increase in postactivation exhaustion in myasthenics. Borenstein and Desmedt (30) speculate that the exercise produces depletion of the ACh transmitter and that the anoxia impairs the resynthesis and/or packaging into vesicles of new transmitter in the motor nerve endings. This increases the range and precision of the measurement, permitting identification of myasthenia in muscles with no overt clinical weakness.

Curare

Another procedure recommended for detecting myasthenia in the minimally affected patient is a regional curare test (52), which consists of the intravenous administration of 0.2 mg of tubocurarine into an ischemic arm followed by repetitive supramaximal percutaneous stimulation of the median or ulnar nerve. In seven of 14 patients with clinically restricted ocular myasthenia gravis, a decrease in the amplitude of the initial evoked potential and a decrement of greater than 10% in the amplitude of the succeeding three to five potentials were produced at stimulation rates of 3, 5, and 15 pulses per sec. The authors suggest that all myasthenic patients with ocular symptoms or signs undergo periodic regional curare tests; however, some laboratories consider the test potentially hazardous (27).

OTHER DISORDERS AFFECTING THE NEUROMUSCULAR JUNCTION

Botulism

The toxin of botulinus bacteria has the same effect on the neuromuscular junction as the removal of calcium ions. This toxin inhibits the release of ACh from the nerve terminal causing a considerable decrease in EPP amplitude. As a consequence, the evoked responses are low in amplitude with a small decrement at low rates of stimulation. Exercise produces only a small facilitation.

Single fiber electromyographic investigation of botulinum poisoning has shown increased jitter and some blocking. Electromyographic examination may show short duration motor unit potentials as well as fibrillation potentials.

Neurogenic Atrophy

A decrement of the evoked responses at low rates of stimulation may be observed at times in amyotrophic lateral sclerosis. Poliomyelitis and syringomyelia may also show responses similar to myasthenia gravis.

Myasthenic Syndrome

The myasthenic syndrome associated with intrathoracic neoplasms is not a common condition. The incidence in total pulmonary neoplasms is 1%, with a greater occurrence of 6% in the oat cell carcinoma (53). The important clinical symptoms which may serve to differentiate this syndrome from myasthenia gravis are: (a) predilection for muscles of the extremities, especially pelvic and thigh—the ocular muscles and face are infrequently affected; (b) diminished or absent deep tendon reflexes; (c) initial muscle contraction is weak, increasing in strength over the first 1 to 1.5 min; and (d) poor response to prostigmine.

Electrophysiological Studies in Myasthenic Syndrome (32, 54, 55)

The EMG recorded with concentric needle electrodes from a weakly contracting muscle is similar to that seen in myasthenia gravis in that it presents considerable variation in amplitude of the recurring motor unit potential. With careful observation it can be seen that the initial unit is low in amplitude but shows a progressive increment over a period of time.

With single supramaximal stimulation, the muscle action potential which is evoked is consistently smaller than normal. On repetitive stimulation there are two distinct responses, recorded at slow and fast rates, respectively. At a rate less than 10 per sec, the first potential is smaller than normal and is followed by four to 10 decreasing potentials, as seen in myasthenia gravis. The recovery that follows is usually considerably greater than observed in myasthenia gravis. If a control tetanus is applied, the postactivity facilitation may be over 600%. With faster rates of stimulation, the early decrement is absent. Instead, a progressive increment immediately commences and only gives way to a late exponential fall with prolonged stimulation.

In Figure 9.9 the modified Eaton-Lambert test shows small initial potential, the remarkable facilitation, and the subsequent profound postactivity

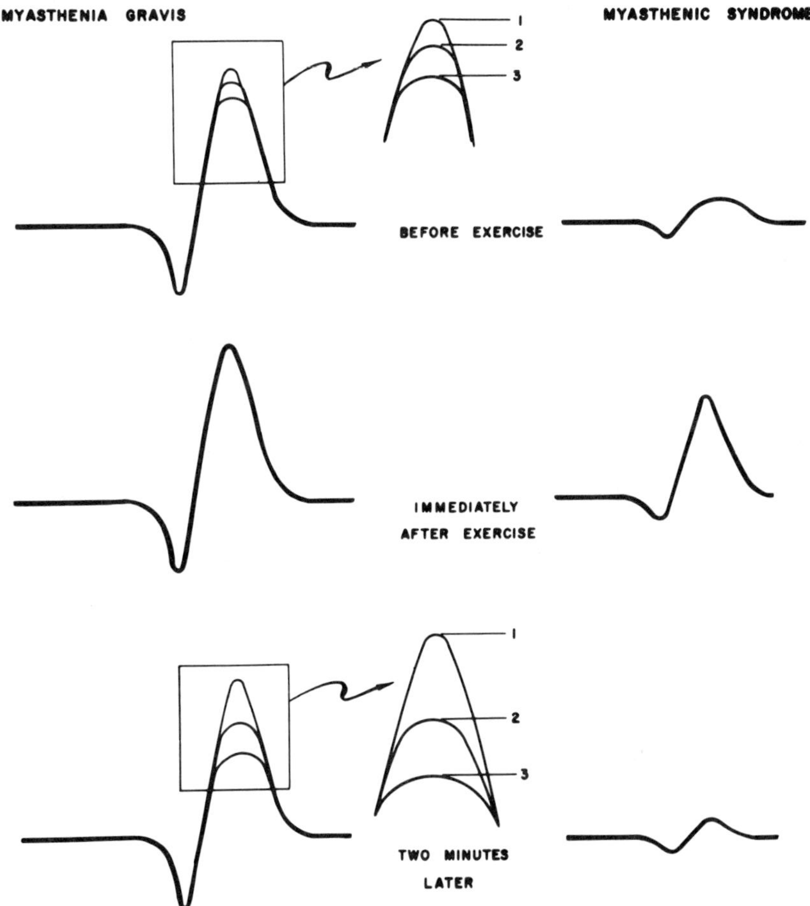

FIG. 9.9. Modified Eaton-Lambert test. Comparison is made of myasthenia gravis and myasthenic syndrome.

depression in the myasthenic syndrome. These features are quite distinct from the recordings in myasthenia gravis, which are presented for comparative purposes.

There is a difference in the nature of the defect of neuromuscular transmission in the myasthenic syndrome associated with carcinoma from that operative in myasthenia gravis (56). When MEPP and EPP potentials are recorded from intercostal muscle specimens of patients with myasthenic syndrome, the former are of normal amplitude; however, the latter, in response to a nerve impulse, are diminished. The number of quanta of ACh released with the nerve impulse is decreased. This type of defect is like that produced by botulinum intoxication, neomycin, or lowered Ca^{2+} concentra-

TABLE 9.2. Comparison of Features of "New" Myasthenic Syndrome, Eaton-Lambert Syndrome, and Myasthenia Gravis*

Features	New Syndrome	Lambert-Eaton Syndrome	Myasthenia Gravis
Clinical			
Weakness and fatigability	+	+	+
Increased strength during beginning of voluntary contraction	−	+	−
Hyporeflexia	+	+	−
Bulbar symptoms	+	−, (+)	+, (−)
Improved by anticholinesterase drugs	−	±	+
Improved by guanidine	−	+	±
Sometimes associated with carcinoma	−	+	−
Circulating antibodies to AChR	−	−	+
Electromyographic			
Repetitive response to single nerve stimulus	+	−	−
Decrementing EMG at slow rate of stimulation	+	+	+
Incrementing EMG at rapid rate of stimulation	−	+	−, (+)
Postactivation facilitation and exhaustion	+	+	+
Electrophysiological			
Small amplitude MEPP	−	−	+
Increased duration and half-decay time of MEPP	+	−	−
Decreased MEPP frequency	+	−	−
Small EPP quantum content at 1 per sec	+	+	−
Increased EPP quantum content at 40 per sec	−	+	−
Decreased store of immediately releasable quanta	+	−	−
Decreased probability of quantal release	−	+	−
Ultrastructural			
Nerve terminal small relative to postsynaptic region	+	−	−
Absolute decrease in nerve terminal size	1/3 to 1/4 of normal	−	2/3 of normal
Increased synaptic vesicle density	+	−	−
Focal degeneration of junctional folds	+	−	+
Labyrinthine membranous networks in junctional folds	+	−	−
Hypertrophy of postysynaptic area	−	+	−
Degenerating nuclei in junctional sarcoplasm	+	−	−
Cytochemical and biochemical			
Decreased postsynaptic AChR	−	−	+
AChE absent from end-plate	+	−	−
16 S AChE absent from muscle	+		

+, present; −, absent; (+), occasionally present; (−), occasionally absent; ±, variable AchR, acetylcholine receptor; AchE, acetylcholinesterase; 16S AchE, 16S component of AchE.

From A. G. Engel, E. H. Lambert, and M. R. Gomez: A new myasthenic syndrome with end-plate acetylcholinesterase deficiency, small nerve terminals, and reduced acetylcholine release. Ann. Neurol., *1:* 326, 1977.

tion. Repeated nerve stimulation increases the quantum content of the end-plate potential and thereby the subsequent muscle response.

Single fiber electromyography in this disorder reveals jitter and blocking.

Guanidine may be very effective in the treatment of the myasthenic syndrome when cholinesterase inhibitors are unimpressive because of its action to augment the quantum release of ACh. Brown and Johns (57) have noted a worsening of neuromuscular block in patients with severe myasthenia gravis treated with guanidine.

A "New" Myasthenic Syndrome

In 1977, Engel et al. (58) described the symptoms in a patient which they considered represented a third type of neuromuscular transmission defect, after that of myasthenia gravis and the Eaton-Lambert syndrome. The clinical, electromyographic, ultrastructural, cytochemical, and biochemical features of the new syndrome clearly distinguished it from the other two (Table 9.2).

The symptoms in the patient began soon after birth and included generalized weakness increased by exertion, easy fatigability, hyporeflexia, and no response to anticholinesterase drugs or guanidine. The electromyographic examination revealed a decremental response at all frequencies of stimulation and a repetitive response to single nerve stimulation. The MEPP's were normal in amplitude but decreased in frequency; the EPP quantum content was low because the store of quanta immediately available for release was reduced. The nerve terminals were reduced in size, and acetylcholinesterase was absent from the motor end-plates.

The authors consider the basic abnormality to be a congenital defect in the molecular assembly of acetylcholinesterase or in its attachment to the postsynaptic membrane.

REFERENCES

1. Willis, T.: *De Anima Brutorum*. Blaeus, Amsterdam, 1672.
2. Erb, W.: Uber einen neuen, wahrscheinlich bulbaren Symptomenkomplex. Arch. Psychiatr. Nervenkr., *9:* 336–350, 1879.
3. Goldflam, S.: Uber einen scheinbar heilbaren bulbarparalytischen Symptomenkomplex mit Betheiligung der Extremitaten, Dtsch. Z. Nervenheilk., *4:* 312–352, 1893.
4. Jolly, F.: Vortrag in der Gesellschaft der Charitearzte. Klin. Wochenschr., *28:* 660, 1891.
5. Jolly, F.: Uber myasthenia gravis pseudoparalytica. Klin. Wochenschr., *32:* 1–7, 1895.
6. Heuser, J. E., and Reese, T. S.: Evidence for recycling of a synaptic vesicle membrane during transmitter release at the frog neuromuscular junction. J. Cell Biol., *57:* 315–344, 1973.
7. Fertuck, H. C., and Salpeter, M. M.: Localization of acetylcholine receptor by ^{125}I-labeled α-bungarotoxin binding at mouse motor endplates. Proc. Natl. Acad. Sci., *71:* 1376–1378, 1974.
8. Delorenzo, R. J., Freedman, S. D., Yoke, W. B., and Maurer, S. C.: Stimulation of Ca-dependent neurotransmitter release and presynaptic nerve terminal protein phosphorylation by calmodulin and a calmodulin-like protein isolated from synaptic vesicles. Proc. Natl. Acad. Sci., *76:* 1838–1842, 1979.

9. Walker, M. B.: Treatment of myasthenia gravis with prostigmine. Lancet: 1200–1201, 1934.
10. Dale, H. H., and Feldberg, W.: Chemical transmission at motor nerve endings in voluntary muscle? J. Physiol. (Lond.), *81:* 39P, 1934.
11. Elmquist, D., Hofmann, W. W., Kugelberg, J., and Quastel, D. M. J.: An electrophysiological investigation of neuromuscular transmission in myasthenia gravis. J. Physiol. (Lond.), *174:* 417–434, 1964.
12. Grob, D.: Spontaneous end-plate activity in normal subjects and in patients with myasthenia gravis. Ann. N. Y. Acad. Sci., *183:* 248–269, 1971.
13. Simpson, J. A.: Myasthenia gravis: A personal view of pathogenesis and mechanism. Part 1. Muscle Nerve, *1:* 45–56, 1978.
14. Simpson, J. A.: Myasthenia gravis: A new hypothesis, Scott. Med. J., *5:* 419–436, 1960.
15. Smithers, D. W.: Tumours of the thyroid gland in relation to some general concepts of neoplasia. J. Facult. Radiol., *10:* 3–16, 1959.
16. Nastuk, W. L., Plescia, O. J., and Osserman, K. E.: Changes in serum complement activity in patients with myasthenia gravis. Proc. Soc. Exp. Biol. Med., *105:* 177–184, 1960.
17. Fambrough, D. M., Drachman, D. B., and Satyamurti, S.: Neuromuscular junction in myasthenia gravis: Decreased acetylcholine receptors. Science, *182:* 293–295, 1973.
18. Patrick, J., and Linstrom, J.: Autoimmune response to acetylcholine receptor. Science, *180:* 871–872, 1973.
19. Lindstrom, J., and Einarson, B.: Antigenic modulation and receptor loss in EAMG. Muscle Nerve, *2:* 173–179, 1979.
20. Almon, R. R., Andrews, C. G., and Appel, S. H.: Serum globulin in myasthenia gravis: Inhibition of α-bungarotoxin binding to acetylcholine receptors. Science, *186:* 55–57, 1974.
21. Mittag, T., Kornfeld, P., Tormay, A., and Woo, C.: Detection of anti-acetylcholine receptor factors in serum and thymus from patients with myasthenia gravis. N. Engl. J. Med., *294:* 691–694, 1976.
22. Lindstrom, J. M., Seybold, M. E., Lennon, A., Whittingham, S., and Duane, D. D.: Antibody to acetylcholine receptor in myasthenia gravis: Prevalence, clinical correlates and diagnostic value. Neurology, *26:* 1054–1059, 1976.
23. Dalla, S. K., and Schwartz, R. S.: Infectious (?) myasthenia. N. Engl. J. Med., *291:* 1304–1305, 1974.
24. Harvey, A. M., and Masland, R. L.: A method for the study of NM transmission in human subjects. Bull. Johns Hopkins Hosp., *68:* 81–93, 1941.
25. Slomic, A., Rosenfalck, A., and Buchthal, F.: Electrical and mechanical responses to normal and myasthenic muscle. Brain Res., *10:* 1–78, 1968.
26. Özdemir, C., and Young, R.: The results to be expected from electrical testing in the diagnosis of myasthenia gravis. Ann. N. Y. Acad. Sci., *274:* 203–222, 1976.
27. Stålberg, E.: Clinical electrophysiology in myasthenia gravis. J. Neurol. Neurosurg. Psychiatry, *43:* 622–633, 1980.
28. Desmedt, J. E., and Borenstein, S.: The testing of neuromuscular transmission. Handbook Clin. Neurol., *7:* 104–115, 1970.
29. Desmedt, J. F.: The neuromuscular disorder in myasthenia gravis. I. Electrical and mechanical response to nerve stimulation in hand muscles. In *New Developments in EMG and Clinical Neurophysiology*, edited by J. E. Desmedt, vol. 1, pp. 241–304. S. Karger, Basel, 1973.
30. Borenstein, S., and Desmedt, J. E.: New diagnostic procedures in myasthenia gravis. In *New Developments in EMG and Clinical Neurophysiology*, edited by J. E. Desmedt, vol. 1, pp. 350–374. S. Karger, Basel, 1973.
31. Lambert, E. H., Rooke, E. D., Eaton, L. M., and Hodgson, C. H.: Myasthenic syndrome occasionally associated with bronchial neoplasm: Neurophysiologic studies. In *Myasthenia Gravis*, edited by H. A. Viets, pp. 362–410. Charles C Thomas, Springfield, Ill., 1961.
32. Johns, R. J., Grob, D., and Harvey, A. M.: Studies in neuromuscular function. 2. Effects of nerve stimulation in normal subjects and in patients with myasthenia gravis. Bull. Johns Hopkins Hosp., *99:* 125–135, 1956.

33. Pritchard, E. A. B.: The occurrence of Wedensky inhibition in myasthenia gravis. J. Physiol. (Paris), *78:* 3–5, 1933.
34. Jager, K. W., Roberts, D. V., and Wilson, A.: Neuromuscular function in pesticide workers. Br. J. Ind. Med., *27:* 273, 1970.
35. Roberts, D. V., and Wilston, A.: Electromyography in diagnosis and treatment. In *Myasthenia Gravis*, edited by R. Greene, pp. 29–42. Heinemann, London, 1969.
36. Desmedt, J. E.: Nature of the defect of neuromuscular transmission in myasthenic patients: "Post-tetanic exhaustion." Nature, *179:* 156–157, 1957.
37. Harvey, A. M., and Masland, R. L.: The electromyogram in myasthenia gravis. Bull. Johns Hopkins Hosp., *69:* 1–13, 1941.
38. Botelho, S. Y.: Alterations in muscle tension without similar changes in electrical activity in patients with myasthenia gravis. J. Clin. Invest., *34:* 1403–1409, 1955.
39. Reinhold, H., Hainaut, K., and Desmedt, J. E.: "Relative" staircase potentiation of the muscle twitch in the partially curarized normal human muscle. Arch. Int. Pharmacodyn. Ther., *185:* 204–207, 1970.
40. Desmedt, J. E., Emeryk, B., Hainaut, K., Reinhold, H., and Borenstein, S.: Muscular dystrophy and myasthenia gravis: Muscle contraction properties studied by the staircase phenomenon. In *New Developments in EMG and Clinical Neurophysiology*, edited by J. E. Desmedt, vol. 1, pp. 380–399. S. Karger, Basel, 1973.
41. Pinelli, P., and Buchthal, F.: Duration, amplitude and shape of muscle action potentials in poliomyelitis. Electroencephalogr. Clin. Neurophysiol., *3:* 497–504, 1951.
42. Mulder, D. W., Lambert, E. H., and Eaton, L. M.: Myasthenic syndrome in patients with amyotrophic lateral sclerosis. Neurology (Minneap.), *9:* 627–631, 1959.
43. Simpson, J. A.: An evaluation of thymectomy in myasthemia gravis. Brain, *81:* 112–144, 1958.
44. Richardson, A. T.: Electromyography in myasthenia gravis and the other myopathies. In *The Innervation of Muscle*, edited by H. Bouman and W. Woolf, p. 116. Williams & Wilkins Co., Baltimore, 1960.
45. Pinelli, P., Arrigo, A., and Moglia, A.: Myasthenic decrement and myasthenic myopathy: A study on the effects of thymectomy. J. Neurol. Neurosurg. Psychiatry, *38:* 525–532, 1975.
46. Ekstedt, J., and Stålberg, E.: Single fiber electromyography for the study of the microphysiology of the human muscle. In *New Developments in EMG and Clinical Neurophysiology*, edited by J. E. Desmedt, vol. 1, pp. 89–112. S. Karger, Basel, 1973.
47. Stålberg, E., Ekstedt, J., and Broman, A.: Neuromuscular transmission in myasthenia gravis studied with single fiber electromyography. J. Neurol. Neurosurg. Psychiatry, *37:* 540–547, 1974.
48. Blom, S., and Ringqvist, I.: Neurophysiological findings in myasthenia gravis: Single muscle fiber activity in relation to muscular fatigability and response to anticholinesterase. Electroencephalogr. Clin. Neurophysiol., *30:* 477–487, 1971.
49. Elmqvist, D., Hofmann, W. W., Kugelberg, J., and Quastel, D. M. J.: An electrophysiological investigation of neuromuscular transmission in myasthenia gravis. J. Physiol., *174:* 417–434, 1964.
50. Schwartz, M. S., and Stålberg, E.: Single fibre electromyographic studies in myasthenia gravis with repetitive nerve stimulation. J. Neurol. Neurosurg. Psychiatry, *38:* 678–682, 1975.
51. Stålberg, E., and Trontelj, J. V.: *Single Fibre Electromyography*. Mirvalle Press, Surrey, U. K., 1979.
52. Horowitz, S. H., Genkins, G., Kornfeld, P., and Papatestas, E.: Regional curare test in evaluation of ocular myasthenia. Arch. Neurol., *32:* 84–88, 1975.
53. Trojaborg, W., Frantzen, E., and Andersen, I.: Peripheral neuropathy and myopathy associated with carcinoma of the lung. Brain, *92:* 71–82, 1969.
54. Howard, F. M., Jr.: Myasthenic diseases and related physiology. Arch. Phys. Med., *47:* 137–146, 1966.
55. McQuillen, M. P., and Johns, R. J.: The nature of the defect in the Eaton-Lambert syndrome. Neurology (Minneap.), *17:* 527–536, 1967.

56. Elmqvist, D., and Lambert, E. H.: Detailed analysis of neuromuscular transmission in a patient with the myasthenic syndrome associated with bronchogenic carcinoma. Mayo Clin. Proc., *43:* 689–713, 1968.
57. Brown, J. C., and Johns, R. J.: Clinical and physiological studies of the effect of guanidine on patients with myasthenia gravis. Johns Hopkins Med. J., *124:* 1–8, 1969.
58. Engel, A. G., Lambert, E. H., and Gomez, M. R.: A new myasthenic syndrome with end-plate acetylcholinesterase deficiency, small nerve terminals, and reduced acetylcholine release. Ann. Neurol., *1:* 315–330, 1977.

chapter 10

Neuropathy

NERVE LESIONS

Although the electrodiagnostic findings in neuropathic diseases may be quite varied, they can generally be related to the presence of (a) axonal failure, (b) primary damage to myelin, (c) a combination of both lesions, and/or (d) anterior horn cell or neuronal disease (1).

Usually the primary result of demyelination is a defect in conduction, whereas axonal failure means that electrophysiological evidence of motor unit dysfunction, i.e., muscle denervation, can be anticipated (Table 10.1).

Primary Axonal Failure

Because axonal lesions affect the motor unit, the most useful information is derived from electromyographic examination. The essential changes involve the following:

1) The characteristics of the single motor unit action potential: In peripheral neuropathy, the mean duration is increased, whereas the mean amplitude is normal or decreased (2). In motor cell lesions, the mean duration and amplitude are increased. The incidence of polyphasic potentials is increased in the neuropathies.

2) The process of recruitment: In moderate neurogenic paresis, a reduced interference pattern is observed with maximal voluntary effort; in severe paresis, discrete activity is obtained. It is useful to identify maximal motor effort by measuring the frequency of firing when discrete motor unit potentials may be recognized, as in severe paresis (3).

3) Abnormal spontaneous activity: Fibrillation potentials, positive sharp waves, increased insertion activity, and fasciculation potentials are characteristically observed but are not pathognomonic.

Myelin Degeneration

The most sensitive indication of slight to moderate demyelination is obtained by recording sensory nerve action potentials (4). When the re-

TABLE 10.1

Pathological Lesion	Most Prominent Electrophysiological Disturbance
Primary axonal failure	Motor unit potential changes, denervation, etc
Primary myelin degeneration	Conduction defect
Demyelination + axonal failure	Motor unit potential changes + conduction defects

TABLE 10.2

Degree of Involvement	Effect on Conduction
Mild demyelination	Delayed conduction of the sensory nerve action potential Slight diminution of amplitude of the response
Advanced demyelination	Delayed conduction in sensory and motor fibers Moderate reduction of amplitude of evoked response
Demyelination + axonal degeneration	Considerable delay in conduction and greater attenuation of the evoked response
Total axonal degeneration	No conduction

sponses from sensory fibers 6 to 10 μ in diameter are recorded by electronic averaging, slowed conduction and slight reduction in amplitude of the evoked sensory fiber response may be seen, whereas conduction velocity of the fastest motor fibers appears to be unaffected. However, the usual method in current use is appropriate only in measurement of the motor conduction in the fibers 12 to 20 μ in diameter. A method of evaluation of conduction in the slower motor fibers has been described (5), but unreliable results with the procedure in our own laboratory parallel the fact that the method has not been generally accepted.

When the larger diameter, faster conducting motor or sensory axons are affected with a greater degree of demyelination, delayed conduction and diminished amplitude of the evoked potential are characteristic.

Because the amplitude of the response is a function of the number of discharging muscle fibers, it is apparent that concomitant axonal degeneration results in a corresponding greater attenuation of the evoked potential (Table 10.2).

Neuronal (Anterior Horn Cell) Disease

Increase in amplitude and duration of the motor unit action potential is the most significant electrophysiological feature of anterior horn cell disease. When mapping of motor unit territory is included among the tests, then the following changes from normal are noteworthy (6): (a) increased amplitude of motor unit action potential; (b) increased amplitude of the interference pattern during voluntary effort; (c) 30% or more increase in mean duration of motor unit action potential; and (d) 80% or more increase in the territorial area of the motor unit.

Increased insertion activity, fibrillation potentials, positive sharp waves, and fasciculations do not have specificity and are, therefore, unreliable in differentiation of neuronal and axonal lesions. As a matter of fact, these abnormal potentials cannot be used unequivocally to separate neuropathy from myopathy. In addition, abnormality in the pattern of recruitment occurs in all reduction of motor unit activity whether of axonal or neuronal origin.

Myelopathy

Traumatic lesions may occur at all levels distal to the spinal cord—roots, plexi, and peripheral nerves.

At the level of the cord itself, chronic myelopathy is not uncommon. Although the myelopathy is associated with spondylosis, its pathogenesis is not entirely clear; speculation regarding etiology includes restricted movement of the cord and roots owing to epidural and arachnoidal adhesions, nonspecific ischemic changes, and direct compression of the cord by spondylotic bars (7).

Electrodiagnostic examination of these myelopathies in our laboratory has been more often than not completely unproductive of diagnostic information. If the compression is sufficient to cause degeneration of motor neurons, then EMG evidence of motor unit disintegration may be found in a restricted segmental distribution.

When the spondylotic bar extends or arises laterally and encroaches on the spinal roots at the foramina or osteophytes directly extend from adjacent articulations, they may result in localized motor and sensory impairment-radiculopathy. The following case report is illustrative.

Case Report. The patient was a 53-year-old white male with intermittent episodes of paresthesias in both upper extremities associated with a more persistent and progressive difficulty in elevating both arms. The symptoms were of 4 years' duration. Muscle fasciculations and atrophy were noted. Physical examination revealed weakness, atrophy, and gross fasciculations of the muscles of both shoulders and distal arms. The left lower extremity presented a slight impairment of rapid alternating movement, and the patellar and ankle reflexes were just perceptibly increased compared to the right side. Sensory examination revealed hypalgia in the $C_{5, 6, 7}$ distribution bilaterally. He was admitted to University Hospital on December 16, 1968.

Radiography. Degenerative disease involving the entire cervical spine from C_2 down, associated with narrowing of the intervertebral spaces and the foramina by osteophytes.

Myelogram. Multiple degenerative changes with ridging at C_6 and T_1. The contrast dye showed a complete block at the level of C_6-C_7.

Electrical Studies. Conduction determinations—sensory and motor were normal for all nerves examined in the upper and lower extremities. Electromyographic examination of the C_5-C_7 distribution bilaterally showed a continuous spontaneous activity consisting of bizarre high frequency discharges with a background of fibrillation potentials and positive sharp waves. Highly complex fasciculation potentials were consistently observed. The motor unit potentials voluntarily recruited were diminished in number and showed an increase in amplitude and duration. The EMG of the lower extremity muscles revealed no abnormalities.

Surgery December 28, 1968. Cervical laminectomy from C_4 to T_1. Bilateral foraminotomies C_4, C_5, C_6, C_7. Postoperative course and clinical recovery excellent.

Follow-up EMG July 11, 1969. Remarkable reduction in spontaneous activity with complete cessation of bizarre discharges and fasciculations. There were no abnormalities on the right, but the left arm showed occasional fibrillation potentials and positive sharp waves. The interference pattern was reduced, and the units were distinctly hypertrophied.

Root Compression Lesions

There is little doubt that root compression lesions from discogenic disease are one of the most common maladies of bipedal man. Electrophysiological examination may be productively utilized in detection and localization of these lesions, but only if analysis of the laboratory data is based on fundamental anatomic and pathologic facts as well as careful evaluation of the observations.

Anatomic and Pathological Background

Spinal Column and Cord. During development of the spinal cord and its bony enclosure, the cord and column are of equal length until the fetus is 3 months of age. Thereafter, a considerable differential rate of growth causes the column to outstrip the cord with the result that at birth the latter reaches only to the level of the L_3 vertebra. In the full grown adult, the cord terminates at the superior border of L_2. As a consequence of the unequal growth pattern, the points of origin of the spinal nerves are displaced upward (Table 10.3). Spinal nerve L_5, for example, which is located opposite lumbar vertebra 5 in the third fetal month, originates in the adult at the level of T_{11} and descends to exit between L_5 and S_1 (Fig. 10.1). The most caudal roots lie medially, so that at a point opposite the L_4 vertebra, the order of most medial to most lateral spinal nerves is S_2, S_1, L_5, and L_4.

The lumbar spinal nerves emerge through the intervertebral foramen *below* the corresponding numbered vertebra; for example, L_5 emerges between vertebrae L_5 and S_1. In the cervical region, because the C_1 nerve emerges between the atlas and the skull, the remaining cervical nerves all

TABLE 10.3 Tabulation of Representative Root Segments Indicating the Level of the Spinal Column at Which They Form and Their Foramen of Exit

Spinal Segment	Spinal Cord Level at Which Root Originates	Intervertebral Foramen of Exit
C_8	C_6	C_7–T_1
T_6	T_3	T_6–T_7
T_{12}	T_9	T_{12}–L_1
L_5	T_{11}	L_5–S_1
S_1	L_1	S_1–S_2

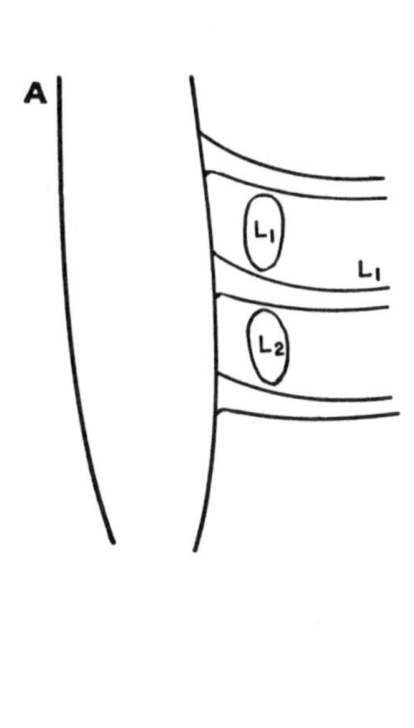

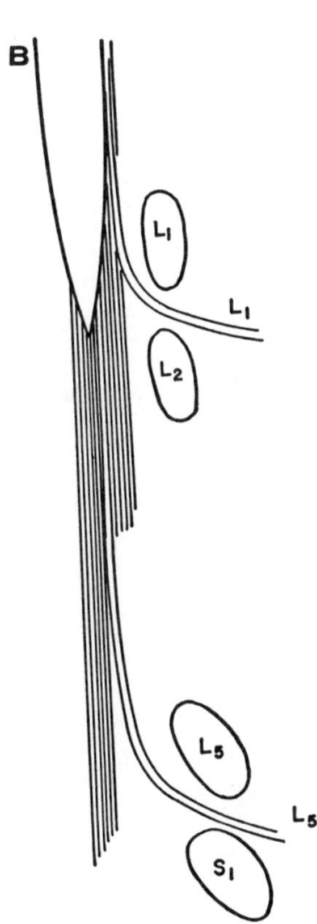

FIG. 10.1. *A*, L_1 root originating and exiting opposite the L_1-L_2 interspace in the 3-month-old fetus. *B*, in the adult, L_1 originates at the level of the T_{9-10} vertebra and descends to exit at the L_1-L_2 foramen. The L_5 spinal nerve originates opposite T_{11} and exits between L_5-S_1 vertebra. The roots which originate most caudally occupy a medial position with respect to those arising at a higher segment.

present *above* the corresponding vertebra; for example, C_5 descends and crosses one vertebral space to its foramen of exit between C_4-C_5. The C_8 root exits between C_7 and T_1.

The spinal nerves, formed by the fused anterior and posterior roots, leave the foramen and immediately divide into anterior and posterior primary rami (Fig. 10.2). The anterior divisions participate in the formation of the limb plexus and, therefore, the ultimate specific peripheral nerve supply to each muscle. The posterior primary rami innervate the back muscles, so that these axial muscles as well as those of the appendages may be used in electromyographic study of root lesions.

The Intervertebral Disc. The anulus fibrosus which encloses the nucleus pulposus of the disc consists of coarse collagen fibers which are subject to metaplasia and other degenerative changes with advancing age. Rupture of the anulus may then ensue under a variety of traumatic circumstances, sometimes quite minor in character. The disc is amply reinforced by the tough anterior longitudinal ligament of the spine but is less efficiently aided by the relatively weaker posterior longitudinal ligament. The lateral expansions of this structure are particularly flimsy. The most common herniation of the nucleus pulposus, therefore, is through the torn anulus in a posterolateral projection. Because the midportion of the ligament is itself not invulnerable, midline herniation does occur, but less frequently (Fig. 10.3).

Myotome. With regard to the segmental architecture of the developing human limb muscles, the term myotome is used. A myotome, by definition, is a group of muscles supplied by a single spinal segment. For example, the C_5 myotome is represented in the arm by the deltoid, biceps brachii, brachialis, and brachioradialis muscles. Because a single muscle receives innervation from more than one spinal segment, these muscles are also

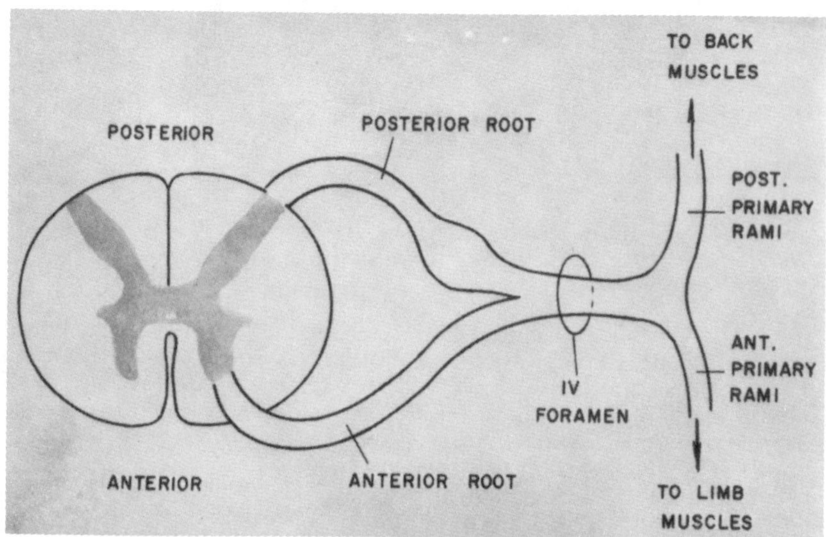

FIG. 10.2. Typical spinal nerve showing formation of anterior and posterior primary rami. The anterior distributes to the limb muscles, the posterior to the back muscles.

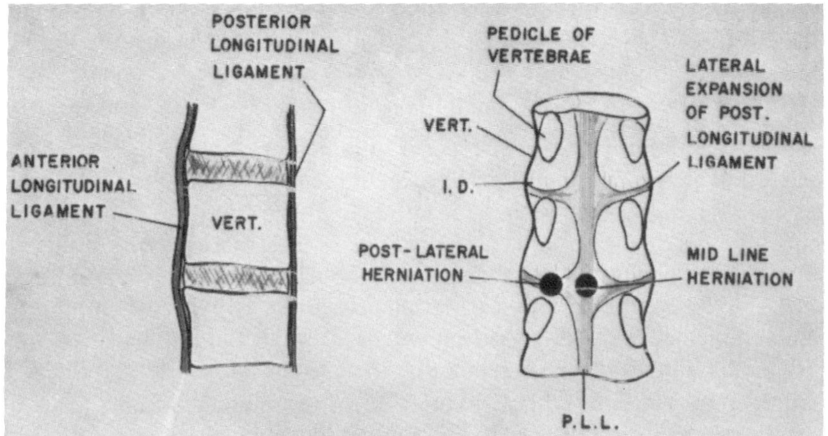

FIG. 10.3. Anterior and posterior longitudinal ligaments of the spine. The thin lateral expansions of the posterior ligament are shown on the *right*.

TABLE 10.4 Myotomic Distribution in Selected Muscles of the Extremities*

Upper Extremity	Muscle Segment	Lower Extremity	Muscle Segment
Infraspinatus, supraspinatus	$\mathrm{C_5C_6}$	Quadriceps femoris	$\mathrm{L_2}\mathit{L_3L_4}$
Deltoid	$\mathrm{C_5C_6}$	Anterior tibial	$\mathrm{L_4L_5S_1}$
Biceps	$\mathrm{C_5C_6}$	Peroneus longus	$\mathrm{L_4}\mathit{L_5}\mathrm{S_1}$
Brachioradialis	$\mathit{C_5C_6}$	Extensor hallucis	$\mathrm{L_4L_5S_1S_2}$
Triceps	$\mathrm{C_6C_7C_8T_1}$	Extensor digitorum brevis	$\mathrm{L_4L_5S_1S_2}$
Extensor carpi radialis	$\mathrm{C_6C_7C_8}$	Abductor hallucis	$\mathrm{S_1}\mathit{S_2}$
Flexor carpi radialis	$\mathrm{C_6C_7C_8}$	Posterior tibial	$\mathit{L_5}\mathrm{S_1S_2}$
Pronator quadratus	$\mathrm{C_8}\mathit{T_1}$	Gastrocnemius	
		Medial belly	$\mathrm{S_1S_2}$
		Lateral belly	$\mathrm{L_5S_1S_2}$
Flexor carpi ulnaris	$\mathrm{C_7C_8T_1}$	Soleus	$\mathrm{S_1S_2}$
Abductor pollicis brevis	$\mathrm{C_8T_1}$	Biceps femoris	
		Short head	$\mathrm{L_5S_1S_2}$
		Long head	$\mathrm{S_1S_2}$
Abductor digiti quinti	$\mathrm{C_8T_1}$	Gluteus maximus	$\mathrm{L_5S_1S_2}$
		Tensor fasciae latae	$\mathrm{L_4L_5S_1}$

* No attempt is made to include all possible roots but rather to emphasize major representations.

included in the C_6 myotome. Within each muscle, the fibers from a single segment do not terminate in one muscle fascicle but arborize to innervate fibers in adjacent bundles as well. In Table 10.4 are enumerated those muscles and their roots most commonly examined in identification of segmental lesions involving the extremities. Regretfully, there is not yet universal acceptance of root distribution for all muscles, but there is sufficient agreement on at least several in the upper and lower limbs to permit accurate identification of the involved spinal segment.

EMG Examination

The EMG abnormalities which occur in radiculopathy are those typically observed in neuropathic disease. However, these may not be overwhelmingly present, so that diligent search for subtle changes from the normal state frequently may be required. Compression of the motor roots results in irritation and/or degenerative changes of the nerve fibers. Increased insertional activity is probably the earliest manifestation of hyperirritability. An increased incidence of polyphasic potentials is also a relatively early finding. With increased severity, fasciculation potentials and bizarre high frequency discharges may occur. When compression of the motor elements leads to axonal degeneration, fibrillation and positive sharp potentials correlate with the denervation of muscle fibers. In review, then, one may see increased insertional activity, increased polyphasic action potentials, fasciculation action potentials, bizarre high frequency discharges, and fibrillation and positive sharp potentials.

It is misleading to accept the occurrence of fibrillation potentials as the only criterion for establishing the diagnosis. The irritative responses appear rather early and are reliable indices of disease; this is especially true of fasciculation action potentials. Fibrillation potentials require at least several weeks to make their appearance if they are to appear at all! The interval of 21 days which is cited throughout the literature is only an average time; they may appear in 2 weeks or may not be seen in some individuals until after 4 weeks. In the paraspinal muscles, they may be recorded at the end of 8 to 10 days.

The key to EMG identification of discogenic disease lies in the detection of abnormalities in a distinct pattern-affection of muscles in a myotome which receive their ultimate segmental innervation through different peripheral nerves. An example of such an arrangement for the L_5 myotome may be tabulated as shown in Table 10.5.

Abnormal findings in several of the muscles enumerated under the L_5 myotome (i.e., peroneus longus, tibialis posterior, and tensor fasciae latae) would quickly differentiate the lesion from a peripheral mononeuropathy. Because the number of fibers from the spinal segment which distribute to

TABLE 10.5

L_5 Myotome	Peripheral Nerve
Peroneus longus	Peroneal
Tensor fasciae latae	Superior gluteal
Tibialis posterior	Tibial
Biceps femoris (short head)	Peroneal portion of sciatic

each muscle is disproportional, it follows that the EMG abnormalities are not equally intense in all muscles of the myotome. The major root innervation to the tibialis anterior is L_4. With a compression of this root little or no findings may be observed in the quadriceps ($L_{2,3,4}$); whereas the tensor fasciae latae may show only a 1+ to 2+ occurrence of fibrillation potentials, the tibialis anterior presents a 4+ incidence. Examination, therefore, should be carried out so that all muscles under investigation are adequately surveyed; emphasis is placed on muscles with the major segmental contribution.

This approach holds as well for the upper extremity. Here the deltoid receives its major root supply from C_5 but shares C_6 with biceps, brachioradialis, and flexor carpi radialis. A patient with an axillary nerve lesion shows abnormalities isolated to the deltoid muscle if EMG is carried out on the enumerated muscles. With a C_5 radiculopathy, however, abnormality may very well be evident in the biceps and the brachioradialis. In addition, the EMG study of the supra- and infraspinatus muscles yields corroborative evidence of C_5 disease.

EMG examination of the paraspinal muscles is a useful procedure in investigation of disc pathology and has apparently been successfully employed by several investigators (8–10). This is particularly true during the 7- to 14-day period after onset of clinical symptoms when increased insertional activity, positive sharp waves, and fibrillation potentials may be present in the paraspinal muscles but absent in the limbs.

The innervation of the sacrospinalis muscle mass is quite diffusely overlapped, so that specific identification of one particular segment is certainly questionable (11). Examination of the deeper small rotator muscles, like the multifidus, affords better localization but is technically more demanding. Because herniations of the dural sleeve at the intervertebral foramen are not extremely unusual, the subarachnoid space may be inadvertently entered by such deep probing. A more practical problem in examining the back muscles relates to the greater difficulty in attaining sufficient relaxation of the patient so that the electrical silence of complete repose may be achieved. This is especially a problem in the cervical region when the muscle action potential of the paraspinal muscles are frequently of short enough duration to be confused with abnormal spontaneous activity (fibrillation action potentials) (Fig. 10.4).

Examination of the muscles of the back may be of critical value in differentiation of a plexus from a root lesion (i.e., intraspinal) because the plexi form from the more distal portion of the anterior rami. If the axial muscles are involved, the lesion must be a proximal one (Fig. 10.5).

In some instances, however, when the interest lies in detection of the presence or absence of a lesion rather than in its localization, the study of the axial muscles may be helpful. This is particularly true when the involved segments do not have appendicular representation, for example, in compression of the dorsal and first lumbar segments.

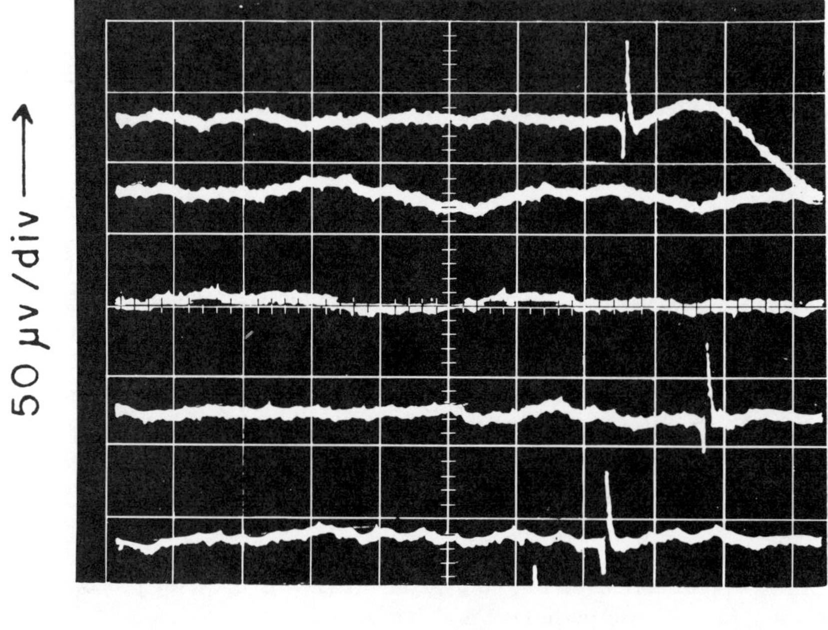

FIG. 10.4. Normal EMG recording of motor units under voluntary control in the cervical paraspinal muscles. Because of their short duration they may be easily confused with fibrillation potentials.

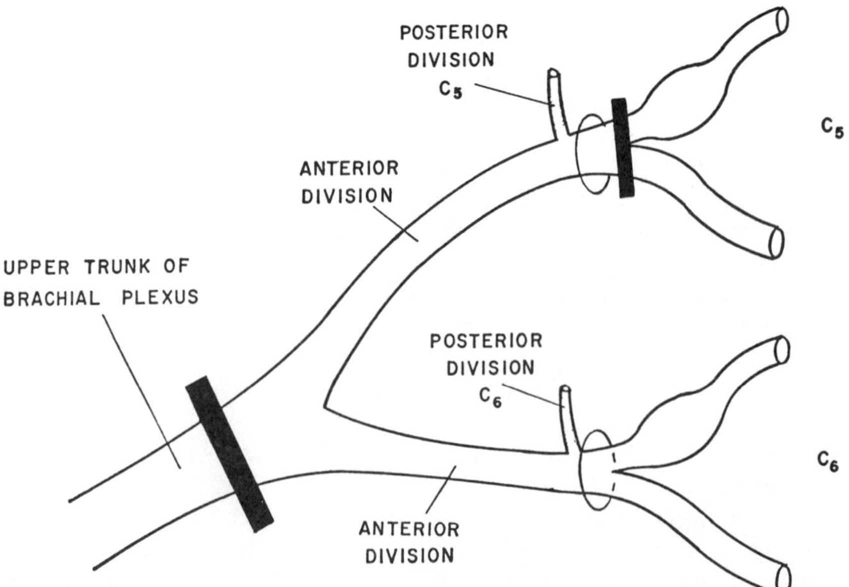

FIG. 10.5. Intraspinal lesion with affection of outflow to posterior division of C_5. Plexus lesion spares back muscles because the trunk nerve forms from the anterior primary divisions.

Conduction Velocity

Conduction velocity studies of the peripheral nerves generally contribute few positive data in electrodiagnosis of discogenic disease because they are usually normal. However, in some cases of compression severe enough to cause significant axonal degeneration, the amplitude of the evoked responses may be notably reduced. The determination is nevertheless important in completeness of differential diagnosis. Denervation limited to the anterior compartment muscles of the leg associated with a motor conduction velocity of 22 m per sec for the peroneal nerve points to peripheral neuropathy rather than to radiculopathy. It is noteworthy to observe that conduction in the distal sensory nerve fibers is unimpaired in root compression, so that the finding of a normal evoked sensory nerve action potential of the digital nerves of the index fingers favors C_{5-6} radiculopathy rather than a peripheral median neuropathy. In both cases the patient's chief complaint may be "numbness" of the second digit.

Recently a new procedure has been developed to apply to continuing evaluation of a C_8T_1 root lesion in suspected cases of thoracic outlet syndrome in contrast to the conventional method of stimulation of Erb's point (12). Stimulation is done with a monopolar electrode (the cathode) inserted approximately 1 cm lateral to and 1 cm above the C_7 spinous process. As soon as the transverse spinous process is felt, a needle is directed slightly laterally. The other stimulating electrode may be a skin electrode placed about 6 inches from the cathode. Employing pulsation of 0.5-msec duration, supermaximal responses are recorded from the abductor digiti quinti. The distance from cathode to recording electrode is measured with the arm in 90° abduction at the shoulder, complete extension at the elbow, and a neutral position of the forearm and wrist.

In 1967 Caldwell et al. (13) reported on a series of nine patients with root lesions of the dorsal region of the cord in whom diagnosis was established by demonstration of conduction delays in the intercostal nerves of the involved segment. Stimulation and recording were carried out with needle electrodes, the former placed as close as possible to the roots and the latter in the intercostal muscles in the midaxillary line. Because the procedure was attended by considerable pain, general anesthesia was required. Morbidity involved a single incidence of pneumothorax. Aside from procedural aspects, the method presents some theoretical problems. In general, root compression by disc herniation does not cause conduction defect in the periphery. If nerve compression does cause delay (such as tardy ulnar palsy), the slowing is segmental across the compressed zone with the usual finding of normal impulse conductions proximally and distally to the lesion. Electromyographic examination of the intercostal muscle in the mildly sedated patient is quite simple and can be carried out with his full cooperation to give essential diagnostic data. Because the most informative electrical changes involve abnormal spontaneous discharges, the EMG pattern from quiet intercostal muscles in the patient instructed to hold his breath is an easier and sufficient method of study.

Interpretation of EMG Findings

The detection of a root compression lesion by EMG examination is less of a chore than is localization of the lesion. The difficulties stem from the fact that the EMG findings identify the *root* but not the vertebral level.

The problems introduced by such anatomic variations as a prefixed or postfixed brachial plexus can be quite complex and confusing. A more common situation concerns herniation of a disc at the L_{4-5} or L_5-S_1 interspace (Fig. 10.6). The usual posterolateral herniation at the L_{4-5} interspace causes impingement on the L_5 root. The L_4 root lays lateral and superior to the disc so that, unless the herniation is huge, the root is spared. A midline protrusion at L_{4-5}, however, may cause the greatest damage to the medially located S_1 root. In recapitulation, the identification of EMG abnormalities in the S_1 segment may reflect a posterolateral herniation at L_5-S_1 or a midline protrusion at the L_4-L_5 interspace. There is also a "lateral" syndrome involving the L_5-S_1 disc. With large lateral protrusions the L_5 root may become involved, rather than the usual S_1 compression seen at that interspace. It is equally important to note that multiple roots may be compressed by a single disc herniation. The number affected is dependent on the exact site and size of the herniation.

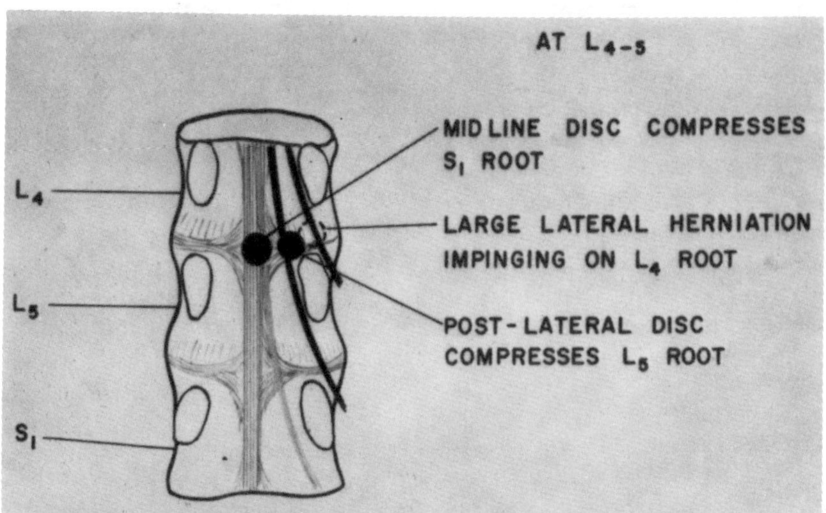

FIG. 10.6. Specific location of disc herniation and root affected. Midline disc affects S_1. Moderate-sized postlateral herniation impinging on the usual L_5 root while large lateral herniation compresses L_4.

It is of interest in interpreting laboratory data to compare the accuracy of EMG studies with contrast myelography as verified at the time of laminectomy. Some reports in the literature have enthusiastically favored EMG. As an example, Shea and Woods (14) reported that electrical studies were accurate in over 90% of cases vs. 79.8% for myelography. In an extensive monograph on lumbar root compression syndromes, Knuttson (15) presents values of 78.6 and 75.2% for EMG and myelography, respectively. The latter percentages are within the range experienced in our department. Although both methods obviously yield significant diagnostic information, it is not suggested that they are mutually exclusive. With EMG, for example, specific affected roots may be identified, but the myelogram is superior in identifying the exact vertebral level.

It has been our experience that in involvement of the L_5-S_1 interspace, the margin of accuracy favors electromyography over radiographic examination. This observation has been made by other investigators and is attributed to the anatomic configuration of the dural sac, which is often tapered in the lumbar sacral region to produce a larger space into which herniations may occur without affecting the column of dye. In general, it can be stated that some root compressions which are missed by either EMG or X-ray study are conclusively demonstrated by the alternate method, so that both procedures are complementary in the solution of the basic problem—establishing an accurate diagnosis.

With regard to the cervical spine, there are no great differences in basic concepts of EMG study. The fact that the difference between level of origin and exit of the roots from the spinal column is almost insignificant in comparison to the lumbosacral region does improve the correlation of EMG and level of disc protrusion.

Myelography of the cervical region presents the annoying feature of excessive false positive X-rays. In a review of 50 cases at the New York University Hospital, for example, nine showed abnormal radiographic findings in the cervical spine which were totally unrelated to the patient's complaints. In two patients examined for complaints referable to the upper spine, there were unrelated myelographic abnormalities in the lumbosacral spine. Corresponding to these observations, Trowbridge and French (16) reported an incidence of 14 false positive lumbar myelograms in a series of 25 patients studied for cervical and upper extremity symptoms. As has been observed, EMG is far from infallible, but false positive results are not one of the pitfalls of a carefully executed examination.

An exceedingly common lesion involving the cervical region is the descriptive "whiplash" injury. The mechanisms involved in the peripheral neurological trauma include stretching, hemorrhage, edema involving roots, foraminal narrowing due to fractures or subluxation, and acute herniation of the nucleus pulposus. Strain of the cervical ligaments seems to be the most common result of this type of injury and explains the frequent cure by "remunerative settlement." Reynolds et al. (17) studied 17 patients (who were clinically and radiologically negative) by EMG examination of the trapezius, sternocleidomastoid, levator scapulae, and scalenus anterior muscles and found evidence of motor unit disintegration in the majority of the subjects. They consider these findings indicative of injury of the C_2, C_3, C_4 roots or to the terminal branches of the accessory nerve. The majority of patients with whiplash injury examined in our laboratory have not shown any EMG abnormality.

The 70 to 80% correlation value between electromyography and myelographic examination pertains to patients who come to surgery; it has no relationship to the incidence of positive EMG findings in the total number of patients referred with diagnosis of root compression. In fully 40 to 50% of the latter patients, the EMG examination is normal. This is true even when deep tendon reflexes are diminished or absent! The explanation of these observations rests on the fact that the most common symptom of root compression encountered in clinical practice is *pain*—not motor impairment (and not every referred pain means radiculopathy)! Because the sensory root, therefore, must be the most commonly affected structure, it can be anticipated that EMG examination of motor distribution will often turn out to be unfruitful. Hence, the electrodiagnostic report must be carefully phrased to avoid the *misleading* appellations of "negative" or "normal." An acceptable and simple format could read as follows:

Case Report. F. E., female, age 47.

History. Second severe attack of low back pain with posterolateral radiation into left leg. Complete bed rest 6 weeks before admission to hospital with insignificant relief of symptoms.

Physical Examination. SLR (straight leg raising) impaired. AJ (ankle jerk) 1+ compared to 4+ on contralateral limb. Vague sensory findings. No motor weakness.

EMG. Quadriceps, anterior tibial, extensor hallucis longus, extensor digitorum brevis, abductor hallucis, and hamstrings normal.

H Reflex. Normal response on right, could not be evoked at all on left side.

Myelogram (Fig. 10.7). Marked indentation of the radiopaque column from the anterior and left side of L_5-S_1. A similar type of protrusion to a lesser degree is noted between L_4-L_5, possibly from disc protrusion into spinal canal.

Surgical Findings. Extruded disc L_5-S_1. At L_4-L_5 there were bilateral protruded discs. Roots at each foramen were compromised by adhesions (and extruded material at L_5-S_1).

Surgery. Partial laminectomy L_4-L_5, L_5-S_1 with dissection of discs between L_4-L_5 and L_5-S_1. Partial foramenotomy L_5-S_1 left, L_4-L_5 bilaterally.

Postoperative Status. Complete relief of symptoms—2-year follow-up.

Comment. Case F. E. is illustrative of disc compression without motor

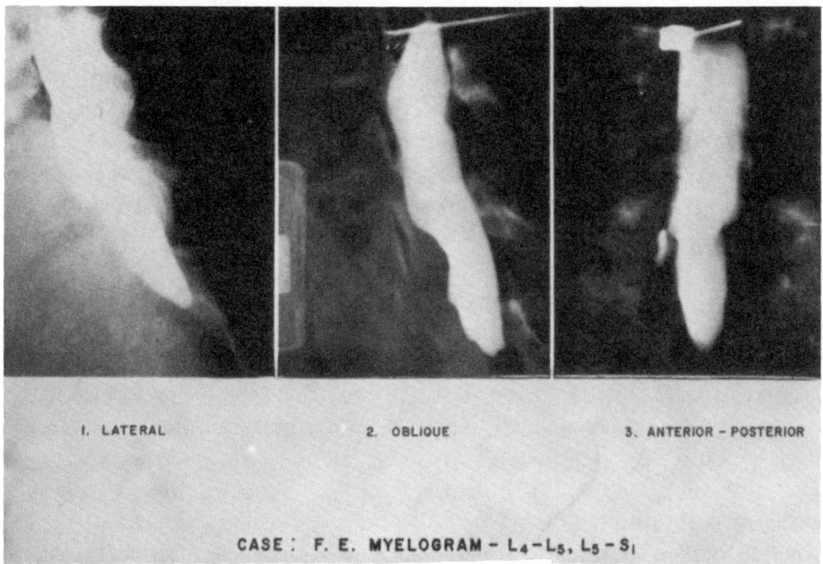

FIG. 10.7. The lateral view of the myelogram shows a slight indentation which cannot be considered abnormal. The defect becomes more apparent in the oblique view and leaves no doubt of the presence of a large lateral compressive lesion at L_5-S_1 on the frontal view. EMG studies were not abnormal.

defect. The only significant electrophysical finding was the inability to evoke an H reflex on the affected side.

The Hoffmann or H reflex is a monosynaptic event which is usually evoked in the leg by stimulating the mixed peripheral nerve and the posterior tibial in the popliteal space and recording both a direct (M) and indirect (H) motor response from the soleus or gastrocnemius muscles with surface or subcutaneous electrodes. (See Chapter 11 for a comprehensive review of the H reflex.) In a small series of patients studied in this department, no statistically valid difference could be found between the involved and uninvolved limb with regard to attenuation of amplitude or measurement of change in the reflex time. Only under one circumstance could the test result be regarded as significant—that is, when no reflex response could be evoked at all!

It seems that measurement of the H reflex in evaluation of sensory root lesions is worthy of continued and more intensive evaluation (18).

In regard to compressive radiculopathy, the findings in patients who have undergone surgery at some time before examination are another point of interest. Because many of these individuals have an "unstable spine," it is not unusual to encounter them again. In most patients EMG abnormalities disappear after compression has been relieved. Knuttson (15) reports the disappearance of EMG stigmata in about 75% of patients examined 1 year postoperatively.

Examination of the paraspinal muscles at the level of the operative site is not advisable in the evaluation of possible recurrences after surgery. Mack (19) reported the persistence of denervation 183 days (range 97 to 293) postoperatively, and Blom and Lemperg (20) detected fibrillation potentials in 37 of 40 patients at the end of 6 months after operation and in 10 of 12 patients at the end of 1 year.

In most instances, however, the reappearance of EMG abnormalities may be regarded as evidence of renewed compression. This is especially significant if the segmental distribution is different from that observed before operation.

Case Report. J. P., male, age 48.

History. 1950 auto accident—injury to back with herniation of disc L_4-L_5. Laminectomy with complete recovery. July 1966, second auto accident—no apparent injuries. June 1967, third accident—low back injury with moderately severe intermittent attacks until recent increasing severe pain.

EMG Studies. February 26, 1967—muscles examined: left quadriceps, left anterior tibialis, left extensor hallucis longus, left extensor digitorum brevis, left gastrocnemius, left soleus, and left biceps femoris (short head).

Comment. There are no abnormalities indicative of denervation. There is, however, increased insertional activity in the gastrocnemius and soleus which is indicative of some hyperirritability in these muscles of the S_1-S_2 distribution. Advice reexamination in 4 to 8 weeks if radicular symptoms persist.

Reexamination March 21, 1969. Clinically, patient's symptoms were progressive during the 1-month interval (Table 10.6).

Significant Findings. Partial denervation of the latter group of segmentally innervated muscles.

Comment. There is now definite evidence of a S_1 (S_2) segmental neuropathy on the left consistent with motor root compression.

Case J. P. is illustrative of several important features: (a) EMG abnormalities are significant in evaluation of recurrences in root compression

TABLE 10.6

Electromyography	Findings
Left extensor hallucis Left extensor digitorum brevis Left gluteus Left medial hamstrings	Normal
Left gastrocnemius (medial belly) Left soleus Left biceps femoris (long head)	Increased insertional activity; profuse fibrillation potentials and positive sharp waves at rest; normal motor units on volition

disease. (b) The only abnormality evident during an exhaustive initial examination was increased insertional activity. Muscle action potentials associated with denervation were not observed until after 1 month of progressive clinical symptoms.

Some information regarding the $S_{2,3,4}$ spinal segments may be gained from electromyographic examination of the anal sphincter. This easily accessible muscle derives its root distribution through the inferior hemorrhoidal branch of the pudendal nerve. Because this is in common segmentally with the external urethral sphincter, urological dysfunction (i.e., enuresis) may be clinically prominent. The examination is performed with the patient in a modified lithotomy position, and the needle electrode is inserted into the muscle through the perianal skin adjacent to the mucocutaneous junction. It is sometimes quite helpful to insert a gloved finger into the anus so as to guide more accurately the electrode into place and at the same time permit clinical evaluation of tone at rest and during volitional contraction.

Normally the sphincter is maintained in a tonic state, so that in the normal and the partially denervated muscle the detection of abnormal spontaneous activity is always difficult and sometimes borders on educated guesswork. Bailey et al. (21) and Waylonis and Krueger (22) developed a system of arbitrary grading of the extent of recruitment under maximal contractions. As usual there is the inherent weakness of requiring the patient's complete cooperation and the problem of the validity of assigning grades 1+ to 4+. Some experienced electromyographers can derive useful clinical appraisal of sphincter tone during relaxation and contraction. However, the significance of the EMG findings seems to be directly dependent on the severity of the denervating lesion. Fibrillation potentials and positive sharp waves are really only absolutely identifiable when residual sphincteric tone is extremely poor or nonexistent.

In summary, anal sphincter electromyography is technically simple to perform but somewhat difficult to interpret. Objectivity is more attuned to the advanced case and considerably more nebulous in the mild to moderately affected patient. The course of recovery in the sphincter muscle seems to follow the general pattern of the neuropathies; polyphasic potentials are often the first evidence of reinnervation.

Plexus Lesions

Perhaps more than any other problem in clinical neurology and clinical electrodiagnosis, the identification of plexus lesions requires a strong background in the details of the patterns of innervation by spinal segments. This concise knowledge includes the anatomic organization of the roots and trunks, the cutaneous segmental representation, the dermatomes, and the myotomic arrangement of the muscles. These subjects have been adequately reviewed in standard texts (23, 24) and to some degree in the previous section on radiculopathy. The lesions may involve transection (missile or knife), tearing, or traction injury without loss of continuity. The exact nature of the trauma, as revealed in history taking, is of considerable importance in differential diagnosis. Involvement of two different peripheral nerves or a trinerve lesion almost axiomatically requires diagnosis of plexus disease unless an appropriate injury exists—i.e., multiple fractures of the arm and forearm may affect median, ulnar, and radial nerves although the plexus itself remains intact.

The electrodiagnostic determinants are characteristically neuropathic and are only meaningful if the segmental involvement is searched for and identified. There are several features worthy of comment.

Mild traction injuries of the brachial plexus which leave the nerves in continuity are less serious and offer better prognosis for recovery. These lesions exhibit the characteristics of conduction blocks. Motor and sensory conduction is normal, and abnormal EMG findings are absent or sparse except for the impairment of voluntary motor unit activation.

When the lesion is more advanced and includes axonal degeneration, evidence of disruption of the motor unit becomes obvious. Extensive Wallerian degeneration is incompatible with impulse conduction, so that sensory nerve action potentials and motor responses are severely attenuated or are not evoked.

The avulsion of roots after traction injuries may be differentiated from more distal lesions because it takes place at the level of the spinal canal proximal to the dorsal root ganglia. Because the distal peripheral sensory fibers maintain anatomic and functional continuity with their dorsal root cells, the capacity to conduct is not disturbed in spite of severe clinical loss of sensibility.

A method to determine specifically whether the sensory root proximal to the ganglia has actually been avulsed has been proposed by Zalis et al. (25). They suggest recording the evoked somatosensory potential from the scalp overlying the contralateral parietal area of the brain in response to stimulation of the median and ulnar nerves in the affected limb. If the afferent loop is broken by a root avulsion, the cerebral response cannot be evoked.

Among the disturbances at the thoracic outlet are included the costoclavicular syndrome, the anterior scalene syndrome, cervical rib and bands, etc. In all such lesions the neurovascular bundle to the arm may be compressed, especially the lower trunk of the brachial plexus with it major outflow through the ulnar nerve. Woods and Shea (26), in an early report (1955) of 66 patients with the diagnosis of scalene syndrome, noted widespread evidence of denervation in the entire brachial plexus distribution in 50% of the subjects. Gilliatt et al. (27) reviewed the clinical and electrophysiological findings in the cervical rib syndrome and found some patients to have a reduction or absence of sensory nerve action potential of the fifth digit and a reduced number of motor units in the frequently atrophied abductor pollicis brevis. Fibrillation potentials were rarely encountered.

When the compression of the bundle primarily affects the neural elements, electrical stimulation at the root of the neck and at a more distal point in the brachium may reveal slowed conduction in the most proximal portion of the ulnar nerve as it passes through the upper aperture of the thorax.

Most of the plexus injuries involving the lower extremities which have been seen in our laboratory have followed severe trauma with multiple pelvic fractures or have been of oncogenic origin. In several patients, reticulum cell sarcomata of the retroperitoneum have been identified as the etiological factor in mild, painless paresis of a limb. The progress of the disorder has often been insidious. The EMG abnormalities diffusely but incompletely involve the segmental distribution of all portions of the limb—distal and proximal, anterior and posterior.

Peripheral Nerves

Examination of peripheral nerves is one of the most valuable areas in which electrophysiological methods are used. The electrodiagnostic laboratories which functioned as part of the network of peripheral nerve centers established at university medical centers and at specially organized military hospitals during World War II and the Korean conflict convincingly demonstrated the contributions of these services toward accurate diagnosis and meaningful prognosis. As a matter of interest, a detailed follow-up study of 3656 World War II peripheral nerve injuries was reported in 1956 as a Veterans Administration Medical Monograph (28).

The methods used in evaluation of peripheral nerve lesions are quite varied in degree of complexity.

Percutaneous Nerve Stimulation

There is no doubt that percutaneous stimulation of accessible peripheral nerves is at the same time one of the simplest and most remarkably informative electrodiagnostic procedures. It quickly answers the question of whether the peripheral neuromuscular system is excitable. The subcutaneous positions of representative peripheral nerves where surface stimulation is most feasible are shown in Figure 10.8. The characteristic low threshold of peripheral nerves makes stimulation with current of high voltage and brief duration a painless and tolerable experience to patients, which is especially valuable in children. The visible contraction in each muscle innervated by a specific nerve provides rapid evidence of continuity and the total or partial nature of the injury. An absent or weak response is nonspecific; the lesion may exist anywhere along the peripheral neuromuscular axis—nerve, neuromuscular junction, or muscle itself. The persistence of excitability in the

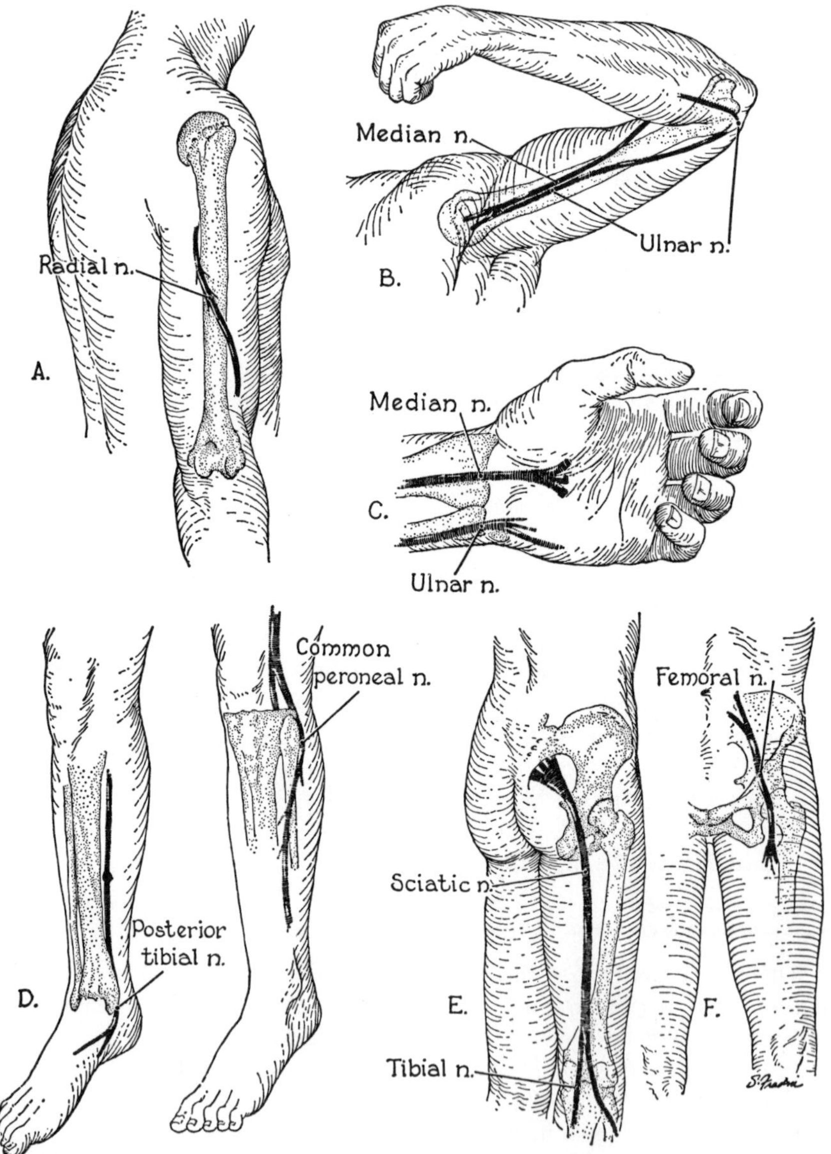

FIG. 10.8. Peripheral nerves commonly used for nerve conduction studies (From H. A. Rusk: *Rehabilitation Medicine*, ed. 2. C. V. Mosby Co., St. Louis, 1964.)

distal stump of a transected nerve for several days has already been alluded to; complete Wallerian degeneration is obviously incompatible with any impulse conduction. The completely degenerated muscle in dystrophic disease is also incapable of responding with a visible twitch.

When this simple method is used to demonstrate block of conduction, it is particularly impressive. Aside from the entrapment neuropathies which occur at specific anatomic sites, block of conduction secondary to trauma may also be encountered in "tourniquet paralysis," although presently this iatrogenic lesion occurs with notably diminished frequency. The radial nerve in the arm, however, may be unintentionally and excessively compressed during surgery on the forearm. The typical pathological lesion of localized segmental demyelination is electrically represented by an absence of response to stimulation above and at the lesion and a normal reaction when the nerve is stimulated distal to the involved segment. In this type of limited pathology, neurapraxia, complete recovery is the general rule. However, neurapraxia may be the first and early response to compression and may yield to axonotmesis, or local axon degeneration, with its sequela of muscle denervation.

Information regarding sensory nerve dysfunction may be gained from simple percutaneous nerve stimulation, but it does require the cooperation of the patient. When a peripheral nerve (e.g., median nerve at the wrist) is stimulated with an intensity of current subthreshold to motor fibers, careful questioning of the subject reveals that at some point he perceives radiating paresthesias into the anatomic distribution of the nerve. The median, of course, will be localized to the lateral three and one-half digits. With the ulnar nerve as well, it is not unusual for the patient to trace the exact anatomic distribution of the digital nerves as he denotes the pattern in which the paresthesias occur.

Conduction Studies

The evaluation of evoked responses in motor and sensory fibers seems to be a natural second step in the procedure of study of peripheral nerve injuries. If segmental demyelination occurs without block, conduction studies may very well show slowed conduction plus some small attenuation of the evoked response even while the visible twitch looks normal. When axonotmesis predominates, the number of functioning axons is reduced and the evoked response is diminished in amplitude. If axonotmesis is complete or the lesion is actually a severance—neurotmesis—then there is an absolute failure of conduction.

During recovery from injury, such as follows in the wake of neurorrhaphy, the reinnervating axons are immature and of small diameter; conduction velocity, therefore, is considerably slower than normal.

Peripheral nerve injuries do not produce any specific EMG abnormalities. The disintegration of the motor unit and the impaired pattern of recruitment described as characteristic of neuropathy are quite applicable. During the course of recovery, perhaps 2 months before clinical evidence, polyphasic motor unit potentials appear. The earliest variety of low amplitude and relatively short duration potentials (formerly called nascent units) gives way to the progressively larger amplitude and longer duration polyphasics and an increasing number of diphasic and triphasic motor unit potentials. They are accompanied by a progressively decreased incidence of fibrillation potentials. The ultimate EMG picture of full recovery may be indistinguishable from normal, but frequently recruitment is not really complete and the amplitude of the potentials is greater than normal. The percentage of polyphasic potentials also often remains at an increased level.

The evaluation of peripheral nerve regeneration is complicated by a delay between the time at which axons physically reach the muscle and the actual return of functional capacity for muscle contraction. Several factors have been held responsible for the terminal delay (29): (a) maturation of each regenerated terminal axon, (b) reconstruction of motor end-plates, and (c) adequate reinnervation by a minimal required number of mature nerve fibers necessary to actuate the motor unit.

The need for knowledge concerning the extent of reinnervation before maturation (which is evident by EMG study) is most acute with regard to the surgical repair of nerve lesions, especially those performed within a military setting. Kline et al. (30, 31) have proposed a solution to the problem by the in vivo study of nerve action potentials stimulated proximally and recorded distal to the site of injury and repair. In studies with primate subjects after nerve transection and repair, they demonstrated that EMG evidence of reinnervation always was accompanied by positive recording of a nerve action potential, whereas the converse was not always true. Nerve action potentials could be recorded weeks before EMG evidence of distal reinnervation.

Vander Ark et al. (32) have apparently found this approach valuable in their postsurgical studies.

NEURONAL INVOLVEMENT

Motor Neuron Disease

Walton's (33) views on classification of motor neuron disease seem to be most appropriate as a background in planning and understanding electrodiagnostic testing. According to his concept the disease involves degeneration of motor neurons at all levels (brain and cord); the separate syndromes depend only upon the sites of maximal stress of the pathological process (Table 10.7).

The symptoms vary with respect to the site or sites of maximal stress, but noteworthy in occurrence are weakness, atrophy, gross fasciculations, tendency to retain deep tendon reflexes, spasticity of the lower extremities, dysarthria, dysphagia, and wasting and fasciculation of the tongue.

The unusually high incidence of amyotrophic lateral sclerosis among

TABLE 10.7

Form	Site of Maximal Stress
Progressive spinal atrophy	Spinal motor neurons
Amyotrophic lateral sclerosis	Spinal motor neurons Lateral columns (corticospinal tract)
Progressive bulbar paralysis	Brain stem

inhibitants of the Mariana Islands is suggestive of a hereditable background, at least in this geographically isolated form. In some cases this variety is even more complex because of additions of Parkinsonian symptoms and dementia to the usual findings of amyotrophic lateral sclerosis (34). Aside from being reported in Guam, familial amyotrophic lateral sclerosis has been noted in an impressive number of kinships (35–37).

Electrodiagnosis

The EMG is classically neuropathic, with the discrete activity pattern (often with giant motor units) a most frequent observation. Widely distributed fasciculation potentials, observed in a warm room with the patient completely relaxed, are also rather commonly seen. The fasciculation may be of simple configuration, resembling a normal motor unit action potential, or may be complex (polyphasic). The fasciculations in chronic motor neuron disease have been noted to discharge at a characteristic slow rate; the overall interval (38) between potentials is equal to 3.5 sec. This observation may be of some value in differentiating motor neuron disease from so-called benign fasciculation even though the essential key in identification of benign fasciculation is still elicitation of a completely normal history and physical examination buttressed by normal electrical testing. Fasciculation potentials are probably of peripheral and central influence, because they persist after transection of the peripheral nerve serving an affected muscle.

That fibrillation potentials are not always present is well known. Wohlfart (39) studied the nerves and muscles obtained at autopsy of six patients and concluded that the gap in muscular innervation is rapidly filled from adjacent motor units so as to minimize denervation and its electrical manifestations. As the disease progresses to include destruction of one-third of the motor fibers, atrophy and paresis appear. These conclusions support the experience of the authors in longitudinal studies of patients; after repeated examinations, fibrillations seem ultimately to appear, sometimes quite abruptly, in many muscles where they were not seen as recently as in the previous 3 to 4 weeks.

Erminio et al. (40) have reported a consistent, appreciable enlargement of motor unit territory in motor neuron disease.

The responses to electrical stimulation include these three interesting and pertinent observations: (a) Sensory nerve action potential studies are normal. (b) Motor conduction may be moderately affected. Distal slowing has been reported by Lambert (41) and proximal segment involvement observed by Ertekin (42). With regard to peripheral nerve function in patients with motor neuron disease, Poole (43) found and Shahani and Russell (44) later confirmed that ischemic and postischemic paresthesias were either mild or absent. Shahani and Russell (44) concluded that the absence of paresthesia in motor neuron disease is related to a relatively high resistance of large sensory fibers to ischemia in this disease. (c) In some patients a myasthenic reaction with decrementation and postexercise facilitation and exhaustion may be demonstrated by repetitive stimulation. The changes are not usually as impressive as they are in myasthenia gravis, nor is the response to Tensilon impressive (45).

With brain stem involvement in motor neuron disease, hypoglossal outflow is affected, so that electromyographic examination of the tongue is often extremely useful. For purposes of the examination the tongue may be divided into quadrants. With patients who have particular difficulty in accomplishing lingual relaxation, insertion of the electrode into the muscle bulk through the undersurface of the tongue seems to be much more tolerable.

Spinal Muscular Atrophy

Spinal muscular atrophy of infancy and young childhood is most commonly known under the respective eponyms of Werdnig-Hoffmann disease and Kugelberg-Welander syndrome. A difference of opinion exists concerning the nosological differentiation of the two clinical variants. Munsat et al. (46) are representative of the investigators who feel that the two cannot be differentiated on clinical, electrophysiological, or pathological grounds; separation of the two on the basis of age of onset or rapidity of course is considered entirely artificial. Buchthal and Olsen (6), on the other hand, accept the opposite viewpoint, that the infantile and juvenile forms are distinct entities. One fact is presently accepted by both: some children with infantile spinal atrophy do have a slowly progressive form which permits long term survival. A few of the symptoms which express the motor neuron pathology may be briefly reviewed as follows:

1) Weakness and paralysis, which may be generalized or especially localized to pelvic girdle and proximal leg muscles in a pattern difficult to differentiate from muscular dystrophy (47, 48) are present. It is obvious, therefore, that spinal muscular atrophy must be considered in differential diagnosis of infantile hypotonia.

2) Fasciculation of skeletal muscles may be seen, although the percentage of patients with clinical fasciculation varies. Buchthal and Olsen (6) regard the paucity in the infantile form as evidence for a separate entity. In this regard, Walton (33) does point out that the normal thick subcutaneous tissue of an infant may dampen and conceal the twitch. In the older patients (juvenile form), fasciculation can be seen in about 50% of the cases.

A suggestion that the presence of fasciculation potentials may be utilized in detection of subclinical cases and in genetic counseling (49) has not been supported by corroborative studies. The proposal has an inherent weakness in that Spira's report was based on observation of two kinsmen (both over the age of 20) in obvious good health except for the presence of fasciculation.

3) Fasciculation of the tongue is considered an important objective finding, with an incidence of 33% by Byers and Banker (50) and 66% by Munsat et al. (46).

4) The Kugelberg-Welander syndrome is generally of very slow progression.

Electrodiagnosis

The EMG shows a neuropathic pattern with prominence of the stigmata of motor neuron involvement, that is, marked increase in amplitude with normal or increased duration of individual motor unit potentials and loss of motor units so that recruitment is impaired. Fibrillation potentials, positive sharp waves, increased polyphasia, and fasciculation potentials are also encountered.

A uniquely electrophysiological feature in the infantile form was reported by Buchthal and Clemmesen (51) in 1941 and reiterated by Buchthal and Olsen in 1970 (6); this feature may be sufficiently significant to consider Werdnig-Hoffman disease and Kugelberg-Welander syndrome absolutely distinct thereby. The specific finding consists of spontaneous activity in the relaxed muscles of the infants, persisting for hours and even during sleep. These potentials discharge at a rate of 5 to 15 per sec, but unlike fasciculation potentials, they can be voluntarily activated. They were recorded in 75% of Buchthal's Werdnig-Hoffman disease patients and were not reported in juvenile spinal muscular atrophy.

In Munsat's study of 24 probands, two patients who showed myopathic electromyograms were associated with microscopic reports of myopathic muscle. In all, six of the 24 patients showed such histological patterns. In general, in attempting to correlate electrophysiological and microscopic observations, it is now quite apparent that histological myopathy is not rare in spinal muscular atrophy (52–54). Drachman et al. (55) have pointed out the overall incidence of histological myopathy in chronic neurogenic diseases, and in an earlier paper Wohlfart et al. (47) reported "slight dystrophy like changes microscopically" in this eponymic disorder.

Conduction velocity is usually normal, although a few studies have revealed a slightly decreased rate. This may be due to preferential attack on the largest motor neurons with their larger diameter axons, leaving fibers of smaller diameter and, therefore, somewhat slower conduction velocity (56).

Poliomyelitis

The electrodiagnostic findings in poliomyelitis typify the abnormalities which can be expected in neuronal lesions. The particular muscles which are affected reflect the characteristic irregular segmental pattern in which poliomyelitis attacks various levels of the spinal cord and the unpredictable degree of destruction of the motor neurons which are attacked. Until EMG evidence of denervation appears 3 to 4 weeks after onset of the disease, the involved muscle may either be electrically silent or show an increased proportion of polyphasic potentials in a generally reduced capacity for motor unit recruitment. Whether the denervation is partial or complete determines the extent of recruitment of voluntary motor unit potentials. The severity and ultimate prognosis may be guided by the persistence of evidence of denervation weighed against the appearance of progressive signs of electrophysiological recovery.

EMG study of partially denervated muscle reveals nothing to distinguish the polio-affected muscle from that which may be seen in other neuronal disorders. If the pathological lesion is partial and irritative rather than destructive, fasciculation action potentials may be observed. The motor unit potentials which persist after the acute phase exhibit the neuropathic pattern of increase in duration and amplitude. The observation of hypertrophied motor units (action potential amplitudes greater than 5 mV) late in the disease is not unusual and undoubtedly reflects extensive nerve terminal arborization and reinnervation of denervated muscle fibers.

During the usual course of recovery, long duration polyphasic potentials appear. Small and then larger sized motor unit action potentials are also observed, accompanied by a progressive decrease in fibrillation potentials. Polyphasic potentials, giant motor units, and a single or partial interference pattern sometimes are seen long after apparent complete clinical recovery. In some polio-affected muscles, fibrillation potentials persist for unusually long periods. In our own studies, these potentials have been recorded 60 years after the acute phase of the disease.

With regard to the polyphasic potentials seen during recovery as compared to those which occur early, Buchthal (57) has suggested that polyphasic motor unit potentials, 15 to 30 msec in duration with many short spikes (in more than 12% of the potentials), seem to be associated with the activation of immature regenerating fibers.

The response to electrical stimulation of the peripheral nerves in polio depends on the extent of axonal degeneration consequent to the neuronal lesion. If destruction is severe, there may be no response at all. In the partial lesion where residual motor units are intact, conduction velocity is normal. This fact is useful in differential diagnosis from most cases of acute polyradiculoneuropathy, in which conduction delays are sometimes quite severe. Normal sensory nerve action potentials are regularly recorded in poliomyelitis unless other lesions supervene. Pressure neuropathy, perhaps due to improper use of wheelchair arms or crutches, can cause such a secondary complication.

In some polio patients, a decrementation of the amplitude of successive motor unit potentials (myasthenic response) may be demonstrated in repetitive stimulation studies. This finding is not unique, because it may be observed in other neuronal lesions, e.g., chronic motor neuron disease.

Syringomyelia

The clinical and electrodiagnostic manifestations in syringomyelia are not difficult to correlate with the pathology peculiar to this disease. The cavitations usually begin at the base of a posterior horn in the cervicothoracic cord and result in sensory loss in the segmental distribution of the upper limb. A dissociation of pain and temperature, with preservation of the other sensibilities, is characteristic. The expansion of the cavity and the gliosis which takes place affect the motor neurons; the spread laterally to involve the corticospinal tracts causes upper motor neuron symptoms in the legs (spasticity).

Electrodiagnosis

Motor conduction is essentially normal. The degeneration of axons secondary to the compression of the anterior horn cells may cause a small decrease in the amplitude of the evoked response.

Sensory conduction is also not abnormal in spite of the profound clinical symptoms. This finding can be anticipated, however, because the pathological lesions affecting the sensory fiber pathway are proximal to the dorsal root ganglia. The peripheral sensory axons, therefore, remain intact.

In electromyography the compression of the anterior horn cells results in changes of the motor unit action potential characteristic of neuronal involvement, i.e., amplitude, duration, etc. Clinical and electrical fasciculations are infrequent and quite limited in distribution when they do occur. The electrical signs of denervation are present to the same variable degree as noted in chronic motor neuron disease, but the distribution is much more restrictive (upper extremities).

POLYNEUROPATHY

The electrodiagnostic features of nontraumatic lesions of the peripheral nerves are almost typified in diabetes mellitus with regard to the inferential relationship between the laboratory observations and the presence of demyelination and/or axonal degeneration. The other specific polyneuropathies also closely follow such a pattern of correlation. As examples: (a) Furadantin's (Eaton Laboratories) primary effect on the axon may be productive of changes in the amplitude of an evoked response plus electromyographic evidence of motor unit degeneration without recordable abnormality of conduction velocity. Isoniazid and thalidomide exhibit a similar preference for attacking the axon (58). (b) Lead intoxication primarily and typically causes segmental demyelination, so that conduction defects are dominant (59). It has been suggested that early toxic effects of lead on the peripheral nerves may be detected by observation of an abnormal ratio of the amplitude of the proximally evoked response to that evoked distally. Temporal dispersion caused by subclinical disease of a few fibers may cause attenuation of the proximally evoked muscle action potential before the conduction velocity becomes abnormal (60).

Diabetic Neuropathy

The clinical signs and symptoms of diabetic neuropathy are protean. They range and vary from symmetrical to asymmetrical, from mononeuritis to mononeuropathy multiplex to polyneuritis, and from almost purely sensory to almost purely motor (amyotrophy) fiber involvement. Patchy demyelination of peripheral nerves appears to be the lesion and site of predilection (61). Motor fibers are less affected than sensory, and the upper limbs appear to become less involved than the lower. Destruction of axon cylinders with Wallerian degeneration is seen in the more severe cases of diabetes (62).

Diabetic amyotrophy (63, 64) is an extremely interesting clinical syndrome in which the pathological changes still remain poorly defined. It is characterized by pain in the thighs, weight loss, asymmetrical but bilateral weakness of pelvic girdle muscles, and abnormal reflexes. Sometimes the shoulder girdle is affected as well. Sensory fiber involvement is not conspicuous. Males are affected more than females. The symptoms are generally self-limiting in duration.

With regard to the underlying pathogenesis of diabetic neuropathy, it is evident that there is no single unifying mechanism (65). Acute mononeuritis is probably vascular in origin, whereas the common distal peripheral polyneuropathy is probably of metabolic etiology. It is also apparent that the peripheral nerves of diabetics are more susceptible to localized injury, especially in anatomic sites of predilection for entrapment neuropathy. Signs of neuropathy can occur before there is other clinical evidence of the metabolic carbohydrate disturbance.

Subclinical neuropathy is most reliably detected by demonstration of an abnormal sensory nerve action potential. Delay in conduction and attenuation of the potential correlate well with the presence of demyelination. Based on studies performed on the median nerve, it appears that sensory impairment occurs earlier than motor impairment (66). In the series of patients reviewed in Lamontagne and Buchthal's study (66), all patients with motor abnormalities also had sensory conduction disturbances, whereas the converse was not true (five of 24 patients had sensory fiber abnormalities and also motor defect).

In our laboratory, evaluation of the evoked response in the sural nerve has yielded early and reliable evidence of affection of sensory fibers in the lower extremities.

The effect on the motor fibers in subclinical neuropathy (diabetes without clinical evidence of neuropathy) is less impressive, with a shift of the mean value toward slower conduction and the amplitude of the response to a low normal value (67).

When diabetic neuropathy is evident clinically, the conduction defects may be quite profound, especially in the lower extremities. Because the extensor digitorum brevis is frequently impossible to identify because of severe atrophy, conduction velocity determinations of the tibial nerve may be useful in yielding quantifiable evidence. When the motor fibers in both upper and lower extremities are affected, the degree of distal slowing is comparable for both limbs, but the delay in the proximal segments of the arm (e.g., median nerve) may be 2 to 3 times greater than the slowing in proximal portions of the peroneal nerve.

Johnson and Waylonis (68) studied the latency of conduction of the facial nerve in 59 patients with diabetes mellitus and found a significant delay (mean 6.0 msec) compared to the mean value of 3.4 msec in normal control. The decrease paralleled a decreased conduction in the motor fibers of the peroneal nerve.

Because demyelination is the lesion of predilection, fibrillation potentials are often quite inconspicuous in mild or moderate peripheral polyneuritis. The mononeuropathies of acute onset are associated with a greater profusion of these potentials related to denervation. With axonal involvement the occurrence of fibrillation potentials and positive sharp waves can be anticipated, and these are more reliable indices of motor neuropathy than are small increases in the number of polyphasic potentials or in the mean action potential duration. Axonal failure, of course, also contributes to diminution of the amplitude of evoked motor unit potentials.

The EMG findings in diabetic amyotrophy are sometimes difficult to differentiate from the case of polymyositis presenting with pain and showing a profusion of abnormal spontaneous activity. The differential diagnosis is established clinically by demonstration of the metabolic defect, serum enzyme studies, and careful clinical and EMG examination which delineates the involvement to proximal asymmetrical muscles. Abnormal motor conduction velocity (femoral, peroneal, ulnar, or median nerves) adds important supportive evidence of a diabetic complication. Occasional cases suggestive of myopathy have been reported (66).

Although the relationship between the duration and the severity of diabetic neuropathy has not yet been really defined, several generalizations seem to be applicable. Gregersen (69) studied the peroneal nerve and reported a notable reduction in motor conduction after less than 5 years; the decreased conduction velocity, however, was only statistically significant in young patients. Kraft et al. (70) longitudinally reviewed peroneal conduction values over a period of 1 to 8 years in diabetics and found a mean drop of 8.8 m per sec. There is also a paucity of reports which clearly demonstrate any improvement in motor conduction values after institution of specific treatment (71, 72). It is interesting to note that in experimental diabetes produced in rats by alloxan injections or pancreatectomy, conduction velocity is rapidly reduced (in approximately 1 week) to 30% of normal for both motor and sensory fibers. Alloxan treatment without onset of diabetes did not change the conduction velocity, and insulin treatment was ineffective in preventing the conduction delay (73).

The existence of chronic neuritis due to hyperinsulinism (74–76) has led to the speculation that in some patients with poorly controlled diabetes with frequent hypoglycemic crises, an existing polyneuropathy may be related to hyperinsulinism rather than to hypoglycemia. Mulder et al. (74) have labeled the syndrome "hyperinsulin neuronopathy" because of their postulation that both the anterior horn cells and the peripheral nerves are affected. Normal conduction velocity, fibrillation potentials, and the reduction in the number of motor unit potentials cannot be used to differentiate, because they occur in both neuronal and axonal lesions. The evidence for peripheral nerve affection was mainly inferred from demonstration of a high threshold, long latency component in the response to nerve stimulation; it was interpreted as representing conduction in immature, small diameter motor fibers regenerated from previously damaged fibers rather than by sprouting from residual intact axons (75).

Porphyria

Because the conduction velocity in the nerves of patients with this hereditable polyneuropathy has generally been reported as normal (77), it has been inferred that the lesion may be exclusively axonal. It is possible, however, that two groups exist: in one axonal failure is primary and demyelination secondary and diffuse; in the other the primary lesion is a segmental and patchy demyelination followed by later involvement of the axon (78).

Zimmerman and Lovelace (79) have reported one patient in whom there was early appearance of slow conduction which rapidly improved, an observation consistent with demyelination. In our laboratory we followed a typical patient with acute intermittent porphyria over a span of 9 years (1962 to 1971). The patient was originally admitted to the psychiatric division with acute depression and a history of alcoholism and barbiturate habituation. Two weeks later an acute flaccid paralysis of all limbs appeared. The clinical diagnosis was then established and confirmed chemically. The evidence of diffuse denervation and motor unit disintegration was readily observed in

EMG studies. Motor and sensory conduction studies were normal except for an isolated finding in the ulnar nerve (forearm) which showed a conduction velocity of 40 m per sec (May 1, 1962). The left ulnar was 50 m per sec. The conduction of the involved nerve changed to 45 m per sec on August 9, 1962, to 51 on October 4, 1962, and to 57 m per sec on November 8, 1962. All EMG studies at this late date were normal. There is a strong resemblance between this patient and the subject of Zimmerman and Lovelace's study. The preponderance of electrophysiological evidence, however, does favor a preferential axonal involvement. Examination of the same patient during severe recurrences in August 1967 and February 1970 showed severe and diffuse evidence of denervation in muscles of all four limbs. The motor conduction in the median, ulnar, and peroneal nerves was never abnormal. In spite of severe complaints of loss of sensibility in both hands, every examination of the sensory nerve action potentials (1962 to 1971) was normal.

Neoplasm

Electrodiagnostic evidence of neuropathy secondary to neoplasm can be quite varied. In patients with clinical evidence of neuropathy, conduction velocity and electromyographic findings may be abnormal, implying axonal degeneration and demyelination. Trojaborg et al. (80) have postulated that the mild terminal type of peripheral neuropathy in cancer and a subclinical form evident in 17 of his 55 cases may be due to a primary axonal degeneration. These patients did not show abnormal conductions but did reveal the same electromyographic evidence of disintegration of the motor unit as seen in idiopathic polyneuropathy.

Idiopathic Polyneuropathy

In patients with nontraumatic polyneuritis which is clinically identifiable (atrophy, altered tendon reflexes), sensory and motor conduction studies usually yield sufficient diagnostic information. The EMG study also demonstrates abnormality of motor unit function, with the presence of abnormal spontaneous activity the most consistent finding. Thage et al. (81) reported that the typical patient with polyneuropathy showed fibrillation potentials (29 of 30 patients), positive sharp waves, reduced interference pattern, moderate increase of potential duration, attenuated potential amplitude, and an increase of polyphasic potentials. With the use of these EMG criteria, subclinical and latent polyneuropathy may be identified in patients with normal conduction velocity and either no clinical complaints or only clinical evidence of "mononeuropathy." The polyneuropathic nature of the problem, for example, in a patient referred with "carpal tunnel disease" may become obvious with the demonstration of widespread signs of denervation in the distal musculature of the involved and uninvolved limbs.

Alcoholic Polyneuropathy

Segmental thinning and loss of myelin in the most peripheral part of the nerves have been described as the earliest pathological changes in alcoholic neuropathy (82). The lesion may be paranodal in distribution and associated with slowed transmission in the nodal region (83). With progression of the disease process, dorsal root ganglia, anterior horns, and axons of the peripheral nerves show degeneration. These pathophysiological considerations form an excellent inferential background for the results of a study on alcoholic neuropathy. Mawdsley and Mayer (84) reported that conduction velocity in motor and sensory fibers was subnormal in chronic alcoholics, even in subclinical cases. The changes occurred distally first and became more marked and proximal with deterioration. Axonal involvement of the large fibers was manifested as a drop in amplitude of the evoked response. Prolonged H wave latencies were also recorded in the alcoholic patients.

After an analysis of 145 patients with alcoholic polyneuropathy (85), the existence of this disease as a nosological entity was questioned. The conclusion of the investigator was based on the lack of uniformity of microscopic observations and of clinical signs and symptoms.

Uremic Polyneuropathy

The electrophysiological abnormality due to nephrogenic disease is dependent on the incidence and extent of the pathological changes in the peripheral nerves. Asbury et al. (86) have reported demyelination and axonal degeneration. It may be inferred that demyelination is the earliest pathological change, because conduction in 6- to 12-μ sensory fibers appears to be affected first (57). Other investigators (87) have not noted the selective slowing of sensory fiber conduction but report a smaller but significant slowing in the conduction rate in both motor and sensory fibers of the median nerve in the forearm. During the early phases of the disease, the electrical changes may be found when neuropathic manifestations are still subclinical. The deterioration of nerve function (which is also correlated with serum creatinine levels) or its improvement brought about by kidney transplant or sufficient dialysis may be followed by serial conduction velocity determinations. As demyelination involves longer and greater numbers of segments of the nerve and axon degeneration ensues, the conduction rates and the amplitude of the evoked responses become more abnormal.

Abnormalities of the motor unit potential and signs of denervation are due to the axonal involvement. The marked diminution in amplitude of evoked muscle action potentials during acute renal failure is a characteristic finding and is due to temporary short duration block of nerve fibers (57).

In an extensive study of chronic renal failure, Nielsen (88) found a significant slowing of nerve conduction in one or more nerve segments in patients with severe insufficiency, that is, with a 24-hr creatinine clearance below 10 ml per min per 1.73 m^2. The impaired conduction appeared in the upper and lower extremities, in motor and sensory fibers, and in distal and proximal segments. Nielsen considered the generalized slowing of the nerve conduction to be an integral part of the uremic syndrome. The major findings were as follows: (a) the motor conduction in the common peroneal nerve was relatively more affected than that of the median nerve, (b) distal and proximal segments of the median nerve sensory fibers were equally involved, (c) the amplitude of sensory action potentials was reduced, primarily owing to increased temporal dispersion and increased incidence of irregularities in the potential shapes, and (d) the electromyographic pattern at maximal effort suggested a moderate to severe loss of motor units in the extensor digitorum brevis muscle, but rarely in the abductor pollicis brevis muscle.

The nerve conduction deteriorated gradually and slowly in all nerve segments in the upper and lower extremities during progressive renal failure, although clinical neuropathy was prevalent in the lower extremities. In contrast, clinical findings usually developed abruptly, the first indication being a sudden rise in vibratory perception threshold (89). During regular hemodialysis and when partial control of uremia was established, a marked decrease in vibratory perception threshold occurred, followed by a slower remission of other clinical findings, as well as no further slowing of nerve conduction, but no significant improvement either. Slowed nerve conduction rapidly improved after successful renal transplantation (90). Recovery was more rapid and complete in distal than in proximal segments, where conduction velocity was still significantly slowed after 2 years. Considering the dissociation between clinical findings and nerve conduction data (91), Nielsen (89) advocates the vibratory perception threshold test as the most valuable for the selection of the optimal time for institution of regular hemodialytic treatment.

The conduction velocity of the facial nerve in patients with chronic renal insufficiency appears to be affected in the same way that the limb muscles are involved. With a normal mean latency of conduction of 4.0 ± 0.5 msec, 40 patients with chronic renal insufficiency showed a mean of 5.5 ± 1.0 msec (92).

Guillain-Barré Syndrome

This syndrome is also identified by other names, of which acute infectious polyneuritis and acute polyradiculoneuritis are most common. With regard to etiology, in spite of frequent association with an infectious-like clinical state, the disease may not be infectious at all but may rather primarily be a demyelinating disorder with pathological changes similar to those produced in experimental allergic neuritis or encephalitis (93). From the viewpoint of electrophysiological examination, the descriptive name "polyradiculoneuropathy" is more useful because the electrodiagnostic findings depend on the site of involvement of the lower motor neuron. The pathological lesion is primarily a multifocal demyelination with a variable degree of secondary axonal and neuronal degeneration. Haymaker and Kernohan (94) and more recently Asbury (95) have carefully documented the clinical and diagnostic features.

With only proximal lesions, the clinical features may closely mimic poliomyelitis. When the lesion is more localized at the level of the roots and consists of demyelination (with block) without axonal degeneration, then the patient may be paralyzed or paretic but conventional conduction in the limb may be normal. During this early stage, however, isolated prolongation of the distal latency, temporal dispersion of the compound muscle action potential, and abnormality of the sensory nerve action potential may be observed. In the well developed case the sensory nerve action potential (e.g., median nerve) may be absent in over 50% of the patients and altered with an incidence approaching 75%. Although evidence of secondary axonal degeneration may be sparce, the recruitment pattern of motor units may be reduced. The pathology is not static, at least over the first few weeks, so the conduction abnormalities and certain electrophysiological evidence of axonal degeneration (e.g., diminished amplitude of the evoked muscle action potential—reduced recruitment) may appear late.

The delay in F wave conduction may be of considerable assistance in detection of the presence of proximal lesions and is useful to identify the presence of low grade multifocal sites of demyelination that are additive in effect to produce a prolonged F response. This is due to the length of neural axis examined with F wave conduction in comparison to the relatively short segment studied in conventional conduction velocity determinations. Regression of the electrophysiological abnormalities with good recovery can be anticipated in 75% of the patients (96), although occasionally slow conduction may persist in spite of apparent full clinical recovery (97).

The seventh cranial nerves are affected in about 50% of the patients, and bilateral involvement is not unusual. In these cases, electrodiagnostic study reveals typical evidence of facial neuropathy, i.e., prolonged latency of conduction. The best prognostic approach to recovery from Guillain-Barré syndrome is probably a factor of the degree of secondary axonal degeneration that ensues. Patients with excessive affection of the motor neuron and axon exhibit a far greater morbidity and mortality compared to those patients in whom abnormal conduction due to multifocal demyelination is the outstanding finding.

Charcot-Marie-Tooth Disease (Peroneal Muscular Atrophy)

Peroneal muscular atrophy is a hereditary neuropathy usually passed as a dominant trait which manifests in childhood or adolescence. Classically it is confined to distal muscles, i.e., commencing with limb muscles below the knees (stork legs) and the intrinsics of the hands. Pes cavus is almost always present. Sensory disturbances are part of the symptom complex. Dyck et al. (98) have demonstrated a quantitatively decreased concentration of Meissner's corpuscles in digital skin pads of patients with sensory impairment. The Roussy-Lévy syndrome is included here because its basic symptomatology can be broadly described as Charcot-Marie-Tooth disease (CMT) plus static tremor of the hands without other characteristic symptoms of cerebellar disease. Chronic degeneration of peripheral nerves and roots, decreased number of anterior horn cells, and posterior column degeneration have been reported as the basic pathological lesions.

The most significant electrodiagnostic finding in CMT is the dramatic slowing of motor conduction velocity which is almost universally present in persons with definitive clinical findings. In our laboratory, the slowing has only been equaled in nerves affected in Hansen's disease (2 m per sec). However, severity of the conduction defect cannot be directly correlated with clinical severity. Sensory nerve action potentials are usually affected later, with delayed conduction, attenuated amplitude, or complete absence of response. Study of the compound action potential of the sural nerve in vivo showed low conduction velocity and decreased amplitude of the α- and δ-components without change in the C fiber's potential (99).

Conduction velocity determinations are a helpful tool in genetic studies of CMT kinships, because apparently normal members of a group may be identified by an abnormal conduction rate. In reviewing large series of patients there is a distinct impression that the conduction defect seems to be more severe in succeeding generations (100). A pilot study performed in our own laboratory has revealed that "apparently" normal persons identified by abnormal conduction studies often show mild, easily overlooked distal weakness of the feet when reexamined physically. In young children the conduction velocity in the leg may be normal at first, but slow progressive increase of the distal motor latency may be the earliest electrophysiological abnormality which is detectable.

The EMG findings are quite varied but are characteristically neuropathic. In long-standing cases, the distal musculature has been so severely affected (i.e., fibrotic) that the muscle is electrically silent.

A similar electrodiagnostic picture is seen in Déjerine-Sottas disease (interstitial hypertrophic neuritis), a recessively inherited, severe, mixed sensory-motor neuropathy. The peripheral nerves are characteristically thickened and may be palpated through the skin (detection of this change in the greater auricular is particularly impressive). Nerve hypertrophy, however, is not pathognomonic, because it also occurs in at least CMT and acromegaly. It is now known that histological observation of onion bulb formations in affected nerves is not specific or pathognomonic of Déjerine-Sottas disease (101).

Familial Dysautonomia (Riley-Day Syndrome)

The children affected with this hereditary disorder commonly show such neurological symptoms as reflex changes, motor incoordination, and hypotonia, in addition to their autonomic system manifestations. In spite of these complaints, the infants who have been examined in our department consistently showed normal motor conduction velocity and sensory nerve potentials. These findings are consistent with studies that indicate that the most significant neuropathological lesions are focal demyelination of dorsal roots and posterior columns of the spinal cord (102).

More recently, Aguayo (103) has reported that phase and electron microscopy studies of biopsied sural nerve (pure sensory) showed a remarkable reduction in the total number of unmyelinated fibers. The total number of myelinated fibers was normal, but those larger than 12 μ were absent. The author suggests that the slightly abnormal conduction in the median, ulnar, and common peroneal nerves of the single patient which he reported could be explained if the absence of nerve fibers of diameter greater than 12 μ were a consistent pathological consequence in all of the peripheral nerves of patients with dysautonomia.

Brown and Johns (104) reported an interesting observation in recording mixed nerve action potentials at the level of the elbow after stimulation of the ulnar nerve at the wrist. In normal individuals the mixed nerve action potential showed a single peak. In seven of nine patients with familial dysautonomia, a distinct abnormality was observed when the intensity of stimulation was increased: a second, larger amplitude potential appeared to produce two distinct peaks in the response. The authors postulate that the two potentials are representative of bimodal fiber populations, differing in threshold and conduction velocity. It should be noted that recording of the sensory action potential in response to digital stimulation rather than to stimulation of the nerve at the wrist did not reveal the late abnormal peak.

Metachromatic Leukodystrophy

Metachromatic leukodystrophy (MLD) is a rare hereditary disorder of lipid metabolism in which the basic pathological defect is the absence or deficiency of an enzyme, cerebroside sulfatase, which splits cerebroside sulfate into cerebrosides and sulfate. In the disease there is excessive deposition of sulfuric acid esters of cerebroside in various organs, with predilection for the central nervous system (CNS) and peripheral nerves. The metachromatic granules may be demonstrated in the urine of patients and histologically after appropriate staining of sural nerve biopsies. The disease occurs in infants, juveniles, and adults (105, 106).

The essential lesion of the peripheral nerves in MLD is segmental demyelination (107, 108) with deposition of metachromatic material in the Schwann cells. It follows then that the characteristic electrical abnormality is impaired impulse conduction (109). In several infants studied in our department, observations reported by Yudell et al. (110) that the conduction velocity is reduced by one-third to one-half were confirmed.

Krabbe's disease or globoid leukodystrophy is generally considered a disorder of CNS myelin, but approximately 13 cases have been reported with segmental demyelination of peripheral nerves. Hogan et al. (111) reported a case with overwhelming CNS involvement where the relatively inapparent peripheral neuropathy was only detected by conduction study and confirmed by biopsy.

Refsum's disease is also an inherited defect of lipid metabolism in which hypertrophic peripheral neuropathy is associated with icthyosis, retinitis pigmentosa, bone pathology, and EKG changes. Abnormal deposits of phytanic acid (3, 7, 11, 15-tetramethyl hexadecanoic acid) have been reported in various tissues (112).

Rheumatoid Neuropathy

Based on clinical symptoms, patients with peripheral neuropathy associated with arthritis fall into two groups (113); in Group I, mild sensory symptoms predominate, and in Group II there is severe sensorimotor involvement. On examination of the sural nerves histologically, Group I showed varying degrees of axonal degeneration and some demyelination, and Group II revealed advanced degeneration of myelinated fibers (114). The major cause of the nerve damage was considered to be occlusive involvement of the vasa nervorum, with segmental demyelination occurring in the least affected nerve and axonal degeneration occurring when the vessels were more severely occluded (115).

The possible electrophysiological findings can be summarized as follows: (a) marked slowing of conduction in motor fibers even when clinical abnormality (aside from sensory) is not apparent; (b) little slowing of motor conduction, although the evoked response is smaller, but extensive signs of motor unit disintegration with marked denervation; and (c) predominantly distal clinical findings, with the possibility of rather widespread EMG abnormalities.

Degenerative and proliferative pathological changes due to arthritis which occur at specific anatomic sites may be the etiological factors in the onset of a compressive or entrapment neuropathy. Perhaps the best example is the development of the carpal tunnel syndrome in the rheumatoid patient.

Leprosy (Hansen's Disease)

The neurological symptoms of leprosy have been recognized since Biblical times, and the histopathological features of granulomatous inflammation and axonal destruction with endoneurial fibrosis were well known in the 1800's (116). The occurrence, at some stage, of segmental demyelination has been recently reaffirmed and demonstrated in teased isolated nerve fibers (117).

Based on the pathological lesions, therefore, conduction defects and motor unit disintegration can be expected when electrodiagnostic studies are performed. The lowest conduction velocity values recorded in our laboratory, 2 m per sec, were seen in a patient with Hansen's disease. In this regard, it may be noted that even in highly urban New York City, in its temperate zone setting, there is a sizable segment of approximately 125 reported patients affected with this malady.

Rosenberg and Lovelace (118) have emphasized the occurrence of the clinical picture of mononeuritis multiplex. These authors and also Granger (119) have reported improvement in nerve conduction after specific chemotherapy. The electrodiagnostic findings may be reviewed in the following "average" case.

Case Report. The patient, C. K., was a 28-year-old black male diplomatic representative from Africa. In January 1965 he noted swelling of the left ankle associated with local tenderness. Neurological examination was negative. The complaint was attributed to tenosynovitis. At the end of February 1965, he reported a sudden onset of left foot drop along with sensory loss in the peroneal distribution. The patient showed no skin lesions anywhere on his body, nor were there any other positive physical findings except for mild hypertension. He was referred for electrodiagnostic evaluation of the "peroneal palsy." The following findings were noted and reported: the left tibial nerve showed a normal distal latency of 2.4 msec and conduction velocity of 47 m per sec; the left peroneal nerve did not respond to stimulation.

Chronaxy findings were as follows: left anterior tibial—sluggish contraction, chronaxy of 32 msec; left peroneus longus—sluggish contraction but chronaxy less than 1 msec; left gastrocnemius—sluggish contraction, chronaxy 5.2 msec; left quadriceps—brisk contraction, chronaxy less than 1 msec.

Electromyographic examinations were conducted on the following muscles: left anterior tibial, extensor digitorum brevis, peroneus longus, abductor hallucis brevis, left gastrocnemius, left posterior tibial, left quadriceps, soleus, middle hamstring, lateral hamstring, and left lumbar paraspinous muscles.

The primary observations were that (a) the left peroneal nerve did not respond to maximal intensity stimulation at the level of head of fibula, and (b) electromyography showed evidence of partial denervation in the left gastrocnemius, posterior tibial, and all anterior compartment muscles.

These findings are consistent with a sciatic neuropathy with major involvement of peroneal outflow or a dual nerve lesion—tibial and peroneal.

The patient was admitted to the University Hospital on April 4, 1965, for a complete study which revealed no findings to explain the presenting complaint. On April 6, 1965, a skin and muscle biopsy was performed and showed the presence of subcutaneous granulomatous lesions. The etiology was established after identification of both intracellularly and extracellularly situated lepra bacilli.

FACIAL NERVE

The evaluation of facial paralysis is considerably facilitated by information derived from electrophysiological testing. Although a considerable number of procedures have been recommended in an attempt to assess the seventh nerve function (examples include quantification of the nasolacrimal reflex, acoustic impedance measurement of the stapedius reflex, and electrogustometry) (120, 121), the choice of methods and interpretation of results may be simplified by posing several questions: (a) What are the excitability characteristics of the facial nerve to electrical stimulation? (b) Is a muscle action potential evoked in the facial muscles in response to stimulation of the nerve, and what is the rate of impulse conduction? (c) What are the excitability characteristics of the facial muscles to direct electrostimulation? (d) What are the EMG observations on examination of the muscles of expression?

Motor Nerve Excitability

Visual observation leaves little doubt that the most uncomplicated test of seventh nerve excitability involves stimulation of the nerve and observation of the contraction of the facial muscles. The stimulus required to evoke a normal response is generally of extremely short duration, 0.1 to 0.2 msec, so that relatively high voltages may be tolerated without complaint by the subject. If each muscle is individually scrutinized, partial paralysis may be easily identified. For example, failure of the frontalis to contract while all other portions respond would be indicative of such a partial lesion. With a complete neuropathy, of course, there would be no perceptible reaction.

Intensity Threshold

Just one step beyond visual observation of muscle contraction in response to stimulation of the nerve is the measurement of the smallest amount of current (threshold) required to evoke a minimal visible contraction of the muscles (122, 123). In practical application, the sound side is examined first, and then the current required on the involved side is measured. In the normal subject the current required to evoke a response ranges from 3.0 to 8.0 ma. If comparison is made between sound and involved side of the face, an increase of greater than 2.0 ma may be considered significant. Safman (124) points out a pitfall in diagnosis and prognosis. He studied the "uninvolved" side of the face of 18 patients with Bell's palsy with EMG and conduction studies and reported evidence of subclinical neuropathy in 14. If these observations are substantiated, comparative studies must be interpreted with greater caution.

The excitability of the facial nerve remains within the normal range for 72 hr after onset of paralysis. Thereafter the alteration in the threshold current is indicative of the pathological state. If the paralysis is due to a physiological block of conduction, neurapraxia, then the threshold of the facial nerve segment distal to the side of block is essentially unchanged and will remain so for the 7 to 14 days during which the studies are performed. With denervation due to partial axonotmesis, a full response of the facial muscles will be attained only when the stimulation current is increased. If complete degeneration has occurred, it will be impossible to evoke any response. In general, those patients with total denervation show complete loss of excitability by the end of the seventh day.

Because the pathological process in Bell's palsy is not a static one (neurapraxia can progress to a partial or complete axonotmesis), it is at least necessary to perform daily determinations in order to ensure accurate diagnosis and prognosis. Neurapraxia is generally not a long term event but may occasionally persist without denervation for several months. On the other hand, Campbell et al. (123), in reporting on 77 patients, noted an erroneous good prognosis for rapid and complete recovery because the favorable outlook was based on the finding that excitability was not lost by the seventh day.

The prognosis for recovery with the neurapraxic and partially denervated patient is excellent and has been variably reported at 80 to 100%. A disturbing feature, however, is the incidence of synkinesis, contracture, etc., in almost all patients who have shown evidence of denervation. Alford et al. (125) have suggested that when the status of the facial paralysis is monitored daily, prompt surgical decompression at the first sign of degeneration may result in prevention of synkinesis. At the moment, nerve excitability testing brings us as close to the time of onset of the lesion as any of the laboratory methods used to evaluate the physiological state of the nerve. To the advocates of surgical therapy, however, there remains the unsolved potent problem of the exact state of affairs during the first 72 hr.

With regard to recovery of facial nerve function as related to threshold of excitation, it is unfortunate that there is no correlation. Clinical recovery frequently takes place long before normal nerve excitability can be demonstrated.

Conduction Studies and Evoked Muscle Action Potentials

When the facial nerve is stimulated at some critical intensity, the depolarization which occurs results in an impulse which travels down the axons to the muscle, where, in turn, a muscle action potential is evoked. The time between the onset of the supramaximal stimulus and the beginning of the evoked muscle action potential is called the latency of response.

It is not extremely rare to detect an electrical response with a needle electrode in the muscle (i.e., orbicularis oris) when no visible contraction is perceived during determination of the intensity threshold of the nerve (126, 127).

The latency to the orbicularis oris in response to stimulation at the angle of the jaw averages 2.5 to 3.0 msec, with a normal upper limit of 4.0 msec. The recording in Figure 10.9 is that of an evoked response recorded with needle electrode showing a delayed conduction of 20 msec. The results of conduction studies parallel the threshold changes, with a somewhat different time course. In the presence of a mild neurapraxia the conduction is unaffected. At the opposite end of the spectrum, with total axonal involvement, the latency begins to show sharp changes at the end of 3 to 4 days, with complete loss of the evoked potential by the end of 7 to 8 days. When the lesion is incomplete, the greatest changes in latency may be seen to occur within 2 to 4 weeks after onset. Certainly, if a normal latency is present 7 to

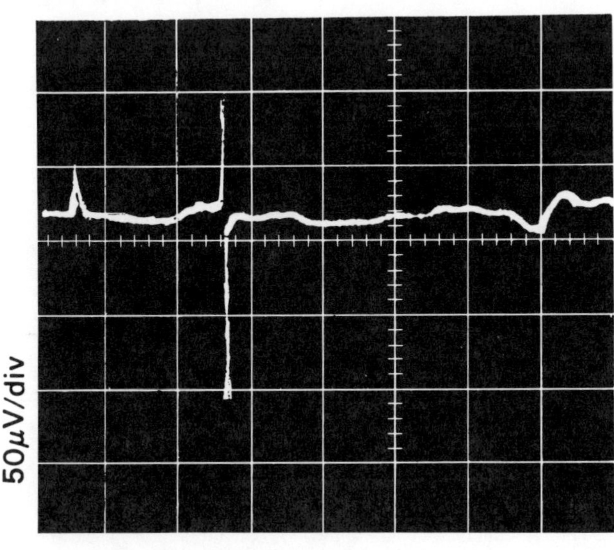

FIG. 10.9. Evoked response. Percutaneous stimulation of facial nerve, recorded with concentric needle electrode at corner of mouth. The latency of response is abnormal, 20 msec. Stimulus artifact is on *left*.

8 days after paralysis appears, the prognosis is usually excellent. Again, this favorable conclusion is not universally applicable because the pathological process involving the facial nerve may be quite progressive over the first few weeks.

During recovery the electrical changes may also lag behind clinical improvement. In spite of good muscle motion, the prolonged latency and the complexity of the action potential may persist.

The ability to evoke a muscle action potential is important in demonstrating that there is continuity of the nerve. This knowledge, of course, is of particular importance when trauma is an etiological factor.

It is also pertinent to note that a delay in conduction in the facial nerve may be part of a subclinical polyneuropathy such as that encountered in diabetes mellitus or uremia. Under these circumstances conduction velocity studies of nerves in the extremities are of assistance in establishing the systemic distribution.

Muscle Excitability Studies

The use of faradic and galvanic currents to determine the "reaction of degeneration" have rightly been made obsolete by the newer methods now

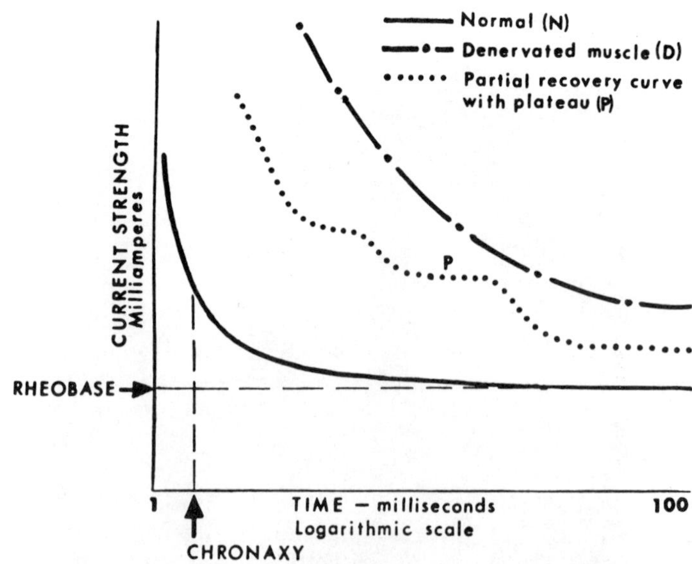

FIG. 10.10. The typical curves relating strength of stimulation vs. duration are presented in this figure. The relatively flat curve is characteristic of the normal state (*N*) and the sharply rising curve shows the typical "shift to the right" of the denervated muscle (*D*). Flattening of the curve with "plateau formation" (*P*) is a most characteristic finding during recovery.

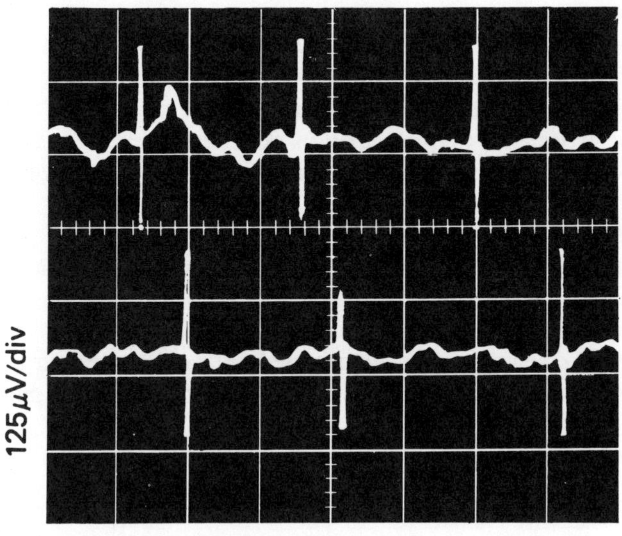

FIG. 10.11. Electromyographic tracing from orbicularis oris. Motor unit potentials are recorded at maximal voluntary effort.

in use. If the subject can tolerate the discomfort, the physical characteristics of the faradic current permit its use as a rough screening procedure of normal response. With regard to galvanic stimulation, the observation of a vermicular response rather than a normal twitch contraction can be of importance in establishing that the muscle is denervated.

As a matter of review, chronaxy determinations depend on the relationship between the stimulus duration and stimulus intensity. The strength-duration (S-D) curve offers statistical advantages over unitary determinations, and at the same time the shape of the curve affords additional prognosticative information. The normal S-D curve is essentially flat, showing a rise near the zero end of the time abscissa (Fig. 10.10). Denervation is characterized by a sharply progressing shift of the curve to the right, a fall in the rheobase, and a rise in chronaxy. Reinnervation is characterized by a shift of the curve to the left, a fall in chronaxy, a rise in rheobase, and the appearance of plateaus. Serial S-D curve studies, therefore, offer excellent diagnostic and prognostic determinations, and may be quite helpful before the EMG findings become significant, but they are of little value in the most immediate onset (first 3 to 4 days).

Electromyography of the facial muscles presents some distinctive features (128, 129).

The duration of the motor unit potentials is quite brief and frequently is within range of the fibrillation potentials seen in denervation (Fig. 10.11).

Because involuntary movements occur with such frequency in facial muscles for a variety of reasons (emotional, etc.), it is sometimes difficult to distinguish the voluntary from spontaneous abnormal activity.

Fibrillation potentials make their appearance in facial muscles after a much shorter interval than they do in skeletal muscle. We have observed them 7 to 10 days after onset, compared to the usual 3 weeks characteristic of the axial musculature.

Because definite changes do not occur until denervation is present, electromyography is not as significant in early prognostic evaluation as we would like it to be. But electromyographic study does make important positive contributions.

Motor unit discharges may be detected with needle electrodes when no visible movement, volitional or in response to electrical stimulation, is apparent.

Voluntary movement due to cross-over innervation may be detected and identified by combining electromyography and stimulation of the ipsilateral and contralateral facial nerves. In one of our patients, a 13-year-old with partial paralysis since 8 months of age, considerable cross-over past the midline to the opposite angle of the mouth was demonstrated by EMG and conduction studies. The distance is consistent with the maximal value of a 3- to 4-cm cross-over from the midline reported by Lefebre and Lerique (130).

This patient was of interest too because of the evidence of an extensive cross-over in a partial lesion. When the left facial nerve (involved side) was stimulated, an evoked response with a latency of 4.3 msec was recorded from the right orbicularis oris at the angle of the mouth. When the right facial nerve was stimulated, a latency of 10.5 msec was recorded from the same muscle. The latency value for stimulation of right facial nerve and response in right orbicularis oris was 3.2 msec.

The presence of fibrillation action potentials and/or positive sharp potentials indicates that the lesion is more than a simple neurapraxia, that the segmental block of conduction in effect has progressed to axonotmesis and has resulted in denervation of some of the muscle fibers. In prognostication, then, the presence of fibrillation potentials denotes greater severity and a more protracted time course of recovery (131).

If the denervation is complete—i.e., there are no voluntary motor unit action potentials and fibrillation and positive sharp potentials are widely observed in the muscle—then prognosis is poor. It is in this category that we find the small percentage of patients left with permanent paralysis or the patients with hemifacial spasm or severe persistent synkinesis.

The observation of polyphasic potentials during the course of serial electromyographic examinations has the same significance as in electromyography of skeletal muscle: polyphasic potentials are usually the first indication of reinnervation. Because the posterior auricular muscle is innervated by the first extracranial branch of the facial nerve, examination of this muscle should be useful in recording earliest signs of reinnervation.

The appearance of polyphasic potentials, coupled with a decreased incidence of spontaneous activity in the form of fibrillations and positive sharp waves, as well as the presence of normal motor units and perhaps some giant motor units is indicative of recovery. The failure of appearance of this pattern points to more serious sequelae.

Electromyographic examination is of value in the early detection of hemifacial spasm and synkinesis (132).

The method is also of value in preoperative and postoperative evaluation. In the treatment of facial paralysis by hypoglossal facial anastomosis, for example, the progress in reinnervation of the muscles of expression and the residual and recovery states of innervation of the tongue may be productively studied by electromyography (133, 134).

UPPER MOTOR NEURON DISEASE

Although this classification, upper motor neuron disease, does not belong under the heading of neuropathy, the presence of some electrodiagnostic findings in these disorders occasionally causes confusion and misdiagnosis. The presence of fibrillation and positive sharp wave potentials, for example, in the electromyographic examination has been considered to be characteristic of lower motor neuron disease since the basic writings of Denny-Brown and Pennybacker (135) and Weddell et al. (136). These potentials are also found in muscle diseases, suggesting that they represent abnormality of the motor unit rather than just denervation. Recently, however, electromyographic evidence of lower motor neuron involvement, in the form of positive sharp waves and fibrillation potentials, in patients with manifest upper motor neuron lesions has aroused considerable interest.

Goldkamp (137), Bhala (138), and Notermans and Blokzijl (139) have reported evidence of denervation in hemiplegic patients, and O'Hare and Abbot (140), Rosen et al. (141), and Nyboer and Johnson (142) have reported similar findings in patients with cervical and high thoracic spinal cord injury. In recent studies, Spielholz et al. (143) observed sustained fibrillation potentials and positive sharp waves in all lower extremity muscles examined in 12 patients with lesions involving the T_{11} to L_1 vertebrae. In addition, these patients had no motor responses to percutaneous nerve stimulation, elevated chronaxies, S-D curves shifted to the right, and no responses to tetanizing currents. All 12 patients showed flaccid paralysis, anesthesia, and absence of any reflex motion throughout the period of study. Taylor et al. (144) found abnormal potentials by 21 days after injury in 22 patients with cervical or high thoracic spinal cord injury; these potentials were present for as long as the patients were followed, 850 days after injury in one case. Motor nerve conduction studies of the peroneal nerve demonstrated that motor conduction velocities were normal for as long as they could be obtained. The amplitude of the evoked muscle action potential diminished progressively with time until no response was obtained after about 4 months after injury.

The fact that the abnormal potentials appear in a bilaterally symmetrical pattern in patients with spinal cord injury and that they also are observed in hemiplegic patients has raised the question as to whether these potentials represent motor unit disease or some other neurophysiological mechanism. Taylor et al. (144) consider the various possible explanations of the origin of the fibrillation and positive sharp waves to fall into five categories: (a) spinal shock, (b) traction injury to roots (mechanical), (c) ischemia of spinal cord, (d) ischemia of muscle, and (e) neurophysiological mechanisms. They reject all of the explanations except the last, which includes the concepts of transneuronal degeneration and of the fibrillation of muscle fibers deprived of neurotransmitter substance. Taylor and his associates suggest that these neurophysiological mechanisms may be the best explanation of the origin of fibrillations and positive sharp wave potentials in spinal cord injury and hemiplegia.

These findings have not been universally accepted. Other studies have either disputed the presence of fibrillations and positive sharp waves in hemiplegic patients (145) or explained them on the basis of coexisting peripheral nerve damage (146).

REFERENCES

1. Simpson, J. A.: Biology and disease of the peripheral nerves. Br. Med. J., *2:* 709–714, 1964.
2. Buchthal, F., and Pinelli, P.: Action potentials in muscular atrophy of neurogenic origin. Neurology (Minneap.), *3:* 591–603, 1953.
3. Willison, R. G.: Electrodiagnosis in motor neurone disease. Proc. R. Soc. Med., *55:* 1024–1028, 1962.
4. Rosenfalck, A., and Buchthal, F.: Demyelination and axonal degeneration. Acta Neurol. Scand., *46* (Suppl. 43): 199, 1970.
5. Hopf, H. C.: Electromyographic study on so-called mononeuritis. Arch. Neurol. (Chicago), *9:* 307–312, 1963.
6. Buchthal, F., and Olsen, P. Z.: Electromyography and muscle biopsy in infantile spinal muscular atrophy. Brain, *93:* 15–30, 1970.
7. Stoops, W. L., and King, R. B.: Chronic myelopathy associated with cervical spondylosis. J.A.M.A., *192:* 281–284, 1965.
8. Johnson, E. W., and Melvin, J. L.: The value of electromyography in the management of lumbar radiculopathy. Arch. Phys. Med., *50:* 720, 1969.
9. Golding, J. S. R.: Electromyography of the erector spinale in low back pain. Postgrad. Med. J., *28:* 401–406, 1952.
10. Gough, J. G., and Koepke, G. H.: Electromyographic determination of motor root levels in erector spinal muscles. Arch. Phys. Med., *47:* 9–11, 1966.
11. Jonsson, B.: Morphology, innervation, and electromyographic study of the erector spinae. Arch. Phys. Med., *50:* 638–641, 1969.
12. Johnson, E. W.: Personal communication.
13. Caldwell, H. W., Crane, C. R., and Boland, G. L.: Determinations of intercostal motor

conduction time in diagnosis of nerve root compression. Arch. Phys. Med., *49:* 515–518, 1968.
14. Shea, P. A., and Woods, W. W.: The diagnostic value of the EMG. Br. J. Phys. Med., *19:* 1–8, 1956.
15. Knuttson, B.: Comparative value of electromyographic, myelographic, and clinical-neurological examinations in diagnosis of lumbar root compression syndrome. Acta Orthop. Scand. (Suppl.)*49:* 1–135, 1961.
16. Trowbridge, W. V., and French, J. D.: "False positive" lumbar myelogram. Neurology (Minneap.), *4:* 339–344, 1954.
17. Reynolds, G. G., Pavot, A. P., and Kenrick, M. M.: Electromyographic evaluation of patients with posttraumatic cervical pain. Arch. Phys. Med., *49:* 170–172, 1968.
18. Visser, S. L.: The significance of the Hoffman reflex in the EMG examination of patients with herniation of the nucleus pulposus. Psychiatr. Neurol. Neurochir., *68:* 300–305, 1965.
19. Mack, E. W.: Electromyographic observations on the postoperative disc patient. J. Neurosurg., *8:* 469–472, 1951.
20. Blom, S., and Lemperg, R.: Electromyographic analysis of the lumbar musculature in patients operated on for lumbar rhizopathy. J. Neurosurg., *26:* 25–30, 1967.
21. Bailey, J. A., Powers, J. J., and Waylonis, G. W.: A clinical evaluation of electromyography of the anal sphincter. Arch. Phys. Med., *51:* 403–408, 1970.
22. Waylonis, G. W., and Krueger, K. C.: Anal sphincter electromyography in adults. Arch. Phys. Med., *51:* 409–413, 1970.
23. Haymaker, W., and Woodhall, B.: *Peripheral Nerve Injuries*, ed. 2. W. B. Saunders Co., Philadelphia, 1953.
24. Sunderland, S.: *Nerves and Nerve Injuries.* Williams & Wilkins Co., Baltimore, 1968.
25. Zalis, A. W., Oester, Y. T., and Rodriquez, A. A.: Electrophysiological diagnosis of cervical nerve root avulsion. Arch. Phys. Med., *51:* 708–710, 1970.
26. Woods, W. W., and Shea, P. A.: The anterior scalene syndrome. West. J. Surg., *63:* 682–685, 1955.
27. Gilliatt, R. W., LeQuesne, P. M., Logue, V., and Summer, A. J.: Wasting of the hand associated with a cervical rib or band. J. Neurol. Neurosurg. Psychiatry, *33:* 615–624, 1970.
28. Woodhall, B., and Beebe, G. W.: *Peripheral Nerve Regeneration.* U.S. Government Printing Office, Washington, D.C., 1956.
29. Sunderland, S.: Rate of regeneration in human peripheral nerves: Analysis of the interval between injury and onset of recovery. Arch. Neurol. Psychiatry, *58:* 251–295, 1947.
30. Kline, D. G., and DeJonge, B. R.: Evoked potentials to evaluate peripheral nerve injuries. Surg. Gynecol. Obstet., *127:* 1239–1248, 1968.
31. Kline, D. G., Hackett, E. R., and May, P. R.: Evaluation of nerve injuries by evoked potentials and electromyography. J. Neurosurg., *31:* 128–136, 1969.
32. VanderArk, G. D., Meyer, G. A., Kline, D. G., and Kempe, L. G.: Peripheral nerve injuries studied by evoked potential recordings. Milit. Med., *135:* 90–94, 1970.
33. Walton, J.: *Disorders of Voluntary Muscle*, p. 418. Little, Brown and Co., Boston, 1964.
34. Eldridge, R., Ryan, E., Rosario, J., and Brody, J. A.: Amyotrophic lateral sclerosis and Parkinsonian dementia in a migrant population from Guam. Neurology (Minneap.), *19:* 1029–1037, 1969.
35. Hirano, A., Kurland, L. T., and Sayre, G. P.: Familial amyotrophic lateral sclerosis. Arch. Neurol. (Chicago), *16:* 227–238, 1967.
36. Poser, C. M., Johnson, M., and Bunch, L. D.: Familial amyotrophic lateral sclerosis. Dis. Nerv. Syst., *26:* 697–702, 1965.
37. Fleck, H., and Zurrow, H. B.: Familial amyotrophic lateral sclerosis. N. Y. J. Med., *67:* 2368–2373, 1967.
38. Trojaborg, W., and Buchthal, F.: Malignant and benign fasciculation. Acta Neurol. Scand., *41*(Suppl. 13): 251–254, 1965.
39. Wohlfart, G.: Collateral regeneration from residual nerve fibers in amyotrophic lateral sclerosis. Neurology (Minneap.), *7:* 124–134, 1957.
40. Erminio, F., Buchthal, F., and Rosenfalck, P.: Motor unit territory and muscle fiber

concentration in paresis due to peripheral nerve injury and anterior horn cell involvement. Neurology (Minneap.), *9:* 657–671, 1959.
41. Lambert, E. H.: Diagnostic value of electrical stimulation of motor nerves. Electroencephalogr. Clin. Neurophysiol., *(Suppl. 22):* 9–16, 1962.
42. Ertekin, C.: Sensory and motor conduction in motor neurone disease. Acta Neurol. Scand., *43:* 499–512, 1967.
43. Poole, E. W.: Ischaemic and post-ischaemic parasthesiae in motor neurone disease. J. Neurol. Neurosurg. Psychiatry, *20:* 225–227, 1957.
44. Shahani, B., and Russell, W. R.: Motor neurone disease: An abnormality of nerve metabolism. J. Neurol. Neurosurg. Psychiatry, *32:* 1–5, 1969.
45. Mulder, D. W., Lambert, E. H., and Eaton, L. M.: Myasthenic syndrome in patients with amyotrophic lateral sclerosis. Neurology (Minneap.), *9:* 627–631, 1959.
46. Munsat, T. L., Woods, R., Fowler, W., and Pearson, C. M.: Neurogenic muscular atrophy of infancy with prolonged survival. Brain, *92:* 9–24, 1969.
47. Wohlfart, G., Fox, J., and Eliasson, S.: Hereditary proximal spinal muscle atrophy simulating progressive muscular atrophy. Acta Psychiatr. (Kobenhavn), *30:* 395–406, 1955.
48. Kugelberg, E., and Welander, L.: Heredofamilial juvenile muscular atrophy simulating muscular dystrophy. Arch. Neurol. Psychiatry, *75:* 500–509, 1956.
49. Spira, R.: A family with Kugelberg-Welander disease; electromyographic findings in subclinical cases. Confin. Neurol., *28:* 423–431, 1967.
50. Byers, R. K., and Banker, B. Q.: Infantile muscular atrophy. Arch. Neurol. (Chicago), *5:* 140–164, 1961.
51. Buchthal, F., and Clemmesen, S. N.: On the differentiation of muscle atrophy by electromyography. Acta Psychiatr. Neurol. Scand., *16:* 143–181, 1941.
52. Dubowitz, V.: Pathology of experimentally re-innervated skeletal muscle. J. Neurol. Neurosurg. Psychiatry, *30:* 99–110, 1967.
53. Pearce, J., and Harriman, D. G. F.: Chronic spinal muscular atrophy. J. Neurol. Neurosurg. Psychiatry, *29:* 509–520, 1966.
54. Kondo, K. B.: "Pseudo-dystrophische" Natur der Amyotrophie bei der Wohlfart-Kugelberg-Welanderschen Krankheit. Acta Neuropathol. (Berl.), *13:* 29–42, 1969.
55. Drachman, D. B., Murphy, S. R., Nigam, M. P., and Hills, J. R.: "Myopathic" changes in chronically denervated muscle. Arch. Neurol. (Chicago), *16:* 14–23, 1967.
56. Gamstorp, I.: Progressive spinal muscular atrophy with onset in infancy or early childhood. Acta Paediatr. Scand., *56:* 408–423, 1967.
57. Buchthal, F.: Electrophysiological abnormalities in metabolic myopathies and neuropathies. Arch. Neurol. Scand., *46(Suppl. 43):* 129–176, 1970.
58. Fullerton, P. M., and O'Sullivan, D. J.: Thalidomide neuropathy: A clinical, electrophysiological and histological follow-up study. J. Neurol. Neurosurg. Psychiatry, *31:* 543–551, 1968.
59. Fullerton, P. M.: Toxic chemicals and peripheral neuropathy: Clinical and epidemiological features. Proc. R. Soc. Med., *62:* 201–204, 1969.
60. Catton, M. J., Harrison, M. J. G., Fullerton, P. M., and Kazantzis, G.: Subclinical neuropathy in lead workers. Br. Med. J., *2:* 80–82, 1970.
61. Dolman, C. L.: The morbid anatomy of diabetic neuropathy. Neurology (Minneap.), *13:* 135–142, 1963.
62. Thomas, P. K., and Lascelles, R. G.: The pathology of diabetic neuropathy. Q. J. Med. (NS), *35:* 489–509, 1966.
63. Locke, S., Lawrence, D. G., and Legg, M. A.: Diabetic amyotrophy. Am. J. Med., *34:* 775–785, 1963.
64. Garland, H., and Taverner, D.: Diabetic myelopathy. Br. Med. J., *1:* 1405–1408, 1953.
65. Locke, S.: Axons, Schwann cells, and diabetic neuropathy. Bull. N.Y. Acad. Med., *43:* 784–791, 1967.
66. Lamontagne, A., and Buchthal, F.: Electrophysiological studies in diabetic neuropathy. J. Neurol. Neurosurg. Psychiatry, *33:* 442–452, 1970.
67. Mulder, D. W., Lambert, E. H., Baston, J. A., and Sprague, R. G.: The neuropathies associated with diabetes mellitus. Neurology (Minneap.), *11:* 275–284, 1961.
68. Johnson, E. W., and Waylonis, G. W.: Facial nerve conduction delay in patients with diabetes mellitus. Arch. Phys. Med., *45:* 131–139, 1964.

69. Gregersen, G.: Motor-nerve function and duration of diabetes. Lancet, *2:* 733, 1964.
70. Kraft, G. H., Guyton, J. D., and Huffman, J. D.: Follow-up study of motor nerve conduction velocities in patients with diabetes mellitus. Arch. Phys. Med., *51:* 207–209, 1970.
71. Gregersen, G.: Variations in motor conduction velocity produced by acute changes of metabolic state in diabetic patients. Diabetologia, *4:* 273–277, 1968.
72. Gregersen, G.: Diabetic neuropathy: Influence of age, sex, metabolic control and duration of diabetes on motor conduction velocity. Neurology (Minneap.), *17:* 972–980, 1967.
73. Eliasson, S. G.: Nerve conduction changes in experimental diabetes. J. Clin. Invest., *43:* 2353–2358, 1964.
74. Mulder, D. W., Bastron, J. A., and Lambert, E. H.: Hyperinsulin neuronopathy. Neurology (Minneap.), *6:* 627–635, 1956.
75. Lambert, E. H., Mulder, D. W., and Bastron, J. A.: Regeneration of peripheral nerves with hyperinsulin neuronopathy. Neurology (Minneap.), *10:* 851–854, 1960.
76. Danta, G.: Hypoglycemic peripheral neuropathy. Arch. Neurol. (Chicago), *21:* 121–132, 1969.
77. Gilliatt, R. W.: Nerve conduction in human and experimental neuropathies. Proc. R. Soc. Med., *59:* 989–993, 1966.
78. Annotations: Neuropathology of acute intermittent porphyria. Lancet. *2:* 1336, 1965.
79. Zimmerman, E. A., and Lovelace, R. E.: The etiology of the neuropathy in acute intermittent porphyria. Trans. Am. Neurol. Assoc., *93:* 294–296, 1968.
80. Trojaborg, W., Frantzen, E., and Andersen, I.: Peripheral neuropathy and myopathy associated with carcinoma of the lung. Brain, *92:* 71–82, 1969.
81. Thage, O., Trojaborg, W., and Buchthal, F.: Electromyographic findings in polyneuropathy. Neurology (Minneap.), *13:* 273–278, 1963.
82. Denny-Brown, D.: Special problems concerning beriberi: The neurological aspects of thiamine deficiency. Fed. Proc., *17(Suppl. 2):* 35–39, 1958.
83. Mayer, R. F., and Denny-Brown, D.: Conduction velocity in peripheral nerve during experimental demyelination in the cat. Neurology (Minneap.), *14:* 714–726, 1964.
84. Mawdsley, C., and Mayer, R. F.: Nerve conduction in alcoholic polyneuropathy. Brain, *88:* 335–356, 1965.
85. Bischoff, A.: Alcoholic polyneuropathy. Dtsch. Med. Wochenschr., *96:* 317–322, 1971.
86. Asbury, A. K., Victor, M., and Adams, R. D.: Uremic polyneuropathy. Trans. Am. Neurol. Assoc., *87:* 100–103, 1962.
87. Jebsen, R. H., and Tenckhoff, H. A.: Comparison of motor and sensory conduction velocity in early uremic polyneuropathy. Arch. Phys. Med., *50:* 124–126, 1969.
88. Nielsen, V. K.: The peripheral nerve function in chronic renal failure. V. Sensory and motor conduction velocity. Acta Med. Scand., *194:* 445–454, 1973.
89. Nielsen, V. K.: The peripheral nerve function in chronic renal failure. VII. Longitudinal course during terminal renal failure and regular hemodialysis. Acta Med. Scand., *195:* 155–162, 1974.
90. Nielsen, V. K.: The peripheral nerve function in chronic renal failure. IX. Recovery after renal transplantation: Electrophysiological aspects (sensory and motor nerve conduction). Acta Med. Scand., *195:* 171–180, 1974.
91. Nielsen, V. K.: The peripheral nerve function in chronic renal failure. VI. The relationship between sensory and motor nerve conduction and kidney function, azotemia, age, sex, and clinical neuropathy. Acta Med. Scand., *194:* 455–462, 1973.
92. Taylor, N., Jebsen, R. H., Tenekhoff, H. A.: Facial nerve conduction latency in chronic renal insufficiency. Arch. Phys. Med., *51:* 259–263, 1970.
93. Wisniewski, H., Terry, R. D., Whitaker, J. N., Cook, S. D., and Dowling, P. C.: Landry-Guillain-Barré syndrome. Arch. Neurol. (Chicago), *21:* 269–276, 1969.
94. Haymaker, W., and Kernohan, J. W.: Landry-Guillain-Barré syndrome: A clinicopathologic report of 50 fatal cases and a critique of the literature. Medicine, *28:* 59–141, 1949.
95. Asbury, A. K.: Diagnostic considerations in Guillain-Barré syndrome. Ann. Neurol., *9 (Suppl):* 1–5, 1981.
96. McFarland, H. R., and Heller, G. L.: Guillain-Barré disease complex. Arch. Neurol. (Chicago), *14:* 196–201. 1966.
97. Pleasure, D. R., Lovelace, R. E., and Duvoisin, R. C.: Prognosis of acute polyradiculoneuritis. Neurology (Minneap.), *18:* 1143–1148, 1968.

98. Dyck, P. J., Winkelmann, R. K., and Bolton, C. F.: Quantitation of Meissner's corpuscles in hereditary neurologic disorders—Charcot-Marie-Tooth disease, Roussy-Levy syndrome. Dejerine-Sottas disease, hereditary sensory neuropathy, spinocerebellar regenerations and hereditary spastic paraplegia. Neurology (Minneap.), *16:* 10–17, 1966.
99. Dyck, P. J., and Lambert, E. H.: Numbers and diameter of nerve fibers and compound action potential of sural nerve: Controls and hereditary neuromuscular disorders. Trans. Am. Neurol. Assoc., *91:* 214–217, 1966.
100. Dyck, P. J., Lambert, E. H., and Mulder, D. W.: Charcot-Marie-Tooth disease: Nerve conduction and clinical studies of a large kinship. Neurology (Minneap.), *13:* 1–11, 1963.
101. Webster, H. deF., Schröder, J. M., Asbury, A. K., and Adams, R. D.: The role of Schwann cells in the formation of "onion bulbs" found in chronic neuropathies. J. Neuropathol. Exp. Neurol., *26:* 276–299, 1967.
102. Fogelson, M. H.: Spinal cord changes in familial dysautonomia. Arch. Neurol. (Chicago), *17:* 103–108, 1967.
103. Aguayo, A. J.: Peripheral nerve abnormalities in Riley-Day syndrome. Arch. Neurol. (Chicago), *24:* 106–116, 1971.
104. Brown, J. C., and Johns, R. J.: Nerve conduction in familial dysautonomia (Riley-Day syndrome). J.A.M.A., *201:* 200–203, 1967.
105. Greene, H. L., Hug, G., and Schubert, W. K.: Metachromatic leukodystrophy. Arch. Neurol. (Chicago), *20:* 147–153, 1969.
106. Austin, J., Armstrong, D., Fouch, S., Mitchell, C., Stumpf, D., Shearer, I., and Briner, O.: Metachromatic leukodystrophy (MLD). Arch. Neurol. (Chicago), *18:* 225–240, 1968.
107. Webster, H. deF.: Schwann cell alterations in metachromatic leukodystrophy: Preliminary phase and electron microscope observations. J. Neuropathol. Exp. Neurol., *21:* 534–541, 1962.
108. Dayan, A. D.: Peripheral neuropathy of metachromatic leukodystrophy: Observations on segmental demyelination and remyelination and the intracellular distribution of sulphatide. J. Neurol. Neurosurg. Psychiatry, *30:* 311–318, 1967.
109. Fullerton, P. M.: Peripheral nerve conduction in metachromatic leukodystrophy (sulfatide lipidosis). J. Neurol. Neurosurg. Psychiatry, *27:* 100–105, 1964.
110. Yudell, A., Gomez, M. R., Lambert, E. H., and Dockerty, M. B.: The neuropathy of sulfatide lipidosis (metachromatic leukodystrophy). Neurology (Minneap.), *17:* 103–111, 1967.
111. Hogan, G. R., Gutmann, L., and Chou, S. M.: The peripheral neuropathy of Krabbe's (globoid) leukodystrophy. Neurology (Minneap.), *19:* 1094–1100, 1969.
112. Kahlke, W., and Richterich, R.: Refsum's disease (heredopathia atactica polyneuritiformis): An inborn error of lipid metabolism with storage of 3,7,11,15-tetramethyl hexadecanoic acid. II. Isolation and identification of the storage product. Am. J. Med., *39:* 237–244, 1965.
113. Chamberlain, M. A., and Bruckner, F. E.: Cited in reference 114.
114. Weller, R. O., Bruckner, F. E., and Chamberlain, M. A.: Rheumatoid neuropathy: A histological and electrophysiological study. J. Neurol. Neurosurg. Psychiatry, *33:* 592–604, 1970.
115. Pallis, C. A., and Scott, J. T.: Peripheral neuropathy in rheumatoid arthritis. Br. Med. J., *1:* 1141–1147, 1965.
116. Virchow, R.: *Die Krankhaften Geschwülste*, vol. 2. Hirschwald, Berlin, 1864.
117. Dayan, A. D., and Sandbank, U.: Pathology of the peripheral nerves in leprosy: Report of a case. J. Neurol. Neurosurg. Psychiatry, *33:* 586–591, 1970.
118. Rosenberg, R. M., and Lovelace, R. E.: Mononeuritis multiplex in lepromatous leprosy. Arch. Neurol. (Chicago), *19:* 310–314, 1968.
119. Granger, C. V.: Nerve conduction and correlative clinical studies in a patient with tuberculoid leprosy. Am. J. Phys. Med., *45:* 244–250, 1966.
120. Jepsen, O.: Topognosis (topographic diagnosis) of facial nerve lesion: Symposium on Management of Peripheral Facial Palsies, Danish Otolaryngological Society. Arch. Otolaryngol. (Chicago), *81:* 446, 1965.
121. Zilstorff-Pedersen, J.: Quantitative measurements of the nasolacrimal reflex: Symposium on Management of Peripheral Facial Palsies, Danish Otolaryngological Society. Arch. Otolaryngol. (Chicago), *81:* 457, 1965.

122. Laumans, E. P. J.: Nerve excitability tests in facial paralysis: Symposium on Management of Peripheral Facial Palsies, Danish Otolaryngological Society. Arch. Otolaryngol. (Chicago), *81:* 478, 1965.
123. Campbell, E. D. R., Hickey, R. P., Nixon, K. H., and Richardson, A. T.: Value of nerve excitability measurements in prognosis of facial palsy. Br. Med. J., *2:* 7, 1962.
124. Safman, B. L.: Bilateral pathology in Bell's palsy. Arch. Otolaryngol. (Chicago), *93:* 55–57, 1971.
125. Alford, B. R., Weber, S. C., and Sessions, R. B.: Neurodiagnostic studies in facial paralysis. Ann. Otol., *79:* 227–233, 1970.
126. Taverner, D.: Electrodiagnosis in facial palsy: Symposium on Management of Peripheral Facial Palsies, Danish Otolaryngological Society. Arch. Otolaryngol. (Chicago), *81:* 470, 1965.
127. Gilliatt, F. W., and Taylor, J.: Electrical changes following section of the facial nerve. Proc. R. Soc. Med., *52:* 1080, 1959.
128. Buchthal, F.: Electromyography in paralysis of the facial nerve: Symposium on Management of Peripheral Facial Palsies, Danish Otolaryngological Society. Arch. Otolaryngol. (Chicago), *81:* 463, 1965.
129. Goodgold, J.: Electrodiagnostic testing. In *Otolaryngology,* vol. 2, *Proceedings of the Centenniel Symposium Manhattan Eye, Ear and Throat Hospital,* edited by W. F. Robbetts, ch. 8, p. 73. C. V. Mosby Co., St. Louis, 1969.
130. Lefebre, J., and Lerique, J.: Contralateral reinnervation of the paramedian muscles during facial palsy. J. Radiol. Electr., *45:* 96–98, 1964.
131. Granger, C. V.: Toward an earlier forecast of recovery in Bell's palsy: Arch. Phys. Med., *48:* 273, 1967.
132. Ghiora, A.: "Spreading galvanic response" (SGR). In *Infranuclear Facial Paralysis, Proceedings of the Third International Congress P.M. & R.*, p. 329, 1960.
133. Kessler, L. A., Moldaver, J., and Pool, J. L.: Hypoglossal-facial anastomosis for treatment of facial paralysis. Neurology (Minneap.), *9:* 118–125, 1959.
134. Thulin, C. A., Petersen, I., and Granholm, L.: Follow-up study of spinal accessory-facial nerve anastomosis with special reference to the electromyographic findings. J. Neurol. Neurosurg. Psychiatry, *27:* 502–506, 1964.
135. Denny-Brown, D., and Pennybacker, J. B.: Fibrillation and fasciculation in voluntary muscle. Brain, *61:* 311–334, 1938.
136. Weddell, G., Feinstein, B., and Pattle, R. E.: Electrical activity of voluntary muscle in man under normal and pathological conditions. Brain, *67:* 178–257, 1944.
137. Goldkamp, O.: Electromyography and nerve conduction studies in 116 patients with hemiplegia. Arch. Phys. Med. Rehabil., *48:* 59–63, 1967.
138. Bhala, R. P.: Electromyographic evidence of lower motor neuron involvement in hemiplegia. Arch. Phys. Med. Rehabil., *50:* 632–637, 1969.
139. Notermans, S. L. H., and Blokzijl, E. J.: Electromyography in patients with lesions of central motor neuron and so-called parietal muscular atrophy. Psychiatr. Neurol. Neurochir., *72:* 557–567, 1969.
140. O'Hare, J. M., and Abbot, G. H.: Electromyographic evidence of lower motor neuron injury in cervical spinal cord injury. Proc. Ann. Spinal Cord Inj. Conf., *16:* 25–27, 1967.
141. Rosen, J. S., Lerner, I. M., and Rosenthal, A. M.: Electromyography in spinal cord injury. Arch. Phys. Med. Rehabil., *50:* 271–273, 1969.
142. Nyboer, V. J., and Johnson, H. E.: Electromyographic findings in lower extremities of patients with traumatic quadriplegia. Arch. Phys. Med. Rehabil., *52:* 256–259, 1971.
143. Spielholz, N. I., Sell, G. H., Goodgold, J., Rusk, H. A., and Greens, S. K.: Electrophysiological studies in patients with spinal cord lesions. Arch. Phys. Med. Rehabil., *53:* 558–562, 1972.
144. Taylor, R. G., Kewalramani, L. S., and Fowler, W. J., Jr.: Electromyographic findings in lower extremities of patients with high spinal cord injury. Arch. Phys. Med. Rehabil., *55:* 16–23, 1974.
145. Alpert, S., Idarraga, S., Orbegozo, J., and Rosenthal, A. M.: Absence of electromyographic evidence of lower motor neuron involvement in hemiplegic patients. Arch. Phys. Med. Rehabil., *52:* 179–181, 1971.
146. Moskowitz, E., and Porter, J. I.: Peripheral nerve lesions in upper extremity in hemiplegic patients. N. Engl. J. Med., *269:* 776–778, 1963.

chapter

11

The Blink, H, and Tonic Vibration Reflexes*

THE BLINK REFLEX

Blinking in response to a tap on the face has been studied clinically since it was first described by Overend in 1896 (1). He described it as a new "cranial reflex" and considered that the afferent stimuli come from cutaneous rather than from deep structures such as periosteum, bone, or muscle. After this original description the blink reflex was described under a multitude of different names according to the area tapped, the muscles which responded, and the mechanism considered to be responsible. In 1945 Wartenberg (2) reviewed the controversy over the nature of this response, which he termed the "orbicularis oculi reflex." He proposed that, in general, all reflexes be divided into "skin-muscle" (superficial or cutaneous) and "deep muscle" depending on where the receptors responsible for them were thought to lie. He felt that the corneal reflex was the superficial reflex of the orbicularis oculi muscle whereas the blink reflex was the "muscle reflex." Wartenberg had the "definite impression" that tapping was effective by its activation of intramuscular receptors directly or indirectly "by transmission of the concussion to the muscle" through bone or other tissues.

An electromyographic investigation of this clinical phenomenon was first undertaken by Kugelberg (3), who found that the blink reflex produced by a single stimulus often consists of two separate bursts of EMG acitivty in

---

* The section on the blink reflex was written by Bhagwan T. Shahani, M.D., D. Phil.(Oxon), and Robert R. Young, M.D., of the Laboratory of Clinical Neurophysiology, Department of Neurology, Harvard Medical School and Massachusetts General Hospital, Boston, Massachusetts.

orbicularis oculi muscle. He considered these two components of the blink reflex to be two different reflexes. The first component has a shorter latency and is more synchronized than the second, and after a tap over a muscle, its distribution is restricted to that muscle. For these reasons, Kugelberg suggested that the first component "is, according to existing evidence, compatible with a myotatic reflex." The relatively asynchronous second component, which has a longer latency and can be evoked by a variety of stimuli, including pinprick, a puff of air to the face, or corneal stimulation, was, therefore, thought to be a cutaneous reflex.

Both Wartenberg's assumption that the receptors for blink reflexes were in muscles and Kugelberg's suggestion that the first component was myotatic were impressions of hypotheses without convincing evidence. This hypothesis was subsequently assumed by others to have been proven (4, 5), despite the fact that facial muscle spindles have not been found on careful examination in man (5, 6); neither have typical muscle spindles been demonstrable in facial muscles in animals (7, 8).

Because of the similarity of two reflex components in orbicularis oculi to those in tibialis anterior muscle during cutaneously evoked flexor reflexes (9–11), it was proposed that adequate stimuli for the first component of the blink reflex are also cutaneous or exteroceptive in nature. This hypothesis was supported by findings that the first component can be produced by an electrical stimulation which does not produce vibration, stretching, or deformation of any mechanoreceptors (9). Moreover, the first component could be evoked when electrical pulses were delivered to discrete areas of the facial skin beneath which neither facial muscles nor putative facial muscle afferents could be found (9). These observations were subsequently confirmed by Penders and Delwaide (12) in man, Lindquist and Mortensson in cat (13), and Shahani and Young (14) in monkey. Other physiological data to support the contention that the first component is cutaneous rather than proprioceptive in nature have appeared (14–17). There is no physiological or anatomic evidence to support the original contention that the first component of the blink reflex is a monosynaptic proprioceptive reflex akin to the H reflex recorded from the triceps surae muscle. In fact, all of the existing experimental evidence leads one to the conclusion that both the first and the second components are parts of a polysynaptic blink reflex which is, in many ways, similar to other cutaneous double component reflexes recorded in man (9, 11, 18).

The afferent arc of the blink reflex is provided by sensory divisions (first and second) of the trigeminal nerve, whereas motor axons in the facial nerve form its efferent arc. Although it has been claimed that the afferent impulses for the second component descend ipsilaterally to the spinal tract of the trigeminal nerve and ascend to make bilateral connections with facial nuclei (19), the experimental evidence at the present time does not conclusively prove existence of such a complex pathway. It is possible that the second component, like the first, is mediated at the level of the pons and that differences in latencies for the two components are due to mechanisms similar to those responsible for the two components of the flexor reflex, which clearly is a segmental spinal reflex. Either gentle mechanical tapping or electrical stimulation in the distribution of the first division of the trigeminal nerve evokes both components of the blink reflex on the ipsilateral side and *only* the second component on the contralateral side (Fig. 11.1*B*). Stimulation over the glabella (central part of the forehead) evokes both components of the blink reflex on both sides (Fig. 11.1*A*) In most clinical studies, blink reflexes have been evoked electrically by small single square wave pulses (duration 0.05 to 0.5 msec and 5 to 100 V amplitude) to the supraorbital nerve near the supraorbital groove. Stimuli are delivered at intervals of 2 to 10 sec. Surface EMG recordings are made by means of two silver EEG electrodes taped to the skin, 1 cm apart, over the outer two-thirds of the inferior orbicularis oculi muscle, 1 cm below the lid margin. After proper amplification, these responses are displayed on an oscilloscope. The data are recorded by photographing either single sweeps or five to 10 superimposed sweeps.

Some Distinguishing Features of the First and Second Components of the Blink Reflex

In order to interpret results of blink reflex studies properly, it is important to recognize certain features which distinguish one of the two components from the other. The first component (sometimes termed R_1) is briefer in duration and relatively more constant in latency, size, and shape than the second component (R_2). The first component is seen only on the side of stimulation, whereas the second component is seen bilaterally. In different normal subjects, values for minimal latency range from 8 to 14 msec for the first and 23 to 44 msec for the second component produced by electrical

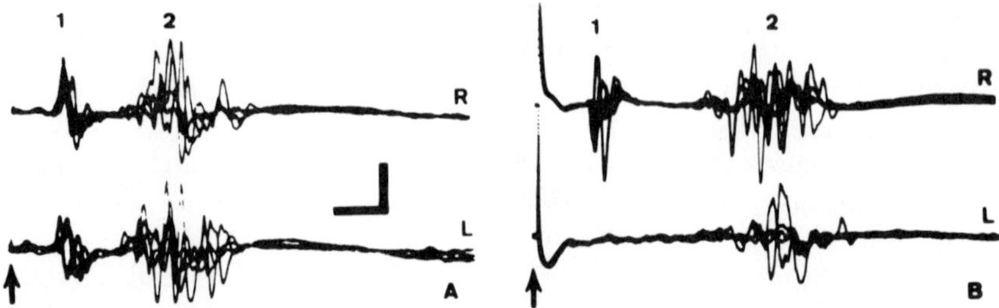

FIG. 11.1. First (*1*) and second (*2*) component of the blink reflex recorded from right (*R*) and left (*L*) orbicularis oculi muscle. In *A*, a mechanical tap on glabella (*arrow*) elicits both components on either side, whereas in *B*, electrical stimulation of the right supraorbital nerve (*arrow*) evokes the first component on the ipsilateral side and the second component bilaterally. Five traces are superimposed. Calibrations: 10 msec and 200 μV.

stimulation over the supraorbital nerve. The minimal latency difference for the first component on the two sides in the same individual is normally less than 1.5 msec. Apprehension results in a marked increase of the amplitude of the second component (11), with diminution in size of the first component. Similarly, there is decrease in the amplitude or disappearance of the first component in light sleep, whereas the second component is then prolonged in its duration (15). With repeated stimulation in a relaxed subject, there is "habituation" of the second component, i.e., successive stimuli result first in a decrease in the amplitude and duration of the response, which may finally completely disappear. The clinically observable blink or movement of the eyelid is related to the second component (11), and it is the disappearance of this reflex component which is observed by the clinician when he notes habituation in the blink after repeated glabellar taps.

Clinical Applications

Lesions of the Peripheral Nervous System

Recording of blink reflexes electromyographically is a simple, reproducible procedure which can be performed in any clinical EMG laboratory. Determinations of values for the minimal latency of the two components on the ipsilateral side and the second component on the contralateral side after stimulation of the supraorbital nerve can be useful in localizing a lesion in the trigeminal and/or facial nerves. Thus, a prolonged latency for first and second components on the ipsilateral side and the second component on the contralateral side suggests a lesion of the afferent arc, i.e., the ipsilateral trigeminal nerve. On the other hand, unilateral delay in the latency of the second component, regardless of the side of stimulation, suggests a lesion of the efferent arc, i.e., the facial nerve. Changes in latency as well as amplitude of the two components of the blink reflex can also be produced by lesions of the central nervous system, a fact which must be recognized whenever one is performing any reflex study for diagnostic purposes. Finally, as mentioned earlier, one must take into consideration various physiological variables which influence reflex studies in a clinical setting.

One of the commonest disorders affecting cranial nerves is a peripheral facial nerve paresis (Bell's palsy). Various electrophysiological studies, including electromyography of facial muscles, nerve conduction studies in the peripheral segments of the facial nerve, and studies of threshold for stimulation of the nerve and/or muscle with chronaxie, rheobase, and strength-duration curves, have been carried out in order to assess the function of the facial nerve. These conventional methods, however, are mainly useful in detecting changes produced by Wallerian degeneration and cannot localize lesions to the *proximal* segment of the facial nerve which is primarily affected in most instances. The blink reflex, on the other hand, reflects conduction along the entire length of the facial nerve, including the most commonly involved interosseus portion.

Depending upon the degree of involvement, there may be prolongation of latency or complete absence of both components of the blink reflex after stimulation on the side of the lesion, with a normal second component appearing on the contralateral side. These changes in the two components can be recorded at a time when conventional electrodiagnostic methods fail to reveal any dysfunction of the facial nerve. On the basis of serial changes in the excitability of distal segments of the facial nerve and blink reflex studies, Kimura et al. (20) divided the patient population with Bell's palsy into two groups: (a) Patients in whom excitability of the distal segments of the facial nerve was retained until blink reflex responses returned showed a good clinical recovery. When the first component of the blink reflex was present, its latency was substantially greater than normal during the first 2 days after the onset, further increased during the latter half of the first week, then remained essentially unchanged up to the fourth week. The latency showed a notable reduction during the second month and became essentially normal during the third and fourth months. (b) On the other hand, patients in whom a direct response to facial nerve stimulation became unelicitable (indicating distal degeneration of the nerve) before reflex responses returned showed a prolonged, usually incomplete clinical recovery. Thus, on the basis of blink reflex studies, clinical observations, and conventional EMG and nerve conduction studies, it may be possible to predict the course of recovery in Bell's palsy.

Significant prolongation of the latency of both components of the blink reflex is observed in generalized peripheral neuropathies in which segmental demyelination is the primary pathology (B. T. Shahani and R. R. Young, unpublished observations). On the other hand, in Friedreich's ataxia, where (in the spinal roots, at least) large diameter sensory fibers are primarily affected, with resultant loss of sensory nerve action potentials and H reflex, the minimal latency for the two components of the blink reflex may be normal (16). Blink reflex studies have also been performed in patients with suspected cerebellopontine angle lesions. On 11 patients with cerebellopontine angle tumors studied by Eisen and Danon (21), either absence or prolongation of latency of the first component was seen in every case. Abnormality of the second component contralateral to the lesion (indicating facial nerve involvement) was found twice.

Lesions of the Central Nervous System

In recent years, blink reflexes evoked by electrical stimulation of the supraorbital nerve or by a mechanical tap on the glabella have been used to assess brain stem and higher central nervous system function in patients with various neurological disorders. In a detailed study of blink reflexes recorded in 260 patients with suspected multiple sclerosis (MS), Kimura (22) found that latency of the first component was prolonged in one or both sides in 66% of the patients with a diagnosis of definite MS, 56% of the patients with "probable MS," and 29% of patients with "possible MS." The most significant finding was that 40% of the patients with no clinical signs of brain stem pathology showed abnormality of the first component. On the basis of these findings, Kimura (22) suggested that "the test can be used to document a clinically silent pontine lesion." However, it must be recognized that prolongation of the latency of the first component in the absence of involvement of the peripheral trigeminal or facial nerve does not necessarily localize the lesion to the pons. Nor can one conclude on the basis of abnormality of the second component with relatively well preserved first component that there is a lesion of the lateral medulla, as suggested by some authors (19). It has been shown that both components of the blink reflex can be altered under different physiological conditions, such as fear or apprehension (11), or sleep and wakefulness (15), as well as by various lesions of the central nervous system rostral to the pons (23). Thus, a prolongation of the latency of the first component may be seen on the involved side in patients during the early phase after a stroke due to a supratentorial lesion.

THE H REFLEX

Hoffman (24) demonstrated in 1918 that submaximal stimulation of the medial popliteal nerve evokes both early and late responses in the calf muscles. Magladery and McDougal (25) in the course of their reflex studies designated the first response the "M" wave and called the second response an "H" wave after Hoffman. A small late response which was observed in other muscles and evoked by supramaximal nerve stimulation was called the "F" wave. Subsequent studies by Magladery and his associates (26, 27) supported Hoffman's view that the H reflex was monosynaptic.

The H wave is easily evoked by percutaneous stimulation with brief electrical stimuli and has a threshold usually lower than that of the M wave (Fig. 11.2). As the stimulus intensity is increased, the amplitude of the H wave increases to a maximum and the M wave appears. An important characteristic of the H reflex response is that it declines as the stimulus is further increased and at the same time the M wave is augmented. The H wave disappears when maximal or supramaximal shocks for the M wave are used (Fig. 11.3). The reduction in the H wave is considered to be due to collision between antidromic and reflexly elicited orthodromic impulses in motor axons.

The reflex nature of the H wave is supported by the fact that the latency is increased if the stimulus site is moved distally. In addition, the response is blocked by ischemia produced proximal to the point of stimulation and also by spinal anesthesia. Although the reflex uses a portion of the neural

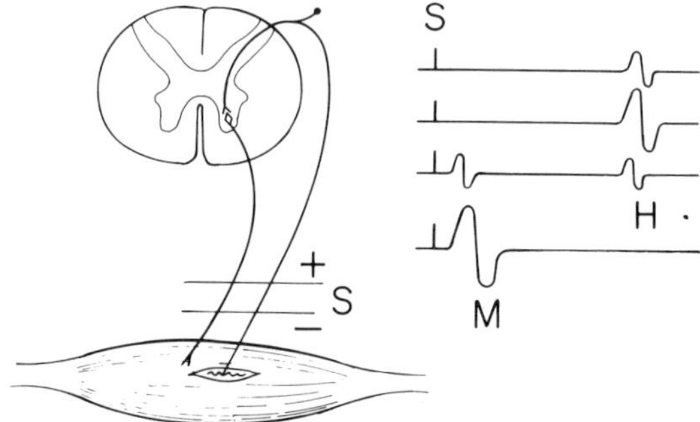

FIG. 11.2. A schematic drawing showing the application of the stimulus (*S*) to a mixed nerve and the response from the muscle. The H wave (*H*) appears, becomes maximum, and then disappears as the stimulus intensity is increased. The M wave (*M*) is maximum in the *bottom* recording.

pathway of the muscle stretch reflex, the two reflexes are not synonymous (28). In the H reflex the afferent fibers are stimulated directly and are free from any direct influence of the fusimotor system, whereas in the stretch reflex the stimulus arises from the muscle spindle receptors.

In normal adults, the H reflexes are commonly observed in the flexor carpi radialis muscle in the arm (29). This latter limitation is not generally accepted. Hohmann and Goodgold (30) reported that they found two normal subjects with unequivocal H waves in their anterior tibial muscles on stimulation of the common peroneal nerve, and Godaux and Desmedt (31) reported recording genuine H reflexes from the masseter muscle. In infants, a similar response was observed in the hand muscles with ulnar nerve stimulation (32), and, with aid of facilitation by active voluntary contration, an H reflex was recorded from the muscles of the hand in normal adults (33, 34). H reflexes can be modified or even induced in muscles when not present at rest. Hoffman (24) first, and others later on (35, 36) observed the inhibition of the H reflex in the calf muscles by contraction of antagonistic muscles. Agonist contraction consistently facilitated the H reflex in the calf muscles (37), and H reflexes have been found in the tibialis anterior muscles in the leg and the extensor digitorum communis muscle in the arm with contraction of the antagonistic calf and flexor carpi radialis muscles, respectively (38). Passive extension of the wrist also induced H reflexes in the extensor digitorum communis muscle (38).

In clinical neurophysiology, H reflex testing has been developed as a convenient method of estimating motor neuron excitability; however, its value in yielding reliable diagnostic data has been controversial. Van der Meulen, during a conference on control of movement and posture, remarked that the H reflex has been overinterpreted in both normal and pathological states (39). He noted that the H reflex activates less than 50% of the available

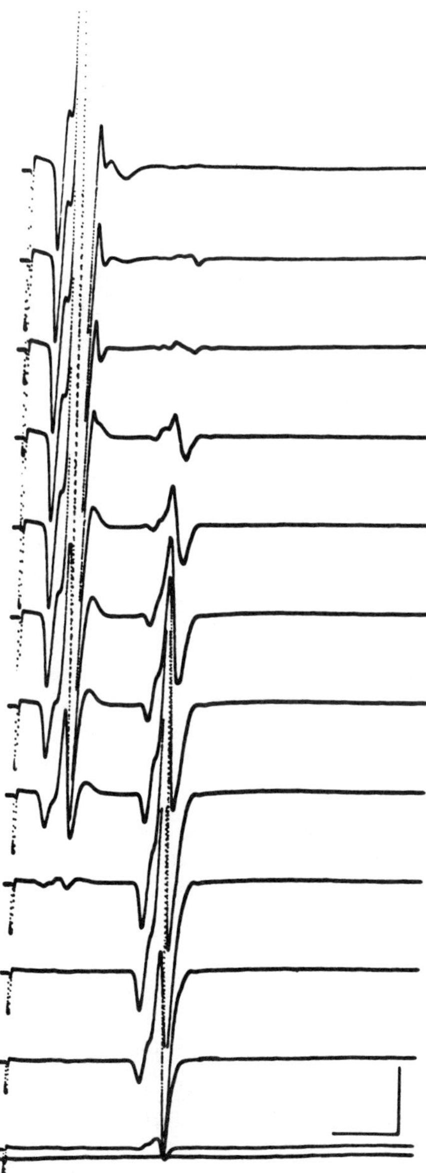

FIG. 11.3. M and H responses recorded from the soleus muscle after stimulation of the tibial nerve at the popliteal fossa. For each trace, the stimulus artifact is on the left followed by the M and H responses. The stimulus is shown decreasing in intensity from *top* to *bottom*. Calibration: horizontal, 10 msec per div; vertical, 1 mv per div.

motor unit pool and is not reproducible until at least a small M response has been elicited. Granit and Burke (39) pointed out that the H reflex, although strongly influenced by presynaptic inhibition, does not distinguish between pre- and postsynaptic inhibition, and that postsynaptic potentials produced by spindle primaries can be easily influenced by conductance changes from adjacent synapses activated by other unrelated input systems. The reflex is susceptible to inhibition and facilitation from many sources, such as active contraction or passive stretch of the calf muscles, contraction of the antagonists, and comfort and state of mind of the patient (35). Nevertheless, under controlled observations it is still possible to record a reproducible series of H reflexes within a reasonable variation. The problem, however, arises in the interpretation of the results.

Upper Motor Neuron Lesions

Because some variables affect both the H and M waves equally, Angel and Hofmann (40) calculated the ratio of the largest H and the largest M amplitudes and considered it to be a measure of that proportion of the motor neuron pool that can be reflexly excited. They found that the ratio was higher than normal in spasticity but unchanged in rigidity. In a recent study of 21 adolescents suffering from cerebral palsy presenting with spasticity of the lower limbs, the H/M ratios of both legs were increased; however, no correlation was found between this increase and the degree of clinical spasticity (41). McComas and Payan (42) demonstrated a reduction in the H/M ratio in patients with Holmes-Adie syndrome, and also showed that the ratio may be unity in healthy subjects, which indicates that the entire motor neuron pool may be excited by an adequate stimulus even without an upper motor neuron lesion. In addition, Matthews (43) demonstrated that intravenous injections of diazepam or chlorproethazine into spastic patients may reduce the size of the ankle jerk without altering the H/M ratio. Táboriková and Sax (44) claimed that the size of the motor neuron pool cannot be estimated from the H/M ratio because a stimulus adequate to elicit an H wave without an M wave may be insufficient to evoke a maximum response from the afferent fibers.

Magladery et al. (27) noted that if the H reflex is elicited by paired stimuli the amplitude varies according to the interval between the stimuli and the stimulus intensity. This method of examining the H reflex recovery cycle (Fig. 11.4), the period during which a test (second) reflex is influenced by a conditioning (first) reflex, was further elaborated by other investigators (45, 46) using identical pulses or pairs of unequal intensity. With identical near-threshold stimuli in normal subjects a low amplitude H reflex can be evoked with stimulus intervals between 5 and 8 msec (early facilitation) which gradually decays as the interval is increased to 20 msec. Between 20 and 80 msec, the reflex is completely inhibited (early depression), except for maxi-

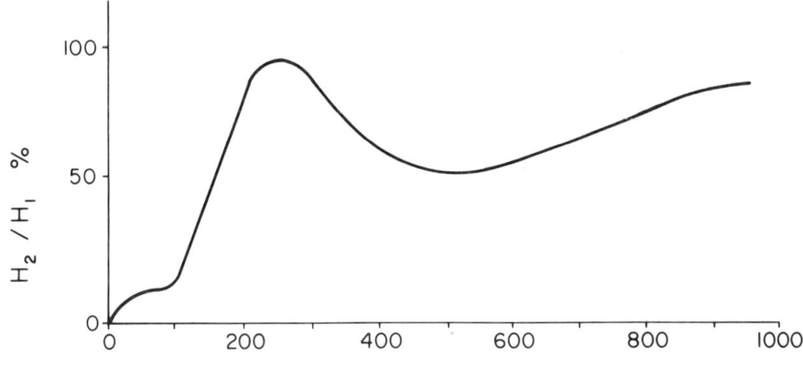

FIG. 11.4. Typical features of a H reflex recovery curve. The ratio of test to conditioning H reflex is plotted against stimulus intervals.

mal stimulation when inhibition is complete up to an interval of 40 msec. As the interval is increased further, the H wave increases (second facilitation) but is followed by a transient decline in amplitude between approximately 300 and 800 msec (late depression). A slow return to normal excitability is attained only with intervals longer than 2 sec.

Physiological explanations of the H reflex recovery cycle after paired stimuli have been controversial, in part because of the complicated interaction of many factors. The relative facilitation of the reflex for a stimulus interval about 200 msec has been attributed to the increased inflow from the spindles after lengthening of the muscle (47) and also to a spinobulbo spinal (long loop) reflex (46, 48). A recent study did not support the long loop reflex as producing the facilitation but instead suggested that it was due to an increase of the central excitatory state of the α-motor neurons during the period of the first subharmonic of the physiological tremor (49). Nevertheless, the H reflex recovery curve after paired stimuli has been used extensively in clinical studies.

Magladery and associates (27) found that the H reflex recovery curves of patients with any type of upper motor neuron lesion were shifted from the normal curve and indicated increased motor neuron excitability. Increased reflex activity has been confirmed in spasticity (45, 48) as well as in Parkinson's disease (50, 51). The H recovery curves approach a normal pattern and the increased excitability is reduced in patients with Parkinson's disease under prolonged treatment with levodopa (L-dopa) (50, 51). Miglietta (52) using paired stimuli, observed that facilitation of the H reflex response was absent in most patients with bilateral upper motor neuron disorders and also in a large number of hemiplegic patients. In many of the latter patients, facilitation was absent not only on the hemiplegic side but on the "normal" side as well. The results of a later study involving the determination of H/M and the H wave recovery curve in hemiplegic patients indicated that motor neuron excitability may be depressed in acute hemiplegia but enhanced in chronic hemiplegia, when the H reflex may also be evoked in the upper limbs.

The amplitude of the H reflex is severely decreased with increasing frequency of stimulation (53). With a stimulus frequency of 3 Hz or less there is no inhibition, but at 4 Hz the H amplitude is 30% of its maximum and at 15 Hz it is only 10% of its peak amplitude (36). The H wave of spinal cord injury patients displayed virtually no low frequency depression on days of diminished spasticity. On days of heightened spasticity H wave amplitude was low, and low frequency depression was evident. The results are compatible with the theory that low frequency depression is mediated by interneuronal circuitry, including possibly the Renshaw cell system (54). With the use of high frequency stimulation (1 to 60 Hz), differences in the frequency depression curves of the H reflexes were recognized in spasticity, rigidity, and cerebellar disturbances (55).

Computation of the H reflex recovery curves after paired stimuli is not routinely performed because the procedure is time consuming and the results have limited clinical usefulness. Computer analysis of the experimental data has been attempted (56), and one program optimally estimates the main feature of the H reflex recovery curve (57), but the fundamental problems of interpretation still remain.

As a new approach, potentiation of the H reflex in paretic muscles during the Jendrassik maneuver was attempted, but this also yielded inconsistent results. Buller (58) found that reinforcement of the H reflex was diminished or absent, whereas Landau and Clare (59) demonstrated that the H reflex could be enhanced provided that the stimulus was submaximal. In normal subjects, the maneuver caused a reduction in H reflex amplitude, and even in the same subject responses varied on different occasions (42). This uncertainty prevents the Jendrassik maneuver from becoming a useful test for the integrity of the descending pathways.

Root Compression Syndrome

Because the H reflex is most easily evoked in normal persons through the S_1 root reflex arc, a few attempts have been made to use it as a tool in detection of root compression syndrome. Drechsler et al. (60) found that the H reflex latency (soleus muscle) was significantly prolonged in both extremities in patients with L_5 and S_1 compression syndrome. In a series of 267 patients with clinical evidence of lumbar root lesions, Notermans and Vingerhoets (61) measured the time interval between the maximal M and H waves for the H reflex over the gastrocnemius and soleus muscles. Patients with a root compression of L_5 and S_1 had an H reflex interval which was more than 2 msec longer in the affected leg or much longer in both legs than the intervals of normal controls. The difference in the M-H interval between left and right legs measured over the same muscle in controls was never more than 1.0 msec.

Braddom and Johnson (62) described a convenient method of eliciting the H reflex and standarized it in 100 normal subjects. With stimulation of the tibial nerve in the midportion of the medial calf muscles, the mean H latency was 29.8 msec (SD = 2.74 msec). A formula for statistical prediction of the H reflex latency was developed that incorporated the simultaneous regression of the latency, leg length, and age on each other, and from this a nomogram was constructed for prediction of the latency in patients with known age and leg length. The H reflex duration and amplitude were less clinically useful than the H reflex latency because of their statistical variability and lack of correlation with age and leg length. In 25 patients with unilateral S_1 radiculopathy, the H reflex on the affected side was either delayed in latency or absent. A difference of 1.5 msec in the H reflex latency of both legs of the same patient was considered objective evidence of S_1 radiculopathy. The authors point out that careful technique and absence of marked leg length discrepancy are essential prerequisites for this to be a meaningful test.

Neuropathy

Magladery and McDougal (25) demonstrated that a sensory nerve conduction velocity could be determined by stimulating the tibial nerve at two locations and recording the latencies of the elicited H reflexes. Liberson (63) used this procedure to study sensory nerve conduction in patients with peripheral neuropathies and found that in some cases of diabetic and alcoholic neuropathy the conduction velocities were slower in the sensory than in the motor fibers.

In another study of peripheral neuropathy (64), the H reflex was absent or had a poor H/M ratio from the gastrocnemius muscle with a comparatively better ratio from the vastus medialis. More recently, Wager and Buerger (65) reported a linear relationship between H reflex latency (when the posterior tibial nerve was stimulated at the ankle) and sensory conduction velocity (calculated for the segment of the posterior tibial nerve between the ankle and the popliteal fossa). Five of 12 diabetic subjects with clinical evidence of neuropathy in the lower extremities had sensory nerve conduction velocities less than 35 m per sec and H reflex latencies greater than 60 msec.

Braddom and Johnson (62) point out that this method may be satisfactory in normal subjects, but that in patients with peripheral neuropathy the H reflex in the foot intrinsics becomes very small in amplitude. It thus becomes difficult to distinguish the H and F waves and measure accurately (even with averaging) the latency. The authors consider H reflex latency measurements to be less valuable clinically in the diagnosis of peripheral neuropathy than carefully performed conduction studies of afferent peripheral nerve fibers.

The F Wave

A potential of low amplitude and a latency greater than the direct motor response can be recorded from the small muscles in the hand or foot upon application of a supramaximal stimulus to a peripheral nerve. Although this was observed earlier by Hoffman (66), Dawson and Scott (67), and Kugelberg (68), it was Magladery and McDougal (25) who first designated this late response the "F" wave. The appellation was based on their recording of responses from "foot" muscles.

Physiology

The nature of the F wave has been a matter of dispute ever since Magladery and McDougal (25) suggested that it was a reflex response involving polysynaptic connections. Dawson and Merton (69), after finding that impulse conduction velocities in motor fibers were the same as those in F wave fibers when measured over long segments of the ulnar nerve, considered that the F wave was due to a small recurrent discharge of a few motor neurons produced by an antidromic volley in the motor fibers. Subsequently, Thorne (70) also obtained evidence that the response was the result of antidromic stimulation of alpha motor neurons. In studies of single motor units of normal subjects he found that those units appearing in the F wave were invariably present in the preceding M wave. Further support came from animal experiments. After section of the dorsal roots in the baboon (71), persistence of the F wave indicated an antidromic component. Similarly, Mayer and Feldman (72) examined a patient with chronic deafferentation of the left upper extremity and found that the response could still be elicited.

The latter concept appears to prevail at the present time, but it has also been suggested that F waves contain both monosynaptic reflex and recurrent responses as well as polysynaptic reflex responses (73). Evidence for this view was derived from cat experiments (74) which indicated that F waves were complex responses in which the contribution of the various components depended on the strength of stimulation and the excitability of the motor neurons. At the higher levels of stimulation, recurrent discharge of motor neurons is the most prominent component, whereas at submaximal stimulation the reflex components are most pronounced (73).

Most investigators today consider the F wave to be a recurrent discharge (or "backfiring") of alpha motor neurons activated by impulses traveling antidromically from the site of peripheral nerve stimulation. It is important to remember here that when a nerve is stimulated, action potentials propagate in both directions from the site of stimulation. Thus, the same alpha motor axon serves as both the afferent and efferent pathway for the F wave. It is not known why recurrent discharges occur, but of all the neurons stimulated, only about 5% are actually involved in the backfiring for an individual F wave (75).

F Wave and H Reflex

A common mistake among students and some investigators is to consider the F wave, like the H reflex, to be a reflex. This is not so. The H response is clearly a reflex involving an arc composed of Ia afferent fibers and efferent (alpha motor) fibers. In contrast, generation of an F wave does not require sensory fibers, only alpha motor axons.

There are several, easily recognized, differences between F wave and H reflex responses (76). The H response, elicited by stimulating the nerve submaximally, is high in amplitude (equal to or often greater than the M response) and is constant in latency, amplitude, and shape for each stimulus. In contrast, the F wave, observed when the stimulus is supramaximal, is small in amplitude (less than 10% of the maximum M amplitude), and the latency as well as the shape can vary from stimulus to stimulus. At times, the F response may not appear with each stimulus.

The F wave is not dependent on the frequency of stimulation, whereas the H reflex is suppressed with increasing frequency of stimulation. Another example of the difference between the two responses is seen in the effect of muscle contraction: agonist contraction consistently facilitates the H reflex recorded from the calf muscles, but the F wave may be inhibited (37).

Procedures

F wave detection and measurement have only recently become part of the routine electrodiagnostic examination. The hesitancy among investigators to employ the F wave as a diagnostic aid has been partly due to the considerable variability, especially the latency, of the response from stimulus to stimulus and to the uncertainty regarding its physiology, i.e., whether or not it is a reflex.

Although these problems still exist, the considerable number of studies published in the last 5 years on physiology and clinical application have increased our knowledge to a point where a workable routine has been established. Actually, the same procedure employed to measure nerve conduction velocity is used to detect F waves—same placement of electrodes and supramaximal stimulation. The difference is in the oscilloscope sweep time used to visualize the late responses; the sweep should be adjusted so that potentials occurring about 25 to 50 msec after the M response can be seen. The latency of the F wave is measured from the onset of the stimulus artifact to the onset of the F wave.

F waves can be found in any muscle, and the stimulus may be applied at any point along the nerve. The basic routine usually involves recording F waves from the median and ulnar nerves with stimulation at the wrist or elbow, and from the tibial and peroneal nerves with stimulation at the ankle or knee. Stimulation of the nerves as proximal as the axilla has been used to evoke an F wave, but there were some difficulties: (a) the high stimulation intensity may simultaneously activate both median and ulnar nerves, and (b) the F wave often is hidden in the terminal portion of the M wave (77, 78). The collision technique was used to separate the two potentials in the latter recording (78).

Most investigators record at least 10 F waves at one stimulus site and measure the shortest latency for all the responses. This is the most consistent measure of the various latencies and is assumed to represent the fastest conducting motor fibers.

The variation in F wave latencies is considered to be due to the different motor units, each with its own axon diameter and conduction velocity, activated by each stimulus. Trontelj and Stålberg (79) demonstrated with single fiber electromyography that there is very little variation in latency of successive F waves recorded from one motor unit. With our present limited knowledge, it is impossible to know whether a specific F wave is conducted along a small diameter (slow conducting) or a large diameter (fast conducting) nerve fiber. It is assumed that the F wave with the shortest latency is conducted along the largest diameter motor fibers. It should be remembered that the beginning of the M response represents the activity of the fastest conducting motor fibers.

The latencies of the F and M responses vary inversely as the stimulating electrode is moved proximally: the F wave latency decreases but the M latency increases. This, of course, follows from the fact that the latency of the F wave includes the conduction time of the motor impulse *to* the spinal cord from the stimulation site and *from* the spinal cord to the muscle. A sample of some typical values (mean latency ± SD) illustrates this difference:

Nerve	*M Wave Latency (msec)*	*F Wave Latency (msec)*
Ulnar		
Wrist	3.4 ± 0.3	31.7 ± 1.8
Below elbow	5.8 ± 0.5	29.2 ± 2.4
Above elbow	7.8 ± 0.6	27.2 ± 2.4
Tibial		
Ankle	4.3 ± 0.7	43.5 ± 3.0
Knee	12.6 ± 0.9	35.4 ± 3.1

In addition to measurements of latency, some investigators have applied the F wave procedure to calculate the conduction velocity in the proximal segments of a motor nerve. This calculation is highly controversial and has been called "not only unnecessary but inaccurate" (80) by its detractors, and "reasonably accurate" (81) by its defenders. The problem stems from the assumptions that must be made regarding the time interval as well as errors in measurement of proximal length.

Conduction velocity is calculated by dividing the time it takes for an impulse to propagate a known distance into that distance. For the F wave conduction velocity, the time interval is calculated in the following manner: The difference in latency between the M response and F wave is the time it takes the impulse to travel to the spinal cord from the site of stimulation and back to that point. A delay or "turnaround" time at the spinal cord motor neuron pool is taken to be 1 msec. Thus, the latency for the proximal segment of the nerve (site of stimulation to spinal cord) may be calculated from the expression: $(F\text{-}M\text{-}1)/2$, where F is the F wave latency, M is the M wave latency, and 1 represents the 1-msec delay (82).

The proximal distances are obtained as follows: For median and ulnar nerves from elbow to spinal cord, surface distance is measured from C_7 spinous process via the axilla and midclavicular point (77, 78); for tibial and peroneal nerve segments, distance is measured from knee to lower border of T_{12} spinous process via greater trochanter of the femur (83, 84).

The conduction velocity in the proximal segment (FWCV) can, thereby, be calculated from the computed proximal latency time and the measured proximal length.

Kimura et al. (82) published values of FWCV obtained in their laboratory. The conduction velocity in the cord-to-elbow segment of the median and ulnar nerves is considered slow if it is less than 50 m per sec (77), whereas motor nerve conduction velocity is slow if it is less than 46 m per sec across the elbow or in the more distal segment. The FWCV in the cord-to-knee segment in peroneal and tibial nerves is considered slow if it is less than 45 m per sec; the motor nerve velocity is slow if it is less than 40 m per sec in the knee-to-ankle segment (83).

Other calculations have been proposed in order to increase the diagnostic yield of F wave determinations. Eisen et al. (85, 86) considered a direct comparison of the M latency vs. the F latency to be the best indication of proximal disease. Kimura and his colleagues (82) also found a direct comparison between F and M responses very useful; but, instead of using F latency, they calculated the proximal conduction time (time from site of stimulation to spinal cord). They defined the F ratio as equal to $(F\text{-}M\text{-}1)/2M$.

Panayiotopoulos (87) has noted that in healthy individuals the latency differences of consecutive F waves may have a limited range because the axons have a limited range of motor nerve conduction velocities. However, in abnormal nerves where some motor axons may be more involved than others, a larger range of conduction velocities may be observed. The term *F chronodispersion* was introduced to denote the dispersion of the relative latencies of statistically significant number of consecutively recorded F waves.

He found that F chronodispersion of the deep peroneal nerve did not exceed 7.5 msec in healthy subjects, while it was greater in uremic patients.

Clinical Value and Findings

Although there may be some uncertainty regarding the clinical usefulness of the F wave conduction velocity determination, there is no disagreement on the value of routine F wave latency measurements. This is especially true since very little extra effort is required to observe the F response during a conventional nerve conduction measurement. Since supramaximal stimulation is already applied, only adjustments in gain and sweep time are necessary to detect the late responses.

The purpose of the F wave determination is to assess the proximal segment of alpha motor axons in upper and lower limbs which are not normally obtainable with conventional nerve conduction measurements. Its use in the clinical examination is relatively new, and the most useful and accurate parameters still remain to be defined. Future studies may demonstrate a utility that is only suggested today: that F waves can be employed in the analysis of central nervous system function (88).

F wave measurements demonstrated slow motor conduction in the Guillain-Barré syndrome (84). Average F ratios within normal limits in this disorder indicated an equal slowing of nerve conduction between proximal and distal segments. In diabetic patients, F wave latencies were increased and conduction velocity decreased for both proximal and distal segments (82, 89). The F ratio results suggest that motor conduction abnormalities in diabetic polyneuropathy are more intense in the distal than in the proximal segments (82).

Severe slowing in both proximal and distal nerve segments was found in Charcot-Marie-Tooth disease (77, 90). F wave determinations have also revealed slow conduction in myotonic dystrophy (90), amyotrophic lateral sclerosis (91), chronic renal failure (92), and alcoholism (93). F responses may be diminished or absent in the first few days after a stroke (88).

Kimura (81) has pointed out that F wave latencies and FWCV are often normal in patients with clinically positive cases of brachial or lumbosacral plexus neuropathy, but at times a delay in the latency may be the only abnormality in these disorders.

THE TONIC VIBRATION REFLEX (TVR)

The response to a tendon tap is well known: a slight extension of the muscle and spindle stretch receptors, a synchronous discharge of the primary endings of the spindles, stimulation and discharge of the motor neurons, quick reflex contraction of the muscle. In contrast, a steady mechanical vibration applied to the muscle belly or tendon elicits an involuntary tonic reflex contraction of the muscle and reciprocal relaxation of its antagonists. The tonic contraction is induced by selective excitation of the primary endings of the muscle spindles, which are extremely sensitive to vibration and can be observed in both upper and lower extremities when a vibrator is applied to either flexor or extensor tendons. This phenomenon, named the tonic vibration reflex by Eklund and Hagbarth (94), in many respects simulates a tonic stretch reflex normally operating during voluntary isometric contraction.

Brown et al. (95) demonstrated that virtually all of the spindle primary endings in the cat soleus muscle can be selectively excited by a high frequency, low amplitude vibration applied longitudinally to the soleus tendon. In man, selective stimulation of the spindle primaries is not possible, and the parameters of the vibrator stimulus must be carefully chosen to minimize spread of the stimulus to the antagonist muscles as well as to reduce involvement of secondary endings and Golgi tendon organs. A vibratory stimulus within the range of 100 to 200 Hz and an amplitude of 1 to 2 mm applied to the tendon has been shown to be most appropriate in man. A small vibrator oscillating at about 150 Hz with an amplitude of 1.5 mm can easily be assembled from a compact cylindrical DC motor equipped with an appropriately large eccentric on the axis and attached with rubber straps over the muscle tendons (96). The response to stimulation can be measured by recording the mechanical tension and the electrical activity developed by the muscles.

The TVR in a normal subject develops after a short latency after onset of vibration and then slowly increases over the next 15 to 30 sec before reaching a plateau. The tonic contraction persists as long as the vibration is maintained. Occasionally, the tonic contraction is preceded by a phasic spike which has been attributed to a vibration-induced equivalent of the tendon jerk (97). The amplitude of the TVR response is a fraction of that developed during a maximal voluntary effort. It can be augmented by reinforcement, for example, using the Jendrassik maneuver or pinna twist. The application of one vibrator to the tendon and one to the muscle belly evokes a stronger reflex contraction than does the application of either one alone (97).

The TVR in normal man can be increased in amplitude by a preceding tetanic stimulation of the muscle nerve, lengthening of the muscle, or cooling of the subject. Tonic neck reflexes and tonic vestibular reflexes can also influence the TVR (94). Suppression of the vibration reflex is observed when the subject is warmed (94) or after administration of drugs such as barbiturates and diazepam (98), and is diminished or absent in patients with damage to the spinal cord. It is noted by Hagbarth (99) that many of the procedures which affect the intensity of the TVR do not alter the response to tendon taps, indicating that the TVR can provide a better index of muscle tone than do phasic myotatic reflexes.

Both the phasic stretch reflex and the H reflex are suppressed during muscle vibration (94, 98, 100). Two explanations have been proposed to account for this suppression: (a) the Ia axons are so busy with impulses initiated by the vibratory stimulus that they are not able to respond to a transient superimposed tendon tap or electric shock—the "busy line" phenomenon (99); and (b) the vibration-induced afferent impulses cause spinal presynaptic inhibition of the Ia afferent terminals (101).

The potentiation of the vibration-induced tonic contraction after a tetanus indicates that the response is mediated at least partially through a monosynaptic reflex. However, it is apparent that the TVR is also dependent upon supraspinal centers for its development. The exact nature of the involvement of the higher centers has been the subject of considerable animal experimentation, especially in the cat. Matthews (102) found that the TVR was present in the decerebrate cat but was abolished by section of the spinal cord at the first cervical segment, demonstrating its dependence on brain stem structures. Gillies et al. (103) observed that the TVR was not affected by section of the dorsal quadrant of the spinal cord but was reduced to 20 to 40% of the control level by a discrete lesion in the ventral column of the cervical spinal cord. The TVR in the cat can be inhibited by stimulation of the contralateral motor cortex, internal capsule, and medial medullary reticular formation. It is facilitated by the lateral vestibular nucleus and vestibulospinal tract, the lateral medullary reticular formation, and the contralateral red nucleus (101). The TVR primarily involves impulses ascending in the dorsal spinocerebellar tract and dorsolateral fasciculus and descending in the vestibulospinal and pontine reticulospinal tracts.

The TVR in Specific Motor Disorders

Spasticity

The TVR may be evoked in spastic patients, but it is lower in amplitude and more abrupt in onset and cessation than in normal individuals (104, 105). In addition, in many spastic patients the vibration reflexes extend to functionally allied muscles acting at neighboring joints, a response which is not obtained in normal subjects. For example, vibration applied to the volar side of the wrist may produce flexion and pronation of movement of the hand in hemiplegic patients as well as elbow flexion and adduction of the whole arm (104).

Vibratory suppression of the tendon jerk and H reflexes of spastic patients is considerably less than in normal subjects. In moderate to severe spasticity, vibration diminishes the TVR by less than 30%, suggesting that the presynaptic inhibitory mechanisms, deprived of supraspinal support, are suppressed in spasticity (101). Another common finding is that vibration potentiates or reduces voluntary power and range of movement depending upon whether the subject tries to contract the muscle vibrated or its antagonist. Thus, in some patients with pronounced weakness and weak or absent TVR the combined effect of vibration and voluntary effort can result in powerful muscle contractions. Potentiation of the active range of motion depends in part upon reciprocal inhibition of antagonistic spastic resistance obtained with the vibration (104). In some patients with spastic hemiplegia, vibratory stimulation can considerably increase the range of motion. Attempts have been made to develop vibrators automatically controlled by myoelectric potentials to assist specific movement patterns in these patients (106).

Parkinson's Disease

The TVR in the rigid muscles of patients with Parkinson's disease does not differ significantly from that of normal muscles (97, 104).

Cerebellar Disorders

The TVR is reduced or absent in patients with cerebellar disease (98, 104).

Spinal Cord Lesions

The TVR is absent in patients with complete spinal transection. From studies in the cat (103), the abolition of the TVR appears to be due to severance of the vestibulospinal and pontine reticulospinal pathways in the anterior column of the spinal cord. Flexor spasms could be induced by vibration in patients with complete or incomplete spinal lesions; however, they may have been caused by cutaneous stimulation (97).

Burke et al. (97) could not demonstrate any relationship between the shape of the TVR and the site of the lesion in the central nervous system. In hemiplegic spasticity, the reflex was essentially similar to that recorded in patients with spinal lesions, but on the clinically normal side of such patients, the TVR appeared to be of normal configuration.

REFERENCES

1. Overend, W.: Preliminary note on a new cranial reflex. Lancet, *1:* 619, 1896.
2. Wartenberg, R.: *The Examination of Reflexes: A Simplification.* Year Book Medical Publishers, Chicago, 1945.
3. Kugelberg, E.: Facial reflexes. Brain, *75:* 385–396, 1952.
4. Rushworth, G.: Observations on blink reflexes. J. Neurol. Neurosurg. Psychiatry, *25:* 93–108, 1962.
5. Gandiglio, G., and Fra, L.: Further observations on facial reflexes. J. Neurol. Sci., *5:* 273–285, 1967.
6. Kadanoff, D.: Die sensible Nervenendigungen in der mimischen Muskulatur des Menschen. Z. Mikrosk. Anat. Forsch., *62:* 1–15, 1956.
7. Bowden, R. E. M., and Mahran, Z. Y.: The functional significance of the pattern of

innervation of the muscle quadratus labii superioris of the rabbit, cat and rat. J. Anat., *90:* 217–227, 1956.

8. Bruesch, S. R.: The distribution of myelinated afferent fibres in the branches of the cat's facial nerve. J. Comp. Neurol., *81:* 169–191, 1944.
9. Shahani, B. T., and Young, R. R.: A note on blink reflexes. J. Physiol. (Lond.), *198:* 103–104, 1968.
10. Shahani, B. T., and Young, R. R.: Human flexor reflexes. J. Neurol. Neurosurg. Psychiatry, *34:* 616–627, 1971.
11. Shahani, B. T., and Young, R. R.: Human orbicularis oculi reflexes. Neurology, *22:* 149–154, 1972.
12. Penders, C. A., and Delwaide, P. J.: Physiologic approach to the human blink reflex. In *New Developments in EMG and Clinical Neurophysiology*, edited by J. E. Desmedt, vol. 3, pp. 538–549. Karger, Basel, 1973.
13. Lindquist, C., and Mortensson, A.: Mechanisms involved in the cat's blink reflex. Acta Physiol. Scand., *80:* 149–159, 1970.
14. Shahani, B. T., and Young, R. R.: The cutaneous nature of the first component of the monkey's blink reflex. Neurology, *22:* 438, 1972.
15. Shahani, B. T.: Effects of sleep on human reflexes with a double component. J. Neurol. Neurosurg. Psychiatry, *31:* 574–579, 1968.
16. Shahani, B. T.: The human blink reflex. J. Neurol. Neurosurg. Psychiatry, *33:* 792–800, 1970.
17. Shahani, B. T., and Young, R. R.: Blink reflexes in orbicularis oculi. In *New Developments in EMG and Clinical Neurophysiology*, edited by J. E. Desmedt, vol. 3, pp. 641–648. Karger, Basel, 1973.
18. Shahani, B. T., Burrows, P., and Whitty, C. W. M.: The grasp reflex and perseveration. Brain, *93:* 181–192, 1970.
19. Kimura, J., and Lyon, L. W.: Orbicularis oculi reflex in the Wallenberg syndrome: Alteration of the late reflex by lesions of the spinal tract and nucleus of the trigeminal nerve. J. Neurol. Neurosurg. Psychiatry, *35:* 228–233, 1972.
20. Kimura, J., Giron, L. T., and Young, S. M.: Electrophysiological study of Bell palsy—electrically elicited blink reflex in assessment of prognosis. Arch. Otolaryngol., *102:* 140–143, 1976.
21. Eisen, A., and Danon, J.: The orbicularis oculi reflex in acoustic neuromas: A clinical and electrodiagnostic evaluation. Neurology, *24:* 306–311, 1974.
22. Kimura, J.: Electrically elicited blink reflex in diagnosis of multiple sclerosis—review of 260 patients over a seven year period. Brain, *98:* 413–426, 1975.
23. Fisher, M. A., Shahani, B. T., and Young, R. R.: Quantitative assessment of excitability at segmental levels of the central nervous system caudal to acute lesions. Neurology, *26:* 366–367, 1976.
24. Hoffman, P.: Über die Beziehungen der Sehnenreflexe zur illkürlichen Bewegung und zum Tonus. Z. Biol., *68:* 351–370, 1918.
25. Magladery, J. W., and McDougal, D. B., Jr.: Electrophysiological studies of nerve and reflex activity in normal man. I. Identification of certain reflexes in the electromyogram and the conduction velocity of peripheral nerve fibres. Bull. Johns Hopkins Hosp., *88:* 265–290, 1950.
26. Magladery, J. W., Porter, W. E., Park, A. M., and Teasdall, R. D.: Electrophysiological studies of nerve and reflex activity in normal man. IV. The two-neurone reflex and identification of certain action potentials from spinal roots and cord. Bull. Johns Hopkins Hosp., *88:* 499–519, 1951.
27. Magladery, R. D., Teasdall, A. M., Park, A. M., and Languth, H. W.: Electrophysiological studies of reflex activity in patients with lesions of the nervous system. I. Comparison of spinal motoneurone excitability following afferent nerve volleys in normal persons and patients with upper motor neurone lesions. Bull. Johns Hopkins Hosp., *91:* 219–244, 1952.
28. Herman, R.: Relationship between the H reflex and the tendon jerk response. Electromyography, *9:* 359–370, 1969.
29. DeSchuytere, J., Rosselle, N., and DeKeyser, C.: Monosynaptic reflexes in man and their

clinical significance. J. Neurol. Neurosurg. Psychiatry, *39:* 555–565, 1976.
30. Hohmann, T. C., and Goodgold, J.: Study of abnormal reflex patterns in spasticity. Am. J. Phys. Med., *40:* 52–55, 1961.
31. Godaux, E., and Desmedt, J. E.: Human masseter muscle: H and tendon reflexes. Arch. Neurol., *32:* 229–234, 1975.
32. Thomas, J. E., and Lambert, E. H.: Ulnar nerve conduction velocity and H reflex in infants and children. J. Appl. Physiol., *15:* 1–9, 1960.
33. Hagbarth, K. E.: Post-tetanic potentiation of myotatic reflexes in man. J. Neurol. Neurosurg. Psychiatry, *25:* 1–10, 1962.
34. Upton, A. R. M., McComas, A. J., and Sica, R. E. P.: Potentiation of "late" responses evoked in muscles during effort. J. Neurol. Neurosurg. Psychiatry, *34:* 699–711, 1971.
35. Mayer, R. F., and Mawdsley, C.: Studies in man and cat of the significance of the H reflex. J. Neurol. Neurosurg. Psychiatry, *28:* 201–211, 1965.
36 Gottlieb, G. L., and Agarwal, G. C.: Effects of initial conditions on Hoffmann reflex. J. Neurol. Neurosurg. Psychiatry, *34:* 226–230, 1971.
37. Fisher, M. A.: Relative changes with contraction in the central excitability state of the tibialis anterior and calf muscles. J. Neurol. Neurosurg. Psychiatry, *43:* 243–247, 1980.
38. Garcia, H. A., Fisher, M. A., and Gilai, A.: H reflex analysis of segmental reflex excitability in flexor and extensor muscles. Neurology, *29:* 984–991, 1979.
39. Granit, R., and Burke, R. E.: The control of movement and posture. Brain Res., *53:* 1–28, 1973.
40. Angel, R. W., and Hofmann, W. W.: The H reflex in normal, spastic and rigid subjects. Arch. Neurol., *8:* 591–596, 1963.
41. Spira, R.: Contribution of the H reflex to the study of spasticity in adolescents. Dev. Med. Child Neurol., *16:* 150–157, 1974.
42. McComas, A. J., and Payan, J.: Motoneurone excitability in the Holmes-Adie syndrome. In *Control and Innervation of Skeletal Muscle: A Symposium*, edited by B. L. Andrew, pp. 182–193. Livingstone, Edinburgh, 1966.
43. Matthews, W. B.: Ratio of maximum H reflex to maximum M response as a measure of spasticity. J Neurol. Neurosurg. Psychiatry, *29:* 201–204, 1966.
44. Táboriková, H., and Sax, D. S.: Motoneurone pool and the H reflex. J. Neurol. Neurosurg. Psychiatry, *31:* 354–361, 1968.
45. Olsen, P. Z., and Diamantopoulos, E.: Excitability of spinal motor neurones in normal subjects and patients with spasticity, Parkinsonian rigidity, and cerebellar hypotonia. J. Neurol. Neurosurg. Psychiatry, *30:* 325–335, 1967.
46. Táboriková, H., and Sax, D. S.: Conditioning of H-reflexes by a preceding subthreshold H-reflex stimulus. Brain, *92:* 203–212, 1969.
47. Paillard, J.: Functional organization of afferent innervation of muscle studied in man by monosynaptic testing. Am. J. Phys. Med., *38:* 239–247, 1959.
48. Yap, C.: Spinal segmental and long-loop reflexes in spinal motoneurone excitability in spasticity and rigidity. Brain, *90:* 203–212, 1969.
49. Masland, W. S.: Facilitation during H reflex recovery cycle. Arch Neurol., *26:* 313–319, 1972.
50. Fujita, S., and Cooper, I. S.: Effects of *l*-dopa on the H reflex in parkinsonism. J. Am. Geriatr. Soc., *19:* 289–295, 1971.
51. McLeod, J. G., and Walsh, J. C.: H reflex studies in patients with Parkinson's disease. J. Neurol. Neurosurg. Psychiatry, *35:* 77–80, 1972.
52. Miglietta, O.: Spinal motoneuron excitability in normal subjects and hemiplegic patients. Arch. Phys. Med. Rehabil., *51:* 696–701, 1970.
53. Cook, W. A., Jr.: Effects of low frequency stimulation on the monosynaptic reflex (H reflex) in man. Neurology, *18:* 47–51, 1968.
54. Ishikawa, K., Ott, K., Porter, R. W., and Stuart, D.: Low frequency depression of H wave in normal and spinal man. Exp Neurol., *15:* 140–156, 1966.
55. Ioku, M., Nakatani, S., Oku, Y., and Jinnai, D.: H-reflex study with high frequency stimulation. Electromyography, *9:* 219–227, 1969.
56. Matsuoka, S., Waltz, J. M., Terada, E., Ikeda, T., and Cooper, I. S.: A computer technique for evaluation of recovery cycle of the H reflex in the abnormal movement disorders.

Electroencephalogr. Clin. Neurophysiol., *21:* 496–500, 1966.
57. Johnson, T. L., Sax, D. S., and Feldman, R. G.: A technique for feature extraction and interpatient comparison of H-reflex conditioning curves. Electroencephalogr. Clin. Neurophysiol., *37:* 188–190, 1974.
58. Buller, A. J.: The ankle-jerk in early hemiplegia. Lancet, *2:* 1262–1263, 1957.
59. Landau, W. M., and Clare, M. H.: Fusimotor function. Part VI. Reflex, tendon jerk, and reinforcement in hemiplegia. Arch. Neurol., *10:* 128–134, 1964.
60. Drechsler, B., Lastovka, M., and Kalvodova, E.: Electrophysiological study of patients with herniated intervertebral disc. Electromyography, *6:* 187–204, 1966.
61. Notermans, S. L. H., and Vingerhoets, H. M.: The importance of the Hoffmann-reflex in the diagnosis of lumbar root lesions. Clin. Neurol. Neurosurg., *1:* 54–65, 1974.
62. Braddom, R. L., and Johnson, E. W.: H reflex: Review and classification with suggested clinical uses. Arch. Phys. Med. Rehabil., *55:* 412–417, 1974.
63. Liberson, W. T.: Sensory conduction velocities in normal individuals and in patients with peripheral neuropathies. Arch. Phys. Med. Rehabil., *44:* 313–320, 1963.
64. Mongia, S. K.: Significance of certain evoked responses in cases of neurogenic disorders. Electroencephalogr. Clin. Neurophysiol., *12:* 191–211, 1972.
65. Wager, E. W., Jr., and Buerger, A. A.: A linear relationship between H-reflex latency and sensory conduction velocity in diabetic neuropathy. Neurology, *24:* 711–714, 1974.
66. Hoffman, P.: *Untersuchungen uber die Eigenreflexe (Sehnenreflexe) Menschlicher Muskeln.* J. Springer, Berlin, 1922.
67. Dawson, G. D., and Scott, J. W.: Recording of nerve action potentials shrough skin in man. J. Neurol. Neurosurg. Psychiatry, *12:* 259–267, 1949.
68. Kugelberg, E.: "Injury activity" and "trigger zones" in human nerves. Brain, *69:* 310–324, 1946.
69. Dawson, G. D., and Merton, P. A.: "Recurrent" discharges from motoneurones. In *XXth International Physiological Congress, Brussels, 1956: Abstracts of Communications*, pp. 221–222. St. Catherine Press, Brussels, 1956.
70. Thorne, J.: Central responses to electrical activation of the peripheral nerves supplying the intrinsic hand muscles. J. Neurol. Neurosurg. Psychiatry, *28:* 482–495, 1965.
71. McLeod, J. G., and Wray, S. H.: An experimental study of the F wave in the baboon. J. Neurol. Neurosurg. Psychiatry, *29:* 196–200, 1966.
72. Mayer, R. F., and Feldman, R. G.: Observations on the nature of the F wave in man. Neurology, *17:* 147–156, 1967.
73. Gassel, M. M.: Monosynaptic reflexes (H reflex) and motoneurone excitability in man. Dev. Med. Child Neurol., *11:* 193–197, 1969.
74. Gassel, M. M., and Wiesendanger, M.: Recurrent and reflex discharges in plantar muscles of the cat. Acta Physiol. Scand., *65:* 138–142, 1965.
75. Fullerton, P., and Gilliatt, R.: Axon reflexes in human motor nerve fibers. J. Neurol. Neurosurg. Psychiatry, *28:* 1–11, 1965.
76. Shahani, B. T., and Young, R. R.: Effect of vibration on the F response. In *The Motor System: Neurophysiology and Muscle Mechanisms*, edited by M. Shahani, pp. 189–195. Elsevier Scientific Publishing Co., Amsterdam, 1976.
77. Kimura, J.: F-wave velocity in the central segment of the median and ulnar nerves: A study in normal subjects and in patients with Charcot-Marie-Tooth disease. Neurology, *24:* 539–546, 1974.
78. Kimura, J., and Butzer, J. F.: F-wave conduction velocity in the Guillain-Barré syndrome: Assessment of nerve segment between axilla and spinal cord. Arch. Neurol., *32:* 524–529, 1975.
79. Trontelj, J. V., and Stålberg, E.: A study of the F response by single fibre electromyography. In *New Developments in Electromyography and Clinical Neurophysiology*, edited by F. E. Desmedt, vol. 3, pp. 318–322. Karger, Basel, 1973.
80. Young, R. R., and Shahani, B. T.: Clinical value and limitations of F-wave determination. Muscle Nerve, *1:* 248–249, 1978.
81. Kimura, J.: A comment on clinical value and limitations of F-wave determination. Muscle Nerve, *1:* 250–252, 1978.
82. Kimura, J., Yamada, T., and Stevland, N. P.: Distal slowing of motor nerve conduction velocity in diabetic polyneuropathy. J. Neurol. Sci., *42:* 291–302, 1979.

83. Kimura, J., Bosch, P., and Lindsay, G. M.: F wave conduction velocity in the central segment of the peroneal and tibial nerves. Arch. Phys. Med., *56:* 492–497, 1975.
84. Kimura, J.: Proximal versus distal slowing of motor nerve conduction velocity in the Guillain-Barré syndrome. Ann. Neurol., *3:* 344–350, 1978.
85. Eisen, A., Schomer, D., and Melmed, C.: The application of F-wave measurements in the differentiation of proximal and distal upper limb entrapments. Neurology, *27:* 662–678, 1977.
86. Eisen, A., Schomer, D., and Melmed, C.: An electrophysiological method for examining lumbosacral root compression. Can. J. Neurol. Sci., *4:* 117–123, 1977.
87. Panayiotopoulos, C. P.: F Chronodispersion: A new electrophysiologic method. Muscle Nerve, *2:* 68–72, 1979.
88. Fisher, M. A., Shahani, B. T., and Young, R. R.: Assessing segmental excitability after acute rostral lesions. Neurology, *28:* 1265–1271, 1978.
89. Panayiotopoulos, C. P., Scarpalezos, S., and Nastas, P. E.: Sensory (1a) and F-wave conduction velocity in the proximal segment of the tibial nerve. Muscle Nerve, *1:* 181–189, 1978.
90. Panayiotopoulos, C. P.: F-wave conduction velocity in the deep peroneal nerve: Charcot-Marie-Tooth disease and dystrophia myotonia. Muscle Nerve, *1:* 37–44, 1978.
91. Argyropoulos, C. J., Panayiotopoulos, C. P., and Scarpalezos, S.: F and M wave conduction velocity in amyotrophic lateral sclerosis. Muscle Nerve, *1:* 470–485, 1979.
92. Panayiotopoulos, C. P., and Scarpalezos, S.: F-wave studies on the deep peroneal nerve. Part 2-1. Chronic renal failure. 2. Limb-girdle muscular dystrophy. J. Neurol. Sci., *31:* 331–341, 1977.
93. D'Amour, M. L., Shahani, B. T., Young, R. R., and Bird, K. T.: The importance of studying sural nerve conduction and late responses in alcoholic subjects. Neurology, *29:* 1600–1604, 1979.
94. Eklund, G., and Hagbarth, K. E.: Normal variability of tonic vibration reflexes in man. Exp. Neurol., *16:* 80–92, 1966.
95. Brown, M. C., Engberg, I. and Matthews, P. B. C.: The relative sensitivity to vibration of muscle receptors of the cat. J. Physiol., *192:* 773–800, 1967.
96. Eklund, G.: Some physical properties of muscle vibrators used to elicit tonic proprioceptive reflexes in man. Acta Soc. Med. Uppsala, *76:* 271–280, 1971.
97. Burke, D., Andrews, C. J., and Lance, J. W.: Tonic vibration reflex in spasticity, Parkinson's disease, and normal subjects. J. Neurol. Neurosurg. Psychiatry, *35:* 477–486, 1972.
98. Lance, J. W., Gail, P. De, and Neilson, P. D.: Tonic and phasic spinal cord mechanisms in man. J. Neurol. Neurosurg. Psychiatry, *29:* 535–544, 1966.
99. Hagbarth, K. E.: The effect of muscle vibration in normal man and in patients with motor disorders. In *New Developments in Electromyography and Clinical Neurophysiology*, edited by J. E. Desmedt, vol. 3, pp. 428–443. Karger, Basel, 1973.
100. Arcangel, C. S., Johnston, R., and Bishop, B.: The Achilles tendon reflex and the H response during and after tendon vibration. Phys. Ther., *51:* 889–902, 1971.
101. Lance, J. W., Burke, D., and Andrews, C. J.: The reflex effects of muscle vibration. In *New Developments in Electromyography and Clinical Neurophysiology*, edited by J. E. Desmedt, vol. 3, pp. 444–462, Karger, Basel, 1973.
102. Matthews, P. B. C.: The reflex excitation of the soleus muscle of the decerebrate cat caused by vibration applied to its tendon. J. Physiol., *184:* 450–472, 1966.
103. Gillies, J. D., Burke, D., and Lance, J. W.: Supraspinal control of tonic vibration reflex. J. Neurophysiol., *34:* 302–309, 1971.
104. Hagbarth, K. E., and Eklund, G.: The effects of muscle vibration in spasticity, rigidity and cerebellar disorders. J. Neurol. Neurosurg. Psychiatry, *31:* 207–213, 1968.
105. Gail, P. De, Lance, J. W., and Neilson, P. D.: Differential effects on tonic and phasic reflex mechanisms produced by vibration of muscles in man. J. Neurol. Neurosurg. Psychiatry, *29:* 1–11, 1966.
106. Hedberg, Å., Oldberg, B., and Tove, P. A.: EMG-controlled muscle vibrators to aid mobility in spastic paresis. In *7th International Conference on Medical and Biological Engineering*, edited by B. Jacobson, p. 197. Almqvist & Wiksell, Stockholm, 1967.

chapter 12

Somatosensory Evoked Potentials*

Recording somatosensory evoked potentials (SEP's) provides noninvasive methods for the evaluation of the nervous system from peripheral receptor to cerebral cortex. Thus, action potentials can be recorded over proximal and distal segments of many peripheral nerves. SEP's to lower limb stimulation which arise in the cauda equina and in spinal cord afferent pathways have been recorded from surface electrodes placed over the spine (1–6), and subcortical and cortical evoked potentials to stimulation of nerves in the lower extremities have been recorded from the scalp (6–9). SEP's to median nerve stimulation which arise in peripheral nerve, subcortical, and cortical structures have also been recorded from the scalp (10–13). Additionally, scalp-recorded SEP's to stimulation of cutaneous mechanoreceptors, dynamic mechanoreceptors, and pain fibers have been obtained (14–19).

Various methods have been used to evoke scalp-recorded SEP's. In most clinical situations, large mixed nerves—such as the median, ulnar, peroneal, or tibial nerves—are stimulated electrically. The advantage to this method is that a maximal number of nerve fibers can be synchronously depolarized, yielding responses which are greatest in amplitude. Stimulation of cutaneous nerves—such as the digital nerves or the sural nerve—is also employed. These responses are smaller than those obtained with mixed nerve stimulation and, therefore, are more difficult to record. Nevertheless, in certain conditions described below this is a preferable method of stimulation. SEP's evoked by electrical stimulation of skin dermatomal regions over the extremities and trunk can also be recorded from the scalp (20, 21).

SEP's to stimulation of mechanical receptors in the finger have been

* This chapter was written by Joan B. Cracco, M.D., Associate Professor, and Roger Q. Cracco, M.D., Professor and Chairman, Department of Neurology, State University of New York, Downstate Medical Center, Brooklyn, New York.

recorded over peripheral nerve and from the scalp (16, 17). This natural form of stimulation permits an evaluation of cutaneous receptors as well as peripheral nerves and central afferent pathways. The disadvantage of this method is that the sensory elements are less synchronously depolarized, which results in lower amplitude potentials because of the greater temporal dispersion of impulses.

Starr et al. (19) have shown that consistent potentials, evoked by stretch of a dynamically responding muscle mechanoreceptor, presumably the muscle spindle primary ending, can be recorded from the scalp. It is known that muscle afferents, including Group Ia muscle afferents, project to sensorimotor cortex in primates (22–24). Burke et al. (25) have shown that stimulation of a mixed nerve evokes a cerebral potential of shorter latency than would be expected were cutaneous afferent activity the responsible input. They concluded that this discrepancy arises because the cerebral potential is generated in part by the activity of fast conducting muscle afferents, presumably Group I afferents. This suggests that SEP latency can vary as a function of the particular type of nerve stimulated in addition to other known variables, including height and limb temperature. It also suggests that stimulation of cutaneous afferent nerves is preferable to stimulation of mixed nerves in studies correlating SEP abnormality with defects in cutaneous sensation since latency of SEP's to mixed nerve stimulation is determined primarily by input from muscle afferent fibers.

Recently, potentials evoked by stimulation of pain fibers have been investigated as a possible method for studying pain physiology. Evoked potentials with latencies greater than 80 msec have been recorded from the scalp to noxious stimuli such as tooth pulp and cutaneous laser stimulation (14, 15, 18).

Since most of the work in the area of SEP's involves electrical stimulation of peripheral nerves, the short and long latency SEP's to stimulation of nerves in the upper and lower extremities will be discussed in the ensuing paragraphs.

MEDIAN NERVE EVOKED POTENTIALS

Short Latency Potentials

Method

Stimulating electrodes are placed over the median nerve at the wrist. The cathode should be situated between the palmaris longus and flexor carpi radialis tendons, 2 cm proximal to the wrist crease. These tendons can be visualized if the subject palmar flexes the wrist against manual dorsiflexion. The anode may be placed either 2 to 3 cm distal to the cathode, lateral to the median nerve, or on the back of the wrist. Electroencephalogram disc, needle, or electromyography stimulating electrodes may be utilized. To reduce discomfort and stimulus artifact, electrode impedances should be kept low, i.e., EEG disc electrodes < 10 Kohms. The stimulus, a square wave electrical pulse of < 0.5 msec duration, should be of sufficient intensity to produce a visible thumb twitch but should be kept below discomfort level. A stimulus rate of 5 to 10 per sec, avoiding an integral of 60 Hz, is used. These rapid stimulus rates do not significantly alter these potentials (13). There is a difference of opinion as to whether increasing the stimulus intensity above motor threshold results in significant increases in amplitude of these responses (13, 26).

Either a constant current or constant voltage stimulator may be used. Whether one is superior to the other is disputable. In a situation where low or constant electrode impedance cannot be maintained, such as intraoperative recordings, a constant current stimulator would be superior since output will vary, within limits, inversely with changes in impedance.

In order to ensure subject safety and to minimize stimulus artifact, the stimulator output must be isolated from ground via a stimulus isolation unit. A ground placed between the stimulus and recording electrodes also helps to reduce stimulus artifact and ensures subject safety in the event of isolation failure.

A bandpass of about 10 to 3000 Hz (−3dB) is commonly used with a sampling rate of 100 μsec or less. The analysis time should be about 25 to 40 msec. Because of the small size of these potentials, averaging 500 to 2000 responses is recommended with at least two separate replications. Tin disc, silver-silver chloride, or gold plate recording electrodes may be used. However, because of the small size of these potentials, it is important that low and stable electrode impedances be maintained throughout the recording.

Recording montages for short latency SEP's have not yet been standardized. Scalp noncephalic reference leads are used to record these potentials in some laboratories (12, 13). The scalp recording electrodes are usually placed over the specific somatosensory receiving area (C_3^1 or C_4^1) which is 2 cm behind C_3 and C_4 for right and left median nerve stimulation, respectively. The shoulder, Erb's point, hand, or knee contralateral to the side of stimulation can be used as the reference site. These recordings may be noisy because of the noncephalic location of the reference electrode, and good recording technique is required. Patients may be sedated when necessary. Using this derivation up to three positive potentials are recorded with peak latencies of about 9 (P_9), 11 (P_{11}), and 13 (P_{13}) msec. P_{11} is not consistently recorded in all normal subjects; therefore, its absence cannot be considered abnormal. P_{13} is bilobed in many normal subjects, the second component (P_{14}) peaking about 1 msec after the first. These are followed by a prominent negative potential peaking at about 20 msec (N_{20}) and a positive potential peaking at about 25 msec (P_{25}) (Fig. 12.1).

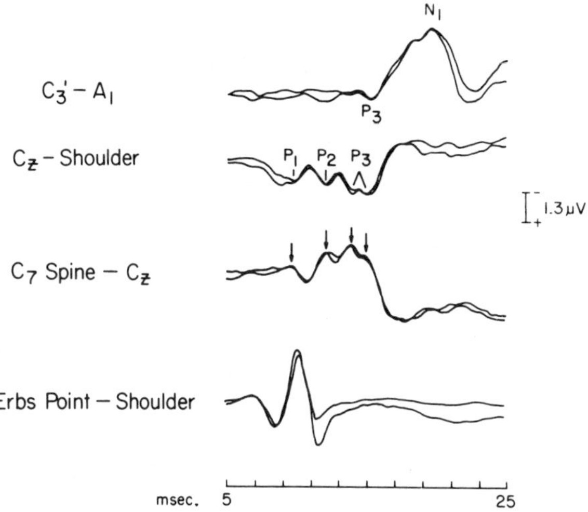

FIG. 12.1. SEP to right median nerve stimulation. Relative negativity in grid I results in an upward deflection. In the C_3-ear recording, a small positive potential (peak latency 15 msec) is followed by negative potential (peak latency 20 msec). In the C_z noncephalic reference lead, three short latency positive potentials are recorded, the third of which is bilobed. In the C_7 spine-C_z lead four negative potentials are recorded which are similar in latency to the above positive potentials (*arrows*). A prominent triphasic potential is recorded over Erb's point. (Note that P_9, P_{11}, P_{13}, and N_{20} are labeled P_1, P_2, P_3, and N_1, respectively.)

Evidence based on studies of patients with focal lesions of the nervous system suggests the following origins for these scalp-recorded short latency potentials (27): P_9, in proximal segments of stimulated median nerve fibers as they course through the brachial plexus from axilla to spinal cord, P_{11} in the dorsal columns of the cervical cord, P_{13} primarily in brain stem lemniscal pathways, and P_{14} in brain stem or diencephalic lemniscal pathways. The volley is thought to arrive in cerebral cortical elements at or before the peak of N_{20}. Subsequent potentials are thought to be cortical in origin. The short latency subcortical positive potentials (P_{11}, P_{13}, P_{14}) are thought to arise in fiber bundles rather than to reflect synaptic activity. This is because the anatomic orientation of cell bodies and dendrites in nuclei would be expected to generate closed fields which might not be recorded in the far field (28). However, the synchronous discharge of axons which are oriented perpendicular to the scalp would be expected to generate an open field of electrical activity which would be recorded in the far field from the scalp as positive events. The short durations of these potentials also favor axonal rather than synaptic events. Arezzo et al. (29) have provided evidence in monkeys which suggests that these short latency potentials arise primarily if not exclusively in fiber tracts.

Some of these short latency potentials can be recorded from leads in which scalp recording electrodes are placed at C_3^1 and C_4^1, and either the ear or frontal scalp is used as the reference site. Using this derivation, the P_{13} P_{14} complex, N_{20}, and N_{25} are recorded, but P_9 and P_{11} are absent or poorly defined (Fig. 12.1). The reason P_9 and P_{11} are not well defined is that these components are similar in amplitude and identical in latency at all cephalic recording locations including the ears and, therefore, undergo cancellation in scalp bipolar and scalp ear leads.

Cervical spine scalp leads are also used to record short latency SEP's (30–32). The cervical electrode is placed over the spine usually at C_7 or C_2 and is linked to a scalp electrode placed at F_z or C_z. Potentials are recorded which are similar in peak latency but opposite in direction to the short latency SEP's recorded in scalp noncephalic reference leads. This would imply that they are negative in polarity if one assumes the cervical electrode is more active than the scalp electrode for these components. Therefore, these components are referred to as N_9, N_{11}, N_{13}, N_{14} (Fig. 12.1).

Recently, Anziska and Cracco (33) compared scalp and cervical spine noncephalic reference recordings with cervical spine scalp recordings in normal subjects and patients with focal lesions of the nervous system. This was done to determine the relative contributions of the cervical spine and scalp recording electrodes to potentials recorded in cervical spine scalp leads and to provide information concerning the generator sources of these potentials. Cervical spine noncephalic reference recordings yielded initially positive di- or triphasic potentials. The initial positive and subsequent negative components had peak latencies of about 9 to 13 msec, respectively. These authors arrived at the following conclusions: N_9 is actually a positive potential which is greater in amplitude over the scalp, where it is recorded as P_9, than it is over the caudal cervical spine. This potential arises in proximal segments of stimulated median nerve fibers. N_{11} is contributed to by both the initial portion of the negative potential recorded by the cervical electrode which arises in the dorsal columns and P_{11} recorded by the scalp electrode which is the far field reflection of the dorsal column volley. N_{13} is also a composite potential which is contributed to by the major portion of the negative potential recorded by the cervical electrode which reflects primarily spinal cord and caudal medullary synaptic activity and the P_{13} potential recorded by the scalp electrode which reflects the medial lemniscal volley recorded in the far field. "N_{14}" was thought to be the P_{14} potential recorded by the scalp electrode since a component at this peak latency was not recorded in cervical spine noncephalic reference leads. P_{14} is thought to arise in brain stem or diencephalic lemniscal pathways.

Comparison of Recording Methods

Scalp-NC recordings are sometimes noisier than cervical spine-scalp recordings. This results from the greater distance between the recording electrodes in scalp-NC leads and the greater likelihood for the NC electrode to record muscle or movement artifact. The N_{11}-N_{13} complex recorded in cervical spine-scalp leads is usually greater in amplitude than P_{11}-P_{13} in scalp-NC leads. This results because of the summation of the negative spinal cord potential recorded by the neck electrode and the positive potentials recorded by the scalp electrode. The greater amplitude of this component in cervical spine-C_z leads is advantageous for clinical use, but the multiple generator sources of this composite potential may complicate the interpretation of brain stem lesions in the presence of an intact spinal cord.

In scalp ear leads the 9- and 11-msec potentials are not well defined because the scalp and ear electrodes are similarly active for these components and they undergo cancellation.

In clinical studies, a recording electrode is often placed over Erb's point ipsilateral to the side of stimulation. This recording consistently yields a well defined, predominantly negative potential (Fig. 12.1). Recording the Erb's point potential is important as a measure of input into the system. The latency of this potential may be subtracted from the latency of potentials recorded in other derivations (cervical spine-scalp, scalp-NC, scalp-ear). This provides information concerning transit times from Erb's point to the generator sources of potentials recorded in each of the other leads. This is preferable to using absolute latencies since variability due to differences in arm length and temperature is eliminated. Interpeak latency differences of potentials recorded in neck-scalp, scalp-NC, and scalp-ear derivations will also provide information concerning transit times between the generator sources of the potentials. These transit times may be abnormally prolonged in patients with neurological disease (27, 34, 35). Absence of components consistently recorded in normal subjects provides additional criteria for abnormality (32, 35–37). Since amplitude shows considerable variability in normals, amplitude changes alone cannot be considered abnormal.

Clinical Applications

Abnormalities of these short latency SEP's have been found in patients with peripheral nerve lesions, lesions of the brachial plexus and the cervical roots, focal subcortical lesions situated along the neuraxis from cervical spinal cord to somesthetic cortex, brain death, and degenerative disease (27, 32, 35, 37–40). By stimulating at two points along the course of a peripheral nerve in the upper extremity and using the peak of the scalp-recorded N_{20} potential as the latency indicator, slowing of conduction velocity within peripheral nerve sensory fibers can be determined (41). In some patients this is possible even when action potentials cannot be recorded over the affected peripheral nerves. The SEP can be recorded from the scalp of these patients presumably because of amplification of the volley within the central nervous system. It is also possible to differentiate severe nonacute lesions of the brachial plexus located distal to the dorsal root ganglion from those located proximal to it. In patients with proximal lesions only N_9 and P_9, which arise in proximal segments of stimulated median nerve fibers, are recorded, whereas in patients with distal lesions no SEP's are recorded (Fig. 12.2). It seems that it may also be possible to localize a lesion within the brachial plexus in some patients by recording SEP's to independent stimulation of multiple peripheral nerves (digital, median, ulnar, and radial) in the upper extremity (42, 43). This method may prove useful in some patients with brachial plexus lesions, particularly those in whom the more simply performed F wave latency determinations fail to provide adequate localizing information.

Information concerning the localization of a lesion in the neuraxis from peripheral nerve to cerebral cortex is provided in some patients by recording these potentials (27, 32, 37). Components originating in structures caudal to the level of the lesion are preserved, whereas components arising in structures at or rostral to the lesion may be absent. Similarly, interpeak latency differences between components arising in neural elements caudal and rostral to the lesion may be increased.

Several studies have demonstrated abnormalities of these short latency SEP's in patients with multiple sclerosis, even in the absence of relevent sensory signs or symptoms (35, 44–46) (Fig. 12.3). Chiappa (47) found that in patients with possible, probable, and definite multiple sclerosis short latency SEP's had a slightly greater incidence of abnormality than visual

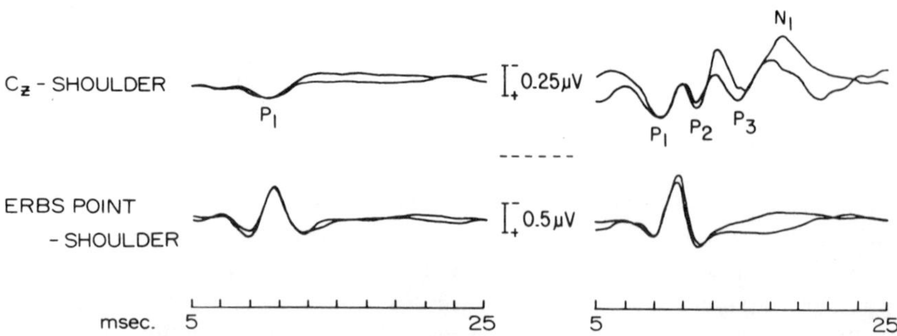

FIG. 12.2. Evoked potentials to right and left median nerve stimulation in a patient with right-sided C_5 to T_1 root avulsion. Initially positive, predominantly negative triphasic potentials are recorded over Erb's point with left and right median nerve stimulation. Normal left median nerve evoked potentials are recorded in the C_z-shoulder lead. Right median nerve stimulation yields only P_9. (Potentials are labeled as in Fig. 12.1). (From B. Anziska and R. Q. Cracco: Short latency somatosensory evoked potentials in patients with focal lesions of the nervous system. Electroencephalogr. Clin. Neurophysiol., *49:* 227–239, 1980.)

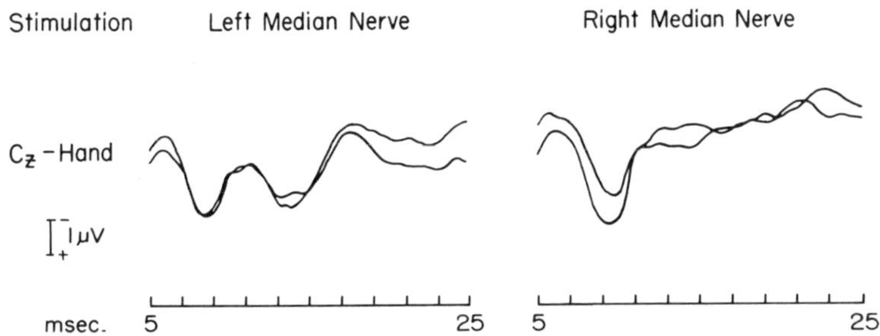

FIG. 12.3. Potentials recorded in a patient with multiple sclerosis. Left median nerve stimulation evoked P_9, P_{13}, and N_{20} potentials. Right median nerve stimulation evoked only a P_9 potential. (From B. Anziska, R. Q. Cracco, A. W. Cook, and E. W. Feld: Somatosensory far field potentials: Studies in normal subjects and patients with multiple sclerosis. Electroencephalogr. Clin. Neurophysiol., *45:* 602–610, 1978.)

evoked potentials and a considerably greater incidence of abnormality than auditory evoked potentials. This is not surprising considering the relative lengths of the pathways involved in the transmission of these three sensory evoked potentials. In patients with multiple sclerosis it is important to demonstrate evoked potential abnormalities in structures or pathways in which abnormalities are not clinically evident so that information concerning the presence of clinically undetected lesions may be provided. A combination of visual, auditory, and SEP studies in these patients is of obvious value in demonstrating the presence of multiple lesions, which is essential in making this diagnosis.

Hume and Cant (48) reported a method for measuring what they termed central somatosensory conduction time. SEP's to median nerve stimulation were recorded simultaneously from cervical spine-scalp and scalp-ear or F_z reference leads. The peak latency difference between the scalp-recorded N_{20} potential and the major component recorded in the cervical spine scalp lead (N_{13}) was thought to reflect central conduction time from caudal brain stem to cerebral cortex. Determinations of this central conduction time in a group of comatose patients at 10 and 35 days after the onset of coma were shown to correlate significantly with the patients' outcome (34).

Longer Latency Potentials

The methods used to record these potentials are similar to those used to record the short latency SEP's with the following exceptions. Rates of stimulation should not be greater than 1 to 2 per sec because at rapid stimulation rates many of these components are significantly attenuated. These potentials are greater in latency, duration, and amplitude than the short latency potentials; therefore, fewer (100 to 200) responses need be summated and longer analysis times (100 to 500 msec) are required. A bandpass of 1 to 1000 Hz is commonly used.

Recording electrodes are usually placed over the specific somatosensory receiving area (C_3^1 or C_4^1). Ear reference recordings are obtained, although frontal scalp locations have also served as reference sites even though these frontal locations are active for these SEP's.

The short latency positive, negative, and positive potentials (P_{13}-P_{14}, N_{20}, P_{25}) recorded in scalp ear leads described in the preceding section are followed by a series of negative and positive components lasting several hundred milliseconds (11, 49, 50) (Fig. 12.4). These longer latency components are widespread in their scalp distribution and show considerable variability both within and across normal subjects. They are sensitive to changes in level of consciousness as well as other ill defined factors (51). These longer latency potentials are thought to arise in cerebral cortical elements and to be mediated primarily by dorsal column and lemniscal

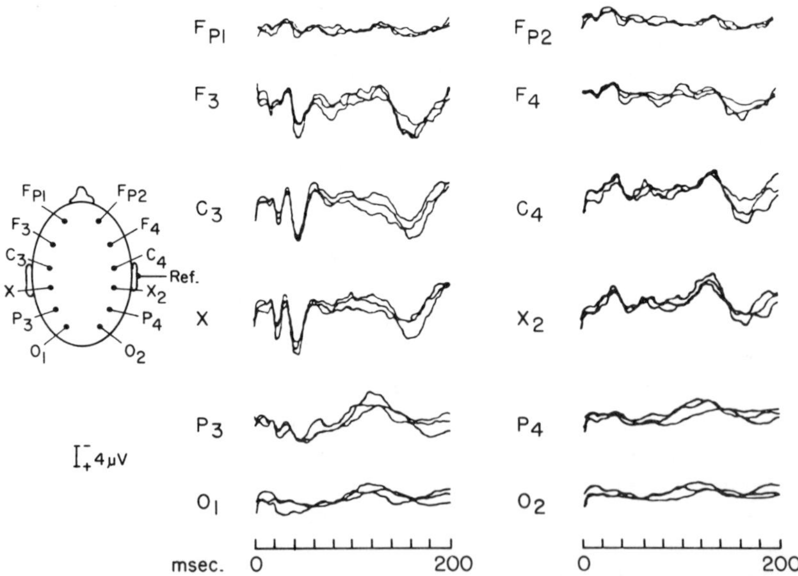

FIG. 12.4. Distribution of the longer latency scalp-recorded somatosensory evoked potentials to right median nerve stimulation in right ear reference recordings. Three recordings are superimposed on each trace. The X scalp electrodes lie over somatosensory cortex. Early components are most prominent overlying somesthetic scalp regions contralateral to the side of stimulation. Later components are more generalized. (From R. L. Calmes and R. Q. Cracco: Comparison of somatosensory and somatomotor evoked responses to median nerve and digital nerve stimulation. Electroencephalogr. Clin. Neurophysiol., *31:* 547–562, 1971.)

pathways (52). Little is known concerning the precise generator sources of these later components.

These SEP's may be reduced in amplitude over the affected hemisphere in patients with focal destructive cerebral lesions (50, 53–56). In these patients the degree of SEP alteration generally correlates well with the severity of sensory impairment, but exceptions have been noted. Abnormal, but inconsistent, alterations in SEP amplitude and waveform have also been observed in epileptic patients. SEP's may be enhanced in some patients with myoclonus or epilepsy (57–59) (Fig. 12.5). These potentials may be absent in some patients with central nervous system degenerative disease (60), and the evaluation of these potentials in severly brain-injured patients is useful in estimating prognosis (61).

For the most part, however, these findings in patients with cerebral dysfunction add little to the information that can be obtained from the clinical evaluation or the electroencephalogram; for this reason, this method has not yet received much enthusiasm in the neurology clinic. There are two important reasons why the recording of these later potentials have limited clinical application. They are quite variable both within and across normal subjects, and they are markedly affected by differences in level of arousal. Because of this variability, it is difficult to define what constitutes an

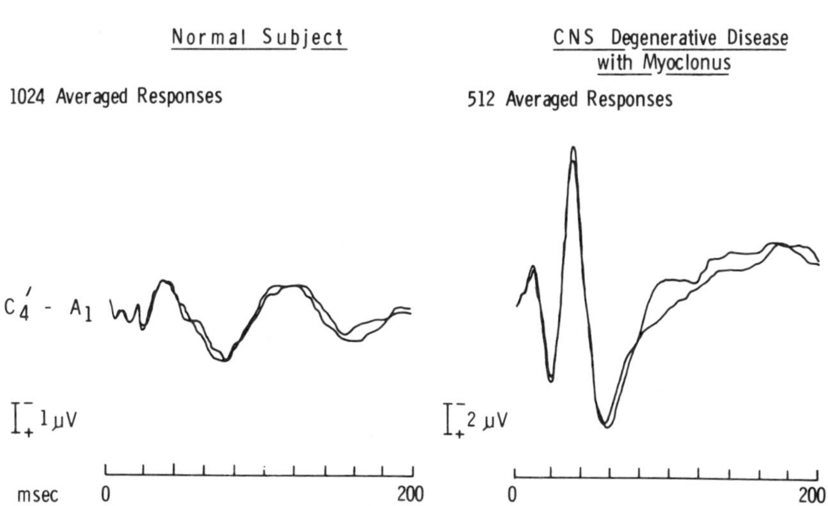

FIG. 12.5. Comparison of cerebral SEP's to median nerve stimulation in a normal child and a child with degenerative disease and myoclonus. The response in the patient is about 10 times greater in amplitude than that in normal subject. (From J. B. Cracco, V. V. Bosch, and R. Q. Cracco: Cerebral and spinal somatosensory evoked potentials in children with CNS degenerative disease. Electroencephalogr. Clin. Neurophysiol., *49:* 437–445, 1980.)

abnormal response. Additionally, little is known concerning the precise generator sources of these components.

Recently Yamada et al. (62) recorded SEP's to simultaneous stimulation of both median nerves. They demonstrated significant latency differences between these potentials recorded over the left and right cerebral hemispheres in patients with multiple sclerosis (63). Some of the problems involved in the clinical application of the longer latency SEP's may be minimized by using this method.

PERONEAL OR TIBIAL NERVE EVOKED POTENTIALS

Scalp-recorded Potentials

Stimulating electrodes are usually placed over the peroneal nerves in the popliteal fossa or tibial nerves at the ankle. The stimulus intensity should be sufficient to produce a visible muscle contraction but below pain threshold. In many laboratories stimulus rates of 1 to 2 per sec are used, and 100 to 300 responses are summated. The frequency response of the recording apparatus is usually 1 to 1000 Hz, and analysis times of 100 to 200 msec are used. A recoding electrode is usually placed at C_z or 2 cm behind C_z since this location overlies the specific somatosensory receiving area for the lower extremity. The reference electrode is usually placed on an ear or at a frontal scalp location.

This evoked response is greater in latency but otherwise similar to the longer latency median nerve evoked potentials (7) (Fig. 12.6). These poten-

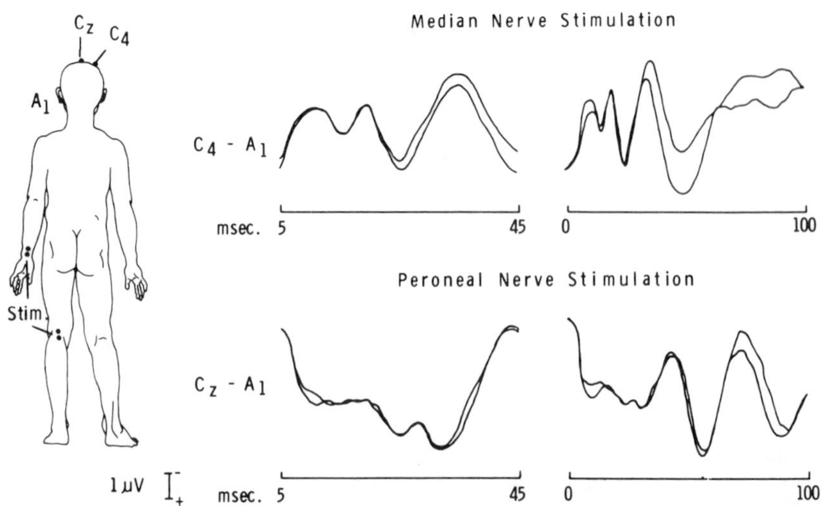

FIG. 12.6. Comparison of longer latency SEP's to median and peroneal nerve stimulation at 40- and 100-msec analysis times. SEP's to peroneal nerve stimulation are greater in latency but similar in waveform to median nerve evoked SEP's.

tials are also variable within and across subjects, and it is, therefore, difficult to define precisely what constitutes a normal or an abnormal response. Nevertheless, these potentials have been found useful in the evaluation of patients with trauma and other lesions of the spinal cord (8). The presence of a scalp-recorded response indicates that there is transmission of the ascending volley across the site of spinal cord pathology. This provides another parameter in the estimation of the completeness of physiological transection of the spinal cord and is particularly useful in patients in whom the clinical evaluation may be difficult or unreliable such as young children and comatose patients. Abnormalities of this response including increases in response latency have also been found in patients with multiple sclerosis (64). Additionally, this method has been employed in monitoring patients during surgery for scoliosis or spinal cord pathology (65, 66). Evoked potential changes induced by the effect of anesthesia or blood pressure would be expected to affect SEP's to stimulation of both upper and lower extremities, whereas changes induced by the spinal surgery would be expected to affect only the lower extremity SEP's. Variations in these peroneal or tibial nerve SEP's have been observed in some patients during these surgical procedures, but this information has been largely anecdotal. The types of changes in SEP configuration which are significant remain to be precisely defined. Therefore, more experience with this method will be required before its value in monitoring surgical procedures can be assessed.

Recently Vas et al. (9), using methods similar to those for recording short latency median nerve SEP's, described short latency SEP's to peroneal nerve stimulation which arise in subcortical and cortical structures. These consist of three positive potentials with peak latencies of about 17, 22, and 27 msec followed by a negative potential peaking at about 34 msec (Fig. 12.7). The first two potentials are thought to arise in the rostral spinal cord and brain stem, respectively. The volley is believed to arrive in cerebral cortical elements about the time of the peak of the third positive potential. Rossini et al. (67) found that by using a frequency bandpass of 150 to 3000 Hz, these short latency SEP's could be fractionated into additional subcomponents

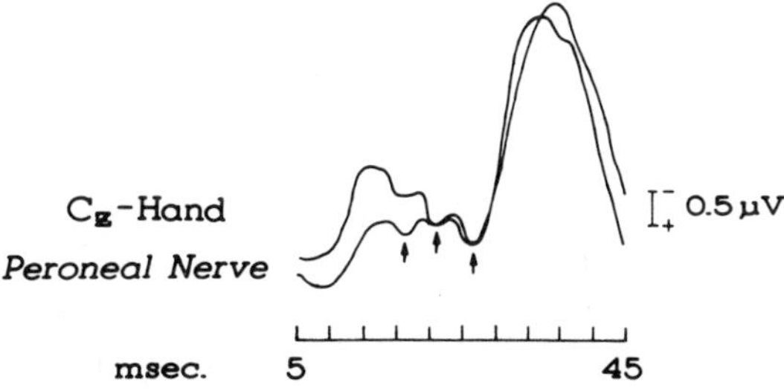

FIG. 12.7. Scalp-noncephalic reference recordings of short latency SEP's to bilateral peroneal nerve stimulation. Three positive potentials with peak latencies of about 17, 22, and 27 msec (*arrows*) are followed by a negative potential peaking at 34 msec.

and up to six positive potentials followed by two negative potentials could be recorded. Although smaller in amplitude than the longer latency potentials, these components are relatively stable and, therefore, may have greater clinical application than the longer latency potentials. Maccabee et al. (68) found that some of these short latency potentials are stable during anesthesia in patients undergoing corrective surgery for scoliosis.

Scalp-recorded SEP's have also been recorded in response to electrical stimulation of the skin over dermatomal regions of the extremities (20, 21). In patients with spinal cord pathology of varied types, stimulation of appropriate dermatomes rostral to the spinal lesion yield normal SEP's, whereas stimulation of dermatomes caudal to the lesion yield abnormal responses.

Spinal Evoked Potentials

Evoked potentials which arise in the cauda equina and in spinal cord afferent pathways can be recorded from surface electrodes attached to the skin over the spine (1, 2). Over rostral spinal cord segments these potentials are very tiny and are recorded with difficulty. The methods are the same as those used for recording potentials from the scalp, except stimulus rates of about 7 to 9 per sec are used, 1000 to 4000 responses are summated, and analysis time is 20 to 40 msec. The frequency response of the recording apparatus is 10 to 3000 Hz. Simultaneous stimulation of multiple nerves, such as both peroneal nerves or both tibial nerves, increases the signal size (69), and this method is routinely employed in some laboratories.

Since recordings over the spine are often obscured by random myogenic activity, this can be minimized by recording when patients are drowsy or sleeping. Recording electrodes are attached to the skin over the spine, and because of the small signal size it is important to maintain low and stable electrode impedances. Bipolar or reference recordings are obtained over various spinal locations. The reference electrode may be placed over the iliac crest, torso, scalp, or sacrum (5, 6, 12). Reference recordings are often considerably noisier than bipolar recordings. If one is recording potentials only over the cauda equina or caudal spinal cord, far fewer responses need be summated since these potentials are much greater in amplitude than those recorded over rostral spinal cord segments. Technically satisfactory recordings have been obtained over this area by summating fewer than 100 responses (5).

These potentials progressively increase in latency from lumbar to cervical recording locations (2–4) (Fig. 12.8). Similar potentials have been obtained from epidural leads in man (70–75). In bipolar surface leads over the lumbar spine, the response consists of initially positive triphasic potentials. This would be expected when recording an impulse traversing a nerve trunk in

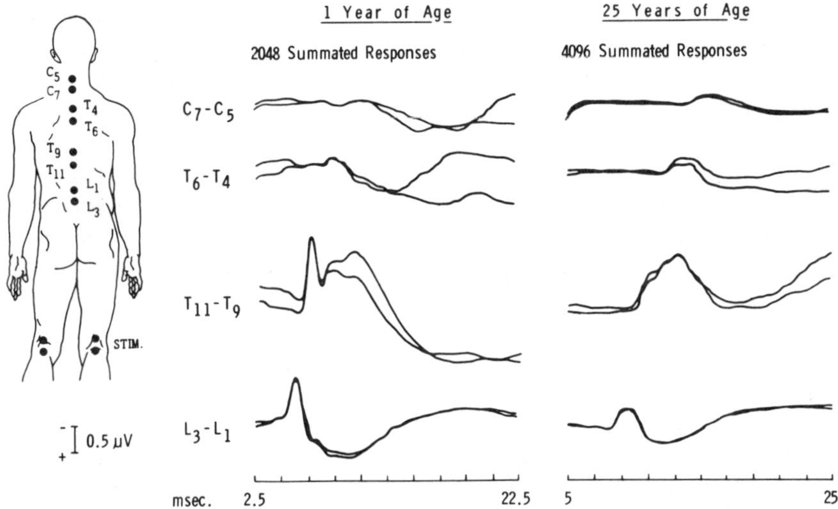

FIG. 12.8. Comparison of bipolar recordings of the spinal response to peroneal nerve stimulation in a 1-year-old infant and an adult. Electrode placement refers to spinous process level. There is a delay of 2.5 msec and 5.0 msec between the stimulus and the averaging process in the infant and adult, respectively. Over the cauda equina (L_3 spine) the response in both the infant and adult consists of triphasic potentials with poorly defined initial positive phases. In the infant, the response over caudal spinal cord (T_{11} spine) consists of a positive-negative diphasic potential followed by a broad negative-positive potential. In the adult it consists of a broad negative potential with two or three inflections. The response over rostral spinal cord in both the infant and adult consists of small, initially positive triphasic potentials with poorly defined positive phases. (From J. B. Cracco, R. Q. Cracco, and R. Stolove: Spinal evoked potential in man: A maturational study. Electroencephalogr. Clin. Neurophysiol., *46:* 58–64, 1979.)

volume and is consistent with potentials arising in the roots of the cauda equina. In leads over the lower thoracic spine which overlie caudal spinal cord segments, the response is often greater in amplitude and duration and more complex in configuration than in more rostral or more caudal leads. In adults this potential usually consists of an initially positive triphasic potential, the negative component of which has several peaks or inflections (2). In infants and young children this response usually consists of a large positive-negative diphasic potential followed by a broad negative and then, at times, by a positive potential (3, 76) (Fig. 12.8). Investigations of similar potentials recorded over caudal cord segments in cats and monkeys suggest that the initial diphasic potential arises in the intramedullary continuations of dorsal root fibers and the subsequent potentials reflect synaptic and postsynatpic activity which is concerned with local reflex mechanisms rather than with the propagation of the response to more rostral levels (77, 78).

Over rostral cord segments the response in children and adults consists of small initially positive triphasic potentials with poorly defined positive phases which progressively decrease in amplitude rostrally (2–4) (Fig. 12.8). This amplitude decrement probably reflects temporal dispersion and the greater distance between the skin recording electrodes and the spinal cord at rostral thoracic and cervical recording sites. Investigations in cats and monkeys suggest that these potentials arise in multiple rapidly conducting afferent pathways including the dorsolateral columns which lie primarily ipsilateral to the stimulated peripheral nerve (77–79). These animal studies also provide evidence which suggests that the peripheral nerve fibers which mediate these potentials recorded at all spinal levels are primarily muscle nerve rather than cutaneous nerve afferent fibers (79).

The onset of the negative potential at each recording site may serve as the latency indicator and be used in determining conduction velocity since this is thought to reflect the approximate time the fastest fibers contributing to a response pass under the recording electrode in reference leads and the recording electrode nearest the approaching volley in bipolar leads (80). Latency differences are greater between equidistant leads placed over caudal spinal cord segments then they are between leads placed over the cauda equina or rostral spinal cord (2, 4). This indicates a decrease in the speed of conduction of the response over caudal cord segments. This slowing probably reflects branching of dorsal root fibers and synaptic activity since this is the region where these fibers undergo synaptic contact in Clark's column and other nuclei.

In normal adults the mean conduction velocity of the response from lumbar to cervical recording locations is about 70 m per sec. Segmental conduction velocities are about 65 m per sec over peripheral nerve and cauda equina (point of peripheral nerve stimulation to L_3 spine), 50 m per sec over caudal spinal cord (T_{12} to T_6 spines), and 85 m per sec over rostral spinal cord (T_6-C_7 spines) (4). In the newborn these segmental conduction velocities are about half those values obtained in the adult. They progressively increase with age. Peripheral conduction velocities are largely within the adult range by 3 years, whereas velocities over the spinal cord do not reach adult values until the fifth year (4) (Fig. 12.9). This suggests that maturation of rapidly conducting spinal afferent pathways proceeds at a slower rate than maturation of rapidly conducting peripheral sensory fibers. Similar findings have been obtained in maturational studies of the scalp-recorded evoked response to median nerve stimulation. Conduction velocities in median nerve reached adult values between 12 and 18 months of age, whereas conduction velocity within central lemniscal pathways did not reach adult values until 5 to 7 years of age (81, 82). The increase in speed of conduction in peripheral nerve and spinal cord is probably related to the increasing fiber diameter and progressive myelination which accompany maturation. However, explanations for the differential rate in maturation of peripheral and central afferent pathways can only be speculative at this time.

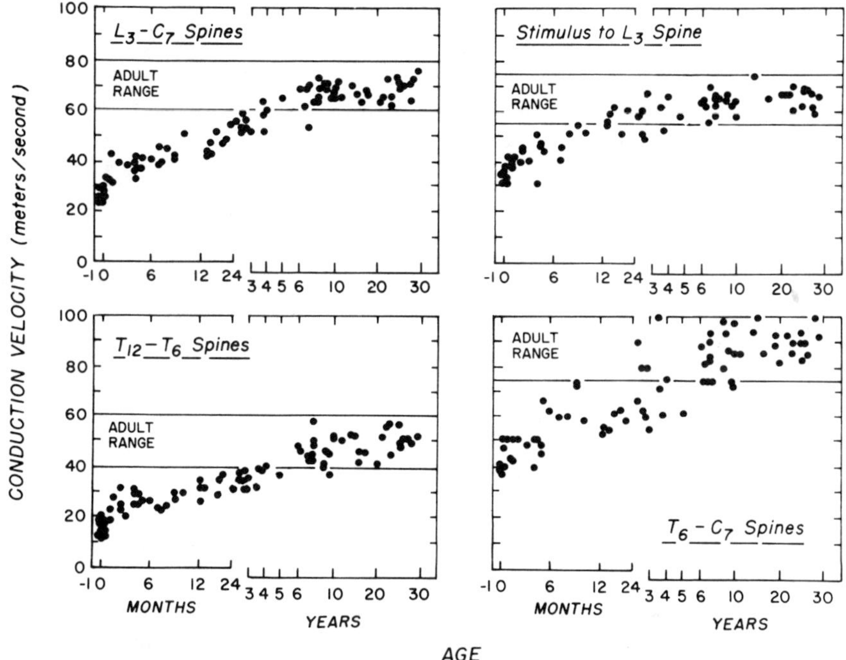

FIG. 12.9. Relationship between age and overall conduction velocity (L_3-C_7 spines) and segmental conduction velocities over peroneal nerve and cauda equina (stimulus to L_3 spine), caudal spinal cord (T_{12}-T_6 spines), and rostral spinal cord (T_6-C_7 spines). Note the change in age scale (from months to years) on the *abscissa*. Infants from -1 to 0 months were premature. All conduction velocities are in the adult range by 5 years of age. Velocities over peroneal nerve and cauda equina increase rapidly during the first year of life, and most values are in the adult range by 3 years. However, velocities over both caudal and rostral spinal cord are not in the adult range until 5 to 6 years of age. (From J. B. Cracco, R. Q. Cracco, and R. Stolove: Spinal evoked potential in man: A maturational study. Electroencephalogr. Clin. Neurophysiol., *46:* 58–64, 1979.)

In adult patients with clinically evident complete spinal cord lesions, evoked potentials recorded from surface electrodes caudal to the lesion are similar to those obtained in normal subjects. No response has been recorded in leads rostral to the lesion (2) (Fig. 12.10). In a study of a group of infants and children with myelodysplasia on whom spinal evoked potentials and cerebral evoked potentials were recorded, there was correlation between the degree of evoked potential abnormality and the clinical status of the patients (3, 76, 83). In a few of these patients it was possible to diagnose caudal displacement of the spinal cord; in these patients the large complex spinal potentials which are normally recorded over the lower thoracic spines were recorded over lumbar spinous processes. In several children with myelomeningocele a positive potential was recorded in leads immediately rostral to the lesion. This potential progressively decreased in amplitude but did not

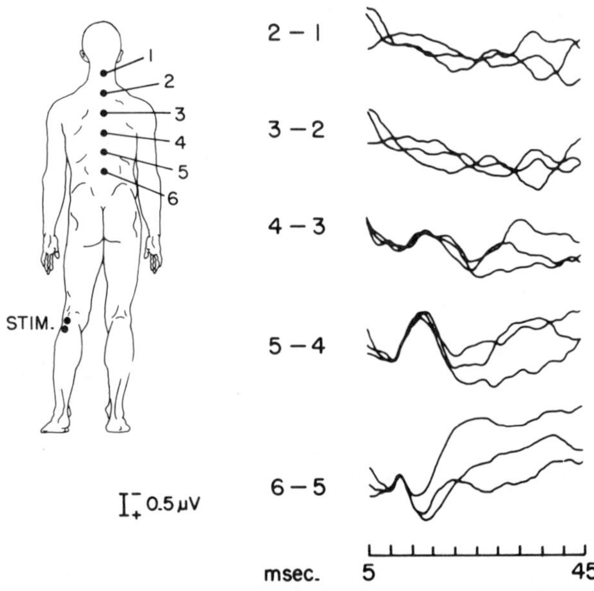

FIG. 12.10. Bipolar recordings of the spinal potential evoked by left peroneal nerve stimulation in a patient with a clinically complete spinal cord lesion at T_8. Potentials caudal to the lesion (*bottom three traces*) are similar to those recorded in normal subjects. No potential is apparent in the lead in which the caudal electrode is placed over the sixth thoracic spine (*trace 3-2*) in relation to the lesion or in the more rostral lead (*top trace*). (From R. Q. Cracco: Spinal evoked response: Peripheral nerve stimulation in man. Electroencephalogr. Clin. Neurophysiol., *35:* 379–386, 1973.)

change in latency rostrally. This is a nonpropagated volume-conducted potential which is consistent with physiological transection of the spinal cord. Similar positive potentials have been recorded rostral to spinal cord transections in cats and monkeys (killed end effect) (77–79).

Spinal- and scalp-recorded SEP's were studied in a group of children with degenerative diseases of the central nervous system (60). The conduction velocity over peroneal nerve was normal. Responses were recorded over the spinal cord in most patients, but conduction velocities over the cord were slowed. Velocities over the spinal cord were slower over rostral cord segments than they were over the caudal cord. This may suggest that a "dying back" process, similar to that known to occur in some peripheral neuropathies, is operative in the spinal afferent pathways of these patients. The short latency evoked potentials to median nerve stimulation which arise within and rostral to the brain stem were absent in most of the patients, as were the longer latency potentials of cerebral cortical origin (Fig. 12.11).

Spinal and peripheral nerve conduction velocities were also found to be slowed in some clinically asymptomatic juvenile diabetics (39). Peripheral

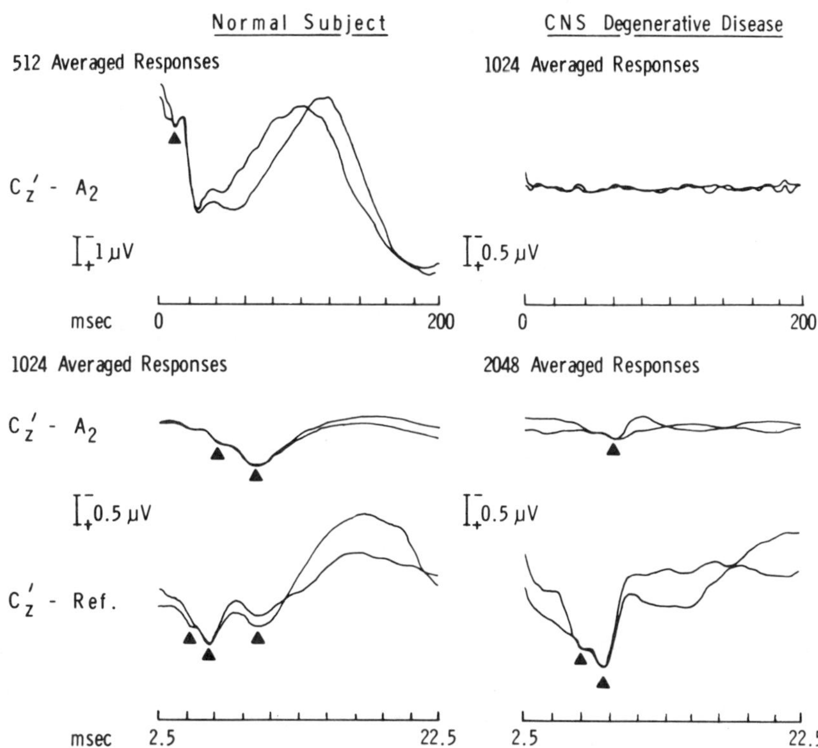

FIG. 12.11. Comparisons of the median nerve evoked short latency (*bottom two traces*) and longer latency (*top traces*) potentials in a normal child and a child with degenerative disease. In the *bottom two traces* the analysis time is 20 msec. In the normal child, three short latency positive potentials are recorded in the C_z-hand reference lead (*arrows*). In the C_z-ear lead only the second two potentials are seen (*arrows*). In the patient, only the first two positive potentials are recorded in the C_z-hand reference lead (*arrows*). Only the second positive potential is seen in the C_z-ear lead (*arrow*). The analysis time in the *top traces* is 200 msec. In the normal child the C_z-ear lead yields prominent longer latency potentials. No response is recorded in the patient. (From J. B. Cracco, V. V. Bosch, and R. Q. Cracco: Cerebral and spinal somatosensory evoked potentials in children with CNS degenerative disease. Electroencephalogr. Clin. Neurophysiol., *49:* 437–445, 1980.)

nerve or spinal conduction velocity alone was slowed in some patients, while in others both peripheral and spinal conduction velocity were slowed. As in the children with central nervous system degenerative disease, spinal conduction velocity over rostral spinal cord segments was chiefly affected.

Dorfman has devised a method by which conduction velocities within spinal cord afferent pathways may be indirectly estimated (84). He used the scalp-recorded SEP's to stimulation of a nerve in the lower extremity and the upper extremity as latency indicators and subtracted out the estimated peripheral conduction time by determining the F wave latencies for the stimulated peripheral nerves. He found slowing in the speed of conduction within spinal cord afferent pathways in normal elderly subjects and in some patients with diabetes and multiple sclerosis (85–87).

CONCLUSION

The recording of SEP's provides a unique opportunity to evaluate the entire neuraxis from cutaneous receptor to cerebral cortex. Information can be obtained concerning receptors, peripheral nerves, spinal cord, brain stem, and cerebral cortex. When these methods are combined with those used in obtaining auditory and visual evoked potentials, it seems that it should be possible to obtain a reliable measure of the physiological integrity of sensory systems in man.

REFERENCES

1. Liberson, W. I., Gratzur, M., Zales, A., and Grabinski, B.: Comparison of conduction velocity of motor and sensory fibers determined by different methods. Arch. Phys. Med., *47:* 17–23, 1966.
2. Cracco, R. Q.: Spinal evoked response: Peripheral nerve stimulation in man. Electroencephalogr. Clin. Neurophysiol., *35:* 379–386, 1973.
3. Cracco, J. B., Cracco, R. Q., and Graziani, L. J.: The spinal evoked response in infants and children. Neurology, *25:* 31–36, 1975.
4. Cracco, J. B., Cracco, R. Q., and Stolove, R.: Spinal evoked potential in man: A maturational study. Electroencephalogr. Clin. Neurophysiol., *46:* 58–64, 1979.
5. Dimitrijevic, M. R., Larsson, L. E., Lehmkuhl, D., and Sherwood, A. M.: Evoked spinal cord and nerve root potentials in humans using a noninvasive recording technique. Electroencephalogr. Clin. Neurophysiol., *45:* 331–340, 1978.
6. Jones, S. J., and Small, D. G.: Spinal and sub-cortical evoked potentials following stimulation of the posterior tibial nerve in man. Electroencephalogr. Clin. Neurophysiol., *44:* 299–306, 1978.
7. Tsumoto, T., Hirose, N., and Nonaka, S.: Analysis of somatosensory evoked potentials to lateral popliteal nerve stimulation in man. Electroencephalogr. Clin. Neurophysiol., *33:* 379–388, 1972.
8. Perot, P. L., Jr.: The clinical use of somatosensory evoked potentials in spinal cord injury. Clin. Neurosurg., *20:* 367–382, 1973.
9. Vas, G. A., Cracco, J. B., and Cracco, R. Q.: Scalp recorded short latency cortical and subcortical somatosensory evoked potentials to peroneal nerve stimulation. Electroencephalogr. Clin. Neurophysiol., *51:*40P, 1981.
10. Dawson, G. D.: Auto-correlation and automatic integration. Electroencephalogr. Clin. Neurophysiol. *4:* (Suppl.) 26–37, 1954.
11. Goff, W. R., Rosner, B. S., and Allison, T.: Distribution of cerebral somatosensory evoked responses in normal man. Electroencephalogr. Clin. Neurophysiol., *14:* 697–713, 1962.
12. Cracco, R. Q., and Cracco, J. B.: Somatosensory evoked potential in man: Far field potentials. Electroencephalogr. Clin. Neurophysiol., *41:* 460–466, 1976.
13. Kritchevsky, M., and Wiederholt, W. C.: Short latency somatosensory evoked potentials. Arch. Neurol., *35:* 706–711, 1978.
14. Chatrian, G. E., Farrell, D. F., Canfield, R. C., and Lettich, E.: Congenital insensitivity to noxious stimuli. Arch. Neurol., *32:* 141–145, 1975.
15. Chen, A. C. N., Chapman, C. R., and Harkins, S. W.: Brain evoked potentials are functional correlates of induced pain in man. Pain, *6:* 365–374, 1979.
16. Pratt, H., Amlie, R. N., and Starr, A.: Short latency mechanically evoked somatosensory potentials in humans. Electroencephalogr. Clin. Neurophysiol., *47:* 524–531, 1979.
17. Pratt, H., Starr, A., Amlie, R. N., and Politoski, D.: Mechanically and electrically evoked somatosensory potentials in normal humans. Neurology, *29:* 1235–1244, 1979.

18. Carmon, A., Friedman, Y., Coger, R., and Kenton, B.: Single trial analysis of evoked potentials to noxious thermal stimulation in man. Pain, *8:* 21–32, 1980.
19. Starr, A., Burke, D., McKeon, B., and Skuse, N.: Stretch-evoked somatosensory potentials in man (Abstract) Neurology, *30:* 372, 1980.
20. Blair, A. W.: Sensory examinations using electrically induced somatosensory potentials. Dev. Med. Child Neurol., *13:* 447–455, 1971.
21. Schramm, J., Oettle, G. J., and Pichert, T.: Clinical application of segmental somatosensory evoked potentials (SEP)—experience in patients with non-space occupying lesions. In *Evoked Potentials: Proceedings of an International Evoked Potentials Symposium Held in Nottingham, England,* edited by C. Barber, pp. 455–464. University Park Press, Baltimore, 1980.
22. Phillips, C. G., Powell, T. P. S., and Wiesendanger, M.: Projection from low-threshold muscle afferents of hand and forearm to area 3a of baboon's cortex. J. Physiol. (Lond.), *217:* 419–445, 1971.
23. Lucier, G. E., Ruegg, D. C., and Wiesendanger, M.: Responses of neurones in motor cortex and in area 3a to controlled stretches of forelimb muscles in cebus monkeys. J. Physiol. (Lond.), *251:* 833–853, 1975.
24. Hore, J., Preston, J. B., Durkovic, R. G., and Cheney, P. D.: Responses of cortical neurons (areas 3a and 4) to ramp stretch of hindlimb muscles in the baboon. J. Neurophysiol., *39:* 484–500, 1976.
25. Burke, D., Skuse, N. F., and Lethlian, A. K.: Cutaneous and muscle afferent components of the cerebral potential evoked by electrical stimulation of human peripheral nerves. Electroencephalogr. Clin. Neurophysiol., *51:*529–588, 1981.
26. Lesser, R. P., Koehle, R., and Lueders, H.: Effect of stimulus intensity on short latency somatosensory evoked potentials. Electroencephalogr. Clin. Neurophysiol., *47:* 377–382, 1979.
27. Anziska, B., and Cracco, R. Q.: Short latency somatosensory evoked potentials in patients with focal lesions of the nervous system. Electroencephalogr. Clin. Neurophysiol., *49:* 227–239, 1980.
28. Lorente de No, R.: *A Study of Nerve Physiology: Studies from the Rockefeller Institute,* vol. 132, ch. 16. Rockefeller University Press, New York, 1947.
29. Arezzo, J., Legatt, A. D., and Vaughan, H. G.: Topography and intracranial sources of somatosensory evoked potentials in the monkey. 1. Early components. Electroencephalogr. Clin. Neurophysiol., *46:* 155–172, 1979.
30. Matthews, W. B., Beauchamp, M., and Small, D. G.: Cervical somatosensory evoked responses in man. Nature, *252:* 230–232, 1974.
31. Jones, S. J.: Short latency potentials recorded from the neck and scalp following median nerve stimulation in man. Electroencephalogr. Clin. Neurophysiol., *43:* 853–863, 1977.
32. Chiappa, K. H., Choi, S. K., and Young, B. R.: Short latency somatosensory evoked potentials following median nerve stimulation in patients with neurological lesions. In *Progress in Clinical Neurophysiology,* edited by J. E. Desmedt, vol 7, pp. 264–281. Karger, Basel, 1980.
33. Anziska, B., and Cracco, R. Q.: Comparison of short latency SEPs to median nerve stimulation: in neck-scalp and scalp noncephalic reference recordings: Origins of components. Electroencephalogr. Clin. Neurophysiol., in press.
34. Hume, A. L., Cant, B. R., and Shaw, N. A.: Central somatosensory conduction time in comatose patients. Ann. Neurol., *5:* 379–384, 1979.
35. Anziska, B., Cracco, R. Q., Cook, A. W., and Feld, E. W.: Somatosensory far field potentials: Studies in normal subjects and patients with multiple sclerosis. Electroencephalogr. Clin. Neurophysiol., *45:* 602–610, 1978.
36. Nakanishi, T., Shimada, Y., Sakuta, M., and Toyokura, Y.: The initial positive component of the scalp recorded somatosensory evoked potentials in normal subjects and in patients with neurological disorders. Electroencephalogr. Clin. Neurophysiol., *45:* 26–34, 1978.
37. Green, J. B., and McLeod, S.: Short latency somatosensory evoked potentials in patients with neurological lesions. Arch. Neurol., *36:* 846–851, 1979.
38. Anziska, B., and Cracco, R. Q.: Somatosensory evoked short latency potentials in brain dead patients. Arch. Neurol., *37:* 222–225, 1980.

39. Cracco, J. B., Castells, S., and Mark, E.: Conduction velocity in peripheral nerve and spinal afferent pathways in juvenile diabetics (Abstract). Neurology, *30:* 370–371, 1980.
40. Goldie, W. D., Chiappa, K. H., Young, R. R., and Brooks, E. B.: Brainstem auditory and short-latency somatosensory evoked responses in brain death. Neurology, *31:* 248–256, 1981.
41. Desmedt, J. E., and Noel, P.: Average cerebral evoked potentials in the evaluation of lesions of the sensory nerves and of the central somatosensory pathway. In *New Developments in Electromyography and Clinical Neurophysiology*, edited by J. E. Desmedt, vol. 2, pp. 353–371. Karger, Basel, 1973.
42. Elleker, G., and Eisen, A.: Segmental sensory stimulation and SEPs—normative data and clinical application (Abstract). Neurology, *30:* 372–373, 1980.
43. Grisolia, J. S., and Weiderholt, W. C.: Short latency somatosensory evoked potentials from radial, median and ulnar nerve stimulation in man. Electroencephalogr. Clin. Neurophysiol., *50:* 375–381, 1980.
44. Mastaglia, F. L., Black, J. L., Cala, L. A., and Collins, D. W. K.: Evoked potentials, saccadic velocities and computerized tomography in diagnosis of multiple sclerosis. Br. Med. J., *1:* 1315–1317, 1977.
45. Small, D. G., Matthews, W. B., and Small, M.: The cervical somatosensory evoked potential (SEP) in the diagnosis of multiple sclerosis. J. Neurol. Sci., *35:* 211–224, 1978.
46. Eisen, A., Stewart, J., Nudleman, K., and Cosgrove, J. B. R.: Short latency somatosensory responses in multiple sclerosis. Neurology, *29:* 827–834, 1979.
47. Chiappa, K. H.: Pattern shift visual, brainstem auditory and short latency somatosensory evoked potentials in multiple sclerosis. Neurology, *30:* 110–123, 1980.
48. Hume, A. L., and Cant, B. R.: Conduction time in central somatosensory pathways in man. Electroencephalogr. Clin. Neurophysiol., *45:* 361–375, 1978.
49. Goff, G. D., Matsumiya, Y., Allison, T., and Goff, W. R.: The scalp topography of human somatosensory and auditory evoked potentials. Electroencephalogr. Clin. Neurophysiol., *42:* 57–76, 1977.
50. Giblin, D. R.: Somatosensory evoked potentials in healthy subjects and in patients with lesions of the nervous system. Ann. N.Y. Acad. Sci., *112:* 93–142, 1964.
51. Cracco, R. Q.: Traveling waves of the human scalp recorded somatosensory evoked response: Effects of differences in recording technique and sleep on somatosensory and somatomotor responses. Electroencephalogr. Clin. Neurophysiol., *38:* 557–566, 1972.
52. Halliday, A. M., and Wakefield, G. S.: Cerebral evoked potentials in patients with dissociated sensory loss. J. Neurol. Neurosurg. Psychiatry, *26:* 211–219, 1963.
53. Liberson, W. T.: Study of evoked potentials in aphasics. Am. J. Phys. Med., *5:* 135–142, 1965.
54. Laget, P., Mamo, H., and Houdart, H.: De l'interet des potentials evoques somesthesiques dans létude des lesions due lobe parietal de l'homme: Etude preliminaire. Neurochirurgie, *13:* 841–853, 1967.
55. Williamson, P. D., Goff, W. R., and Allison, T.: Somatosensory evoked responses in patients with unilateral cerebral lesions. Electroencephalogr. Clin. Neurophysiol., *28:* 566–567, 1970.
56. Kazaki, A., Shiota, K., Terada, C., Itsumi, S., and Hori, P.: Clinical studies on the somatosensory evoked response in neurosurgical patients. Electroencephalogr. Clin. Neurophysiol., *31:* 184–191, 1971.
57. Halliday, A. M.: The incidence of large cerebral evoked responses in myoclonic epilepsy (Abstract). Electroencephalogr. Clin. Neurophysiol., *19:* 102, 1965.
58. Halliday, A. M., and Halliday, E.: Cortical evoked potentials in patients with benign essential myoclonus and progressive myoclonic epilepsy (Abstract). Electroencephalogr. Clin. Neurophysiol., *29:* 106, 1970.
59. Broughton, R., Maier-Ewert, K-H., and Abe, M.: Evoked visual somatosensory and retinal potentials in photosensitive epilepsy. Electroencephalogr. Clin. Neurophysiol., *27:* 373–386, 1969.
60. Cracco, J. B., Bosch, V. V., and Cracco, R. Q.: Cerebral and spinal somatosensory evoked potentials in children with CNS degenerative disease. Electroencephalogr. Clin. Neurophysiol., *49:* 437–445, 1980.

61. Greenberg, R. P., Becker, D. P., Miller, J. D., and Mayer, D. J.: Evaluation of brain function in severe head trauma with multimodality evoked potentials. J. Neurosurg., *47:* 150–162, 1977.
62. Yamada, T., Kimura, J., Young, S., and Powers, M.: Somatosensory evoked potentials elicited by bilateral stimulation of the median nerve and its clinical application. Neurology, *28:* 218–223, 1978.
63. Yamada, T., Shivapouri, E., Wilkinson, J. T., and Kimura, J.: Short and long latency SEPs in multiple sclerosis: Arch. Neurol., *39:* 32P, 1982.
64. Namerow, N. S.: Somatosensory evoked responses in multiple sclerosis patients with varying sensory loss. Neurology, *18:* 1197–1204, 1968.
65. Nash, C. L., Lorig, R. A., Schatzinger, L. A., and Brown, R. H.: Spinal cord monitoring during operative treatment of the spine. Clin. Orthop., *126:* 100–105, 1977.
66. Engler, L. L., Spielholz, N. I., Bernhard, W. N., Danziger, F., Merkin, H. and Wolff, T.: Somatosensory evoked potentials during Harrington instrumentation for scolioses. J. Bone Joint Surg., *60:* 528–532, 1978.
67. Rossini, P. M., Cracco, J. B., and Cracco, R. Q.: Scalp recorded short latency somatosensory evoked potentials (SSEPs) to peroneal nerve stimulation (Abstract). Electroencephalogr. Clin. Neurophysiol., *53:* 32P, 1982.
68. Maccabee, P. J., Pinkhasov, E. I., Tsairis, P., and Levine, D. B.: Spinal and short latency scalp derived somatosensory evoked potentials during corrective spinal column surgery (Abstract). Electroencephalogr. Clin. Neurophysiol., in press.
69. Cracco, R. Q., Cracco, J. B., and Anziska, B. J.: Somatosensory evoked potentials in man: Cerebral, subcortical, spinal and peripheral nerve potentials. Am. J. EEG Technol., *19:* 59–81, 1979.
70. Magladery, J. W., Porter, W. E., Porter, W. E., Park, A. M., and Teasdall, R. D.: Electrophysiological studies of nerve and reflex activity in normal man. IV. The two neuron reflex and identification of certain action potentials from spinal roots and cord. Bull. Johns Hopkins Hosp., *88:* 499–519, 1951.
71. Caccia, M. R., Ubcali, E., and Andreussi, L.: Spinal evoked responses recorded from the epidural space in normal and diseased humans. J. Neurol. Neurosurg. Psychiatry, *39:* 962–972, 1976.
72. Ertekin, C.: Studies in the human evoked electrospinogram. I. The origin of the segmental evoked potentials. Acta Neurol. Scand., *53:* 2–30, 1976.
73. Ertekin, C.: Studies in the human evoked electrospinogram. II. The conduction velocity along the dorsal funiculus. Acta Neurol. Scand., *53:* 21–38, 1976.
74. Shimoji, K., Matsuki, M., and Shimizu, H.: Wave form characteristics and spatial distribution of evoked spinal electrogram in man. J. Neurosurg., *46:* 304–310, 1977.
75. Shimoji, K., Shimizu, H., and Maruzama, Y.: Origin of somatosensory evoked response recorded from the cervical skin surface. J. Neurosurg., *48:* 980–984, 1978.
76. Cracco, J. B., and Cracco, R. Q.: Somatosensory spinal and cerebral evoked potentials in children with occult spinal dysraphism (Abstract). Neurology, *29:* 543, 1979.
77. Cracco, R. Q., and Evans, B.: Spinal evoked potential in the cat: Effects of asphyxia, strychnine, cord section and compression. Electroencephalogr. Clin. Neurophysiol., *44:* 187–201, 1978.
78. Feldman, M. H., Cracco, R. Q., Farmer, P., and Mount, F.: Spinal evoked potential in the monkey. Ann. Neurol., *7:* 238–244, 1980.
79. Sarnowski, R. J., Cracco, R. Q., Vogel, H. B., and Mount, F.: Spinal evoked response in the cat. J. Neurosurg., *43:* 329–336, 1975.
80. Gilliat, R. W., Melville, I. P., Velate, A. S., and Willison, R. G.: A study of normal nerve action potential using an averaging technique (barrier grid storage tube). J. Neurol. Neurosurg. Psychiatry, *28:* 191–200, 1965.
81. Desmedt, J. E., Brunko, E., and Debecker, J.: Maturation of the somatosensory evoked potentials in normal infants and children, with special reference to the early N_1 component. Electroencephalogr. Clin. Neurophysiol., *40:* 43–58, 1976.
82. Desmedt, J. E., Noel, P., Debecker, J., and Nameche, J.: Maturation of afferent conduction velocity as studied by sensory nerve potentials and cerebral evoked potentials. In *New Developments in Electromyography and Clinical Neurophysiology*, edited by J. E. Desmedt,

vol. 2, pp. 52–63. Karger, Basel, 1973.

83. Cracco, R. Q., Cracco, J. B., Sarnowski, R. and Vogel, A. B.: Spinal evoked potentials. In *Progress in Clinical Neurophysiology*, edited by J. E. Desmedt, vol. 7, pp. 87–104. Karger, Basel, 1980.
84. Dorfman, L. J.: Indirect estimation of spinal cord conduction velocity in man. Electroencephalogr. Clin. Neurophysiol., *42:* 26–34, 1977.
85. Dorfman, L. J., and Bosley, T. M.: Age related changes in peripheral and central nerve conduction in man. Neurology, *29:* 38–44, 1979.
86. Dorfman, L. J., Bosley, T. M., and Cummins, K. L.: Electrophysiological localization of central somatosensory lesions in patients with multiple sclerosis. Electroencephalogr. Clin. Neurophysiol., *44:* 742–753, 1978.
87. Gupta, P. R., and Dorfman, L. J.: Spinal somatosensory conduction in diabetics (Abstract). Neurology, *30:* 414–415, 1980.

chapter
13

Ocular Electromyography*

The technique of electromyography of the extraocular muscles was introduced by Björk in 1952 (1). It was subsequently developed and expanded by numbers of investigators concerned with clinical and research aspects of ocular motility. It may be said, in general, that its utility is comparable to that of the technique of peripheral muscle electromyography. Extraocular muscle, however, exhibits peculiar anatomic, pharmacological, and physiological characteristics which make the interpretation of its electromyograms more hazardous than those of peripheral skeletal muscle. It should be pointed out that the safe insertion of needle electrodes into the extraocular muscles requires a certain amount of knowledge of the anatomy of the eye and its adnexae and familiarity with problems of the extraocular muscles. These considerations suggest that the insertion of needle electrodes into the extraocular muscles is properly the task of an ophthalmologist. He may work in association with the peripheral muscle electromyographer or develop his own expertise in this technique. It is clearly a more difficult and demanding task to insert needle electrodes into the extraocular muscles than into the peripheral skeletal musculature. Accidental penetration of the globe could be disastrous.

All of the extraocular muscles are susceptible to investigation by this technique. The inferior oblique muscle is particularly advantageously located, because it may be reached by an insertion through the skin of the lower lid near the medial canthus. No anesthesia is necessary. The needle may be placed in the belly of the inferior oblique with one or two thrusts suitably monitored on the oscilloscope or the audiospeaker. The latter is

* This chapter was written in its entirety by Goodwin M. Breinin, M.D., Professor and Chairman of the Department of Ophthalmology, New York University Medical Center.

particularly helpful because the characteristic sound of units guides one into the active muscle. One is always "working in the dark" with extraocular muscles. Common complications of this technique are corneal exposure and subconjunctival hemmorhage. Care usually prevents the former, but the latter may occur solely through picking up of the conjunctiva with forceps. Although unsightly, it is of no consequence. An antibiotic ointment (and rarely a patch) is required after the procedure. Insertions of the needle into the horizontal recti require topical anesthesia, which is secured by the administration of a few drops of ½% tetracaine or 1% Ophthaine (E. R. Squibb & Sons). The use of a blepharostat (lid retractor) is not necessary for most placements, and its avoidance helps minimize the possibility of corneal exposure.

The conjunctiva overlying the recti muscles is picked up with a fine forceps and the needle electrode is inserted subconjunctivally into the long axis of the muscle. It is guided into the belly of the muscle by visual or auditory monitoring of the oscilloscope and speaker. When suitably placed, the electrode maintains a surprising consistency of position and relation to a given population of motor units, although with marked rotations of the eye it may be displaced and require reinsertion. The superior oblique requires a special needle electrode considerably longer than the standard electrode employed for other placements. The belly of the superior oblique is much less accessible and requires placement through the lid into the upper inner aspect of the orbit running posteriorly until contact is made. The levator palpebrae superioris requires double eversion of the upper lid with insertion through the upper conjunctival cul-de-sac. One must avoid entering the superior rectus.

Needle electrodes designed for extraocular muscle electromyography must be specially prepared. The electrodes used for the peripheral skeletal musculature are much too gross. A 1- to 1½-inch 27- to 30-gauge hypodermic needle with the luer lock removed has been found satisfactory. It is prepared as a concentric electrode in the usual fashion using fine gauge supple wire for the leads to the preamplifier. The technique of preparation of such electrodes is described in *Electrophysiology of the Extraocular Muscle* by Breinin (2). A suitable ground is necessary and can usually be obtained by the application of an ordinary EEG silver grounding electrode to the forehead.

The extraocular muscle motor units differ considerably from those of the peripheral skeletal musculature. They range from 20 to 600 μV in amplitude, averaging about 200 μV in the primary position (straight ahead gaze of the eyes). They are diphasic or triphasic in form, with occasional polyphasic potentials encountered. The duration of the extraocular muscle unit is very short, ranging from 1 to 2 msec with an average of 1.5 msec. The rate of firing is very much higher than that of peripheral motor units, reaching several hundred discharges per second, and these units recruit much faster. The basis for these differences lies in the composition of the anatomic motor units. In contrast to the peripheral skeletal muscle unit, the extraocular muscle unit has a much lower innervation ratio, with one axon distributed to approximately five to 10 muscle fibers. It is probable that this low innervation ratio permits the very rapid, high frequency firing which underlies the very finely graded, exquisitely coordinated movements of the eyes. Brief insertion potentials may be elicited, as well as injury and irritation potentials due to excessive stretching or deformation of the muscle fibers by the electrode.

A profound difference between the extraocular musculature and the peripheral skeletal musculature lies in the existence of constant tonic activity of the extraocular muscle in the alert state. The extraocular muscles fire constantly at high rates of discharge in the primary position, diminishing only as the eye rotates out of the field of action of the given muscle. They do not fatigue, e.g., the lateral rectus fires abundantly with an interference pattern manifested in the primary position. As the eye looks medially, the lateral rectus is progressively inhibited, becoming silent or almost silent only in the most adducted position. The direct antagonist (the medial rectus) at the same time is observed progressively to augment its activity as the eye moves into its field of action, increasing the interference pattern from the primary position into a very high amplitude, high frequency discharge in adduction. If extreme efforts of adduction are made, the activity may actually diminish and abnormal waveforms may be evident. With a pair of electrodes inserted into either direct or contralateral antagonists, it is possible to demonstrate Sherrington's law of reciprocity in its most refined form.

It is important to recognize the peculiar histology and architecture of the extraocular muscle in order to understand the types and characteristics of potentials obtainable by electromyography (3). The extraocular muscle fibers are extremely thin, ranging from 10 to 50 μ in diameter. It is thought that, for the most part, they run from the origin to the insertion of the muscle, although recent work indicates that this is not always true. An extraordinarily interesting development in recent years has been the discovery of the existence of a slow motor system of considerable complexity present in relatively high proportion (perhaps 40%) in the extraocular musculature but not occurring in the levator palpebrae. These fibers show many of the characteristics of the frog slow motor system and have an "en grappe" distributed innervation all along the length of the muscle. These motor endings differ markedly, both anatomically and functionally, from the typical "en plaque" motor end-plates of the usual twitch fiber. The latter occur singly, occasionally doubly, in the proximal one-third of the twitch fiber. The slow fiber shows marked differences from the twitch fiber in both light and electron microscopy, exhibiting the so-called "felderstruktur" consisting of scanty sarcoplasmic reticulum with poorly defined, coalescent myofibrils. There are few triads present in the slow fiber which exhibit an irregular Z line and frequently absent M line. The twitch fiber, the so-called "fibrillenstruktur," on the other hand, shows a regular registration of Z line with abundant sarcoplasmic reticulum surrounding well defined myofibrils and an abundant T-system found in the usual A-I junction. A number of intermediate fiber types have also been described. It is of extraordinary interest that the slow fiber is polyneuronally innervated, as has been clearly demonstrated by microelectrode studies.

The significance of the presence of both slow and twitch fibers has been the subject of much study and speculation. At the present time it is not possible to define conclusively the roles of these elements. Although much disputed, it has been claimed that slow fibers may produce spike potentials hardly distinguishable from those of the twitch fiber. However, the more characteristic monophasic low amplitude potential of a slow fiber often can be obtained by sampling the surface layer of the extraocular muscle, wherein a considerable condensation of such slow fibers tends to occur. These low amplitude monophasic potentials should not be misinterpreted as envelopes due to volume effects and remoteness from the active source. It is usually found that by gently inserting the electrode through the layer of monophasic potentials, the layers of characteristic spikes are encountered. Sampling of the slow fiber layer has only now been recognized as of importance in diagnosis of extraocular muscle function. Although the interior of the muscle is abundantly supplied with slow fibers, it is difficult to recognize these in the midst of all of the spiking activity.

It is thought that the curious pharmacological response of extraocular muscle to acetylcholine and succinylcholine (long lasting contracture) is a function of the slow muscle system.

The characteristic motor unit activity of the extraocular muscle in the waking state can be readily observed to diminish or disappear as the subject falls asleep. A similar waning of the activity is encountered with general, retrobulbar, or local anesthesia (but not with topical anesthesia). It is possible to monitor the state of anesthesia by the firing response of the extraocular muscles. It is obvious, therefore, that general anesthesia cannot be used in routine analysis of extraocular muscle, because the activity disappears. This is a limiting factor in the application of the technique to children and infants, although it is possible in many instances successfully to use this technique with placid or phlegmatic children. The absence of readily available motor points rules out stimulation studies of the extraocular muscle.

APPLICATION

Kinesiology

It is immediately evident that the field of action of a muscle may be determined by its electrical response; such studies have led to the formalization of the role of a given muscle in ocular rotation. In this fashion it has been possible to demonstrate the roles of the vertical recti and obliques in horizontal, vertical, and tertiary (oblique) positions.

Pathology

From the point of view of the general electromyographer, it is important to realize that electromyography of extraocular muscle has a limited practical clinical role. In ordinary strabismus there is nothing to be gained from an electrical assessment of the extraocular muscles. So long as the eye is capable of being rotated into the field of action of a muscle, the EMG shows an abundance of electrical activity. In the presence of palsies of considerable degree, it is readily possible to demonstrate the usual constellation of abnormal electrical potentials and dynamic characteristics which parallel those of the peripheral musculature. Palsies of the extraocular muscles must be of considerable degree, and there must be definite limitation of rotation in order to show such changes. Mild palsies are accompanied by profuse discharge of remaining units, constituting an interference pattern that is not diagnostic. It is often necessary to sample multiply a muscle that shows limitations of action in order to obtain a diagnostic finding. Sampling of a relatively normal muscle simply demonstrates normal activity. Passive movement of the eye does not affect the EMG activity.

Fibrillation

The characteristic fibrillation potential of denervation can be obtained in the extraocular muscle, but such potentials are rarely recognized. Fibrillations so closely resemble normal extraocular motor units that they are frequently indistinguishable. The main characteristic is their failure to recruit on effort and their spontaneity of firing without relation to volition. Their recognition can be facilitated by moving the eye out of the field of the sampled muscle.

Neurogenic Palsy

Paresis of moderate to severe degree is characterized by irregular or sparse recruitment, poorly sustained discharge, and loss of the interference pattern characteristically seen on effort. There is frequently a greater incidence of single unit discharges. In marked paresis the motor units are frequently of decreased amplitude. There may also be a higher incidence of polyphasic and reinnervation units of larger amplitude and longer duration. Giant units are frequently noted in aberrant regeneration of the oculomotor (third nerve). Electrical silence, even in the severer degrees of palsy, is relatively infrequent. Such total silence, however, is encountered in conduction block entities and is often seen in diabetic neuropathy.

Pseudopalsy

Of particular importance in EMG diagnosis are cases of pseudopalsy due to mechanical restriction of the globe. The presence of normal or abundant activity of the extraocular EMG, quite disproportionate to the failure of rotation of the globe, is a characteristic finding. This is analogous to the situation, normally encountered, wherein the muscle recruits in the usual fashion as the patient attempts to rotate the eye into the field of action of the muscle while it is being held immobile by forceps or sutures. Passive movement of the eye does not alter the innervation. The extraocular muscle activity, therefore, follows the effort and not the position of the eye, although in normal, unimpeded rotations the extraocular muscle activity parallels the position of the eye to a very high degree.

A typical example of pseudopalsy occurs in blow-out fracture of the orbit wherein the muscle or muscle fascia is incarcerated in the fracture line so that the globe is mechanically prevented from free rotation. The extraocular EMG helps to determine the existence of normal innervation in such underacting muscles. It is also possible to infer whether the innervation or the muscle itself has been damaged by the trauma creating the blow-out fracture.

Myopathy

The demonstration of extraocular muscle myopathy by the electrical discharge pattern has been an important contribution in the entity known as progressive external ophthalmoplegia (progressive nuclear ophthalmoplegia). It is now well recognized that the pathological changes encountered in this condition center on the extraocular musculature. The characteristic findings of myopathy in the advanced case are those of a relatively abundant, low amplitude, high frequency discharge. In thyroid ophthalmopathy rather similar changes may be encountered, but more frequently a high amplitude, high frequency discharge may be recorded. In many instances there is a mixture of neurogenic and myogenic elements. It is of interest that many early cases of myopathy demonstrate a very high frequency and amplitude discharge which is difficult to distinguish from high normal except by determining the frequency histogram. Pseudotumor of the orbit may also produce a myopathic pattern.

Supranuclear Palsies

It is possible to recognize supranuclear disturbances by the pattern of innervation rather than by alterations of motor units, which tend to be quite normal. However, one may see cogwheel, saccadic augmentation, and inhibition on rotations, which are demonstrated in the EMG very clearly. The presence of innervation in muscles which nonetheless cannot move the eye is a characteristic of the medial longitudinal fasciculus syndrome. It can be shown in the relatively normal discharge of the medial recti in the primary position, although these muscles fail to adduct and demonstrate no augmentation activity on effort. In addition, the reciprocity mechanism can be shown to fail.

Nystagmus

EMG nystagmograms are readily obtained from a pair of extraocular muscles. This technique can demonstrate the existence of very high frequency nystagmus, sometimes existing within only a few motor units.

Myasthenia Gravis

Nowhere is extraocular electromyography better utilized than in the diagnosis of ocular myasthenia gravis. The frequent involvement of the extraocular musculature in this condition makes the technique of considerable importance. The demonstration of fatigue of motor units and the recovery of activity with rest establishes the diagnosis, but often the Tensilon (Roche Laboratories) test will be required to confirm the diagnosis. The intravenous Tensilon test is very readily performed with the needle electrode placed in a muscle clearly showing underaction. The frequency of ptosis often requires that the levator palpebrae be tested. The electrode is slipped through the upper conjunctival fornix into the belly of the levator. A considerable distance is traversed, because there is a very large and broad levator aponeurosis inserting into the lid. While attempting to hold the eye in the field of action of the muscle, 2 mg of the drug are injected intravenously. Usually within seconds a response will be demonstrated. This augmentation of activity may reach to the normal level or may consist of only a very slight but definite recruitment of units. The special importance of this test lies in the fact that a pharmacological EMG response may be demonstrated in the presence of failure of ocular rotation. In these cases the drug does recruit units, but in insufficient amounts actually to turn the eye. The usual clinical test appears to be negative, yet the EMG shows that the muscle is pharmacologically responsive; hence, the test is positive. No such response is seen in the normal muscle or in other palsies. It should be remembered that a myopathic form of myasthenia may also occur. The use of electromyography has proved to be exceedingly valuable in obscure and difficult conditions. Although the first 2 mg of Tensilon are usually effective, it may require a full 10-mg injection to establish adequately the diagnosis of myasthenia gravis or its absence. The injection must be made slowly with atropine available to counteract a cholinergic crisis.

From the foregoing it is apparent that the technique of extraocular electromyography finds the same range of application as does peripheral muscle electromyography. It is of value in neurogenic and myogenic palsies and is extremely valuable in the diagnosis of myasthenia gravis. It is of importance in pseudopalsies due to mechanical limitations of the globe and in congenital anomalies, and it has proved of particular value in determining the physiological characteristics of the extraocular muscle and the kinetics of ocular movements.

REFERENCES

1. Björk, A.: Electrical activity of human extrinsic eye muscles. Experientia, *8:* 226–227, 1952.
2. Breinin, G. M.: *Electrophysiology of the Extraocular Muscle.* University of Toronto Press, Toronto, 1962.
3. Breinin, G. M.: The structure and function of extraocular muscle; an appraisal of the duality concept. Am. J. Ophthalmol., *72:* 1–12, 1971.

appendix

A Glossary of Terms Used in Clinical Electromyography*

ABSOLUTE REFRACTORY PERIOD—See *Refractory Period.*

ACCOMMODATION—The reduced efficacy of a prolonged constant current or a gradually increasing current in generating action potentials from nervous tissue.

ACCOMMODATION CURVE—A curve obtained by plotting the strength of current (in multiples of *Rheobase*) required to produce a response from an excitable tissue against the time required by a slowly rising current pulse to reach that value.

ACTION CURRENT—The electrical current associated with an *Action Potential.*

ACTION POTENTIAL—(Abbr. *AP*). Strictly defined, the all-or-none, self-propagating, nondecrementing voltage change recorded from an excitable cell. The source of the action potential should be specified, e.g., nerve (fiber) action potential or muscle (fiber) action potential. Commonly, the term refers to the nearly synchronous summated action potentials of a group of cells, e.g., *Motor Unit Potential.* To avoid ambiguity in reference to the recording of nearly synchronous summated action potentials of nerve and muscle as done in nerve conduction studies, it is recommended

---

* Compiled by the Nomenclature Committee, American Association of Electromyography and Electrodiagnosis: George H. Kraft, Chairman; Jasper R. Daube; Joel A. DeLisa; Joseph Goodgold; Charles K. Jablecki; Edward H. Lambert; J. A. Simpson; Albrecht Struppler; and David O. Wiechers.

that the terms *Compound Nerve Action Potential* and *Compound Muscle Action Potential* be used, respectively, or the specific named responses, e.g., *M Wave, F Wave, H Wave, R1* and *R2 Waves.*

ACTIVE ELECTRODE—Synonymous with *Exploring Electrode.* See *Recording Electrode.*

ADAPTATION—A transient state at the initiation of an abrupt depolarization in which the impulse frequency first increases and then diminishes before the cell reaches a steady firing frequency.

AFTER DISCHARGE—Repetitive electrical firing that persists after initiation by some other process, usually muscle contraction. It may have variable form and be regular or irregular at long or short intervals.

AFTERPOTENTIAL—Membrane potential following the spike component of an *Action Potential* and not yet returned to a steady resting value. It first has a positive phase (positive afterpotential), which is followed by a negative phase (negative afterpotential).

AMPLITUDE—With reference to an *Action Potential,* the maximum voltage difference between two points, usually base line to peak or peak to peak. By convention, the amplitude of the *Compound Muscle Action Potential* is measured from the base line to the most negative peak. In contrast, the amplitude of a *Compound Sensory Nerve Action Potential, Motor Unit Potential, Fibrillation Potential, Positive Sharp Wave, Fasciculation Potential,* and most other *Action Potentials* is measured from the most positive to the most negative peak.

ANODAL BLOCK—A local block of nerve conduction caused by hyperpolarization of the nerve cell membrane by an electrical stimulus. See *Stimulating Electrode.*

ANODE—The positive terminal of a source of electrical current.

ANTIDROMIC—Said of an action potential or of the stimulation causing the action potential that propagates in the direction opposite to the normal (dromic or *Orthodromic*) one for that fiber—i.e., conduction along motor fibers toward the spinal cord and conduction along sensory fibers away from the spinal cord. Contrast with *Orthodromic.*

ARTIFACT—A voltage change generated by a biological or nonbiological source other than the ones of interest. The *Stimulus Artifact* is the potential recorded at the time the stimulus is applied and includes the *Electrical* or *Shock Artifact,* which is a potential due to the volume conducted electrical stimulus. The stimulus and shock artifacts usually precede the activity of interest. A *Movement Artifact* refers to a change in the recorded activity due to movement of the recording electrodes.

AUDITORY EVOKED POTENTIAL—Electrical waveform of biological origin elicited by a sound stimulus. See *Evoked Potential.*

BACKFIRING—Recurrent discharge of an antidromically activated motor neuron.

BAER—Abbreviation for brain stem auditory evoked response. Synonym: *Brain Stem Auditory Evoked Potential.*

BASE LINE—The potential difference recorded from the biological system of interest while the system is at rest.

BENIGN FASCICULATION—Use of term discouraged. See *Fasciculation Potential.*

BER—Abbreviation for brain stem evoked response. See *Brain Stem Auditory Evoked Potential.*

BIFILAR NEEDLE ELECTRODE—See *Bipolar Needle Electrode.*

BIPHASIC ACTION POTENTIAL—An action potential with two phases.

BIPHASIC SPIKE POTENTIAL—See *End-Plate Activity, Biphasic.*

BIPOLAR NEEDLE ELECTRODE—A recording electrode with two insulated wires side by side in a metal cannula whose bare tips act as the active and reference electrodes. The metal cannula may be grounded.

BIZARRE HIGH FREQUENCY DISCHARGE—See *Complex Repetitive Discharge.*

BIZARRE REPETITIVE POTENTIAL—See *Complex Repetitive Discharge.*

BLINK REFLEX—See *Blink Responses.*

BLINK RESPONSE—Strictly defined, one of the *Blink Responses.* See *Blink Responses.*

BLINK RESPONSES—*Compound Muscle Action Potentials* evoked from the obicularis oculi muscles as a result of brief electrical or mechanical stimuli to the cutaneous area innervated by the supraorbital (or less commonly the infraorbital) branch of the trigeminal nerve. Typically, there is an early compound muscle action potential (*R1 Wave*) ipsilateral to the stimulation site with a latency of about 10 msec and a bilateral late compound muscle action potential (*R2 Wave*) with a latency of approximately 30 msec. Generally, only the *R2 Wave* is associated with a visible twitch of the orbicularis oculi. The configuration, amplitude, duration, and latency of the two components, along with the sites of recording and the sites of stimulation, should be specified. Both *R1* and *R2 Waves* are probably due to a polysynaptic brain stem reflex, the *Blink Reflex*, with the afferent arc provided by the sensory branches of the trigeminal nerve and the efferent arc provided by the facial nerve motor fibers.

BRAIN STEM AUDITORY EVOKED POTENTIAL—(Abbr. *BAEP*). Early (latency less than 10 msec) electrical waveforms of biological origin elicited in response to sound stimuli. See *Evoked Potential.*

BRAIN STEM AUDITORY EVOKED RESPONSE—(Abbr. *BAER, BER*). Synonymous with *Brain Stem Auditory Evoked Potential.*

BREAKTHROUGH VOLUNTARY ACTIVITY—A burst of voluntary activity occurring within the *S-X Interval.*

BSAP—Abbreviation for brief, small, abundant potentials. Use of term is discouraged. It is used to describe a recruitment pattern of brief duration, small amplitude, overly abundant motor unit action potentials. Quantitative measurements of motor unit potential duration, amplitude, numbers of phases, and recruitment frequency are to be preferred to qualitative descriptions such as this. See *Motor Unit Potential.*

BSAPP—Abbreviation for brief, small, abundant, polyphasic potentials. Use of term is discouraged. It is used to describe a recruitment pattern of brief duration, small amplitude, overly abundant, polyphasic motor unit action potentials. Quantitative measurements of motor unit potential duration, amplitude, numbers of phases, and recruitment frequency are to be preferred to qualitative descriptions such as this. See *Motor Unit Potential.*

CATHODE—The negative terminal of a source of electrical current.

CEREBRAL EVOKED POTENTIAL—Electrical waveforms of biological origin recorded over the head and elicited by sensory stimuli. See specific evoked potentials, e.g., *Somatosensory Evoked Potential, Visual Evoked Potential, Auditory Evoked Potential.*

CHRONAXIE—The time required for an electrical current stimulus at a voltage twice the *Rheobase* to elicit the first visible muscle twitch. See *Strength-Duration Curve.*

CLINICAL ELECTROMYOGRAPHY—Loosely used to refer to all electrodiagnostic studies of peripheral nerves and muscle. See *Electrodiagnosis.*

COAXIAL NEEDLE ELECTRODE—See synonym, *Concentric Needle Electrode.*

COLLISION—When used with reference to nerve conduction studies, the interaction of two action potentials propagated toward each other from opposite directions on the same nerve fiber so that the refractory periods of the two potentials prevent propagation past each other.

COMPLEX ACTION POTENTIAL—See preferred term, *Serrated Action Potential.*

COMPLEX MOTOR UNIT POTENTIAL—See preferred term, *Serrated Action Potential.*

COMPLEX REPETITIVE DISCHARGE—Polyphasic or serrated action potentials that may begin spontaneously or after a needle movement. They have a uniform frequency, shape, and amplitude, with abrupt onset, cessation, or change in configuration. Amplitude ranges from 100 μV to 1 mV and frequency of discharge from 5 to 100 Hz.

COMPOUND ACTION POTENTIAL—See *Compound Mixed Nerve Action Potential, Compound Motor Nerve Action Potential, Compound Nerve Action Potential, Compound Sensory Nerve Action Potential,* and *Compound Muscle Action Potential.*

COMPOUND MIXED NERVE ACTION POTENTIAL—A compound nerve action potential is considered to have been evoked from afferent and efferent fibers if the recording electrodes detect activity on a mixed nerve with the electrical stimulus applied to a segment of the nerve which contains both afferent and efferent fibers.

COMPOUND MOTOR NERVE ACTION POTENTIAL—A compound nerve action potential is considered to have been evoked from efferent fibers to a muscle if the recording electrodes detect activity only in a motor nerve or a motor branch of a mixed nerve, or if the electrical stimulus is applied only to such a nerve or a ventral root. The amplitude, latency, duration, and phases should be noted. See *Compound Nerve Action Potential.*

COMPOUND MUSCLE ACTION POTENTIAL—The summation of nearly synchronous muscle fiber action potentials recorded from a muscle commonly produced by stimulation of the nerve supplying the muscle either directly or indirectly. Base line-to-peak amplitude, duration, and latency of the negative phase should be noted, along with details of the method of stimulation and recording. Use of specific named potentials is recommended, e.g., *M Wave, F Wave, H Wave,* and *R1 Wave* or *R2 Wave* (*Blink Responses*).

COMPOUND NERVE ACTION POTENTIAL—The summation of nearly synchronous nerve fiber action potentials recorded from a nerve trunk, commonly produced by stimulation of the nerve directly or indirectly. Details of the method of stimulation and recording should be specified, together with the fiber type (sensory, motor, or mixed).

COMPOUND SENSORY NERVE ACTION POTENTIAL—A compound nerve action potential is considered to have been evoked from afferent fibers if the recording electrodes detect activity only in a sensory nerve or in a sensory branch of a mixed nerve, or if the electrical stimulus is applied to such a nerve or a dorsal nerve root, or an adequate stimulus is applied synchronously to sensory receptors. The amplitude, latency, duration, and configuration should be noted. Generally, the amplitude is measured as the maximum peak-to-peak voltage, the latency as either the *Latency* to the initial deflection or the *Peak Latency* to the negative peak, and the duration as the interval from the first deflection of the waveform from the base line to its final return to the base line. The compound sensory nerve action potential has been referred to as the *Sensory Response* or *Sensory Potential.*

CONCENTRIC NEEDLE ELECTRODE—Recording electrode that measures the potential difference between the bare tip of a central insulated wire in the bare shaft of a metal cannula. The bare tip of the central wire (active electrode) is flush with the bevel of the cannula (reference electrode).

CONDITIONING STIMULUS—A stimulus, preceding a *Test Stimulus,* used to modify the response elicited by the test stimulus alone. See *Stimulus.*

CONDUCTION BLOCK—Failure of an action potential to be conducted past a particular point in the nervous system. In practice, a conduction block is documented by demonstration of a reduction in amplitude of an evoked potential greater than that normally seen with electrical stimulation at two different points on a nerve trunk; anatomic nerve variations and technical factors related to nerve stimulation must be excluded as the source of the reduction in amplitude.

CONDUCTION DISTANCE—See *Conduction Velocity.*

CONDUCTION TIME—See *Conduction Velocity.*

CONDUCTION VELOCITY—Speed of propagation of an *Action Potential* along a nerve or muscle fiber. The nerve fiber studied (motor, sensory, autonomic, or mixed) should be specified. For a nerve trunk, the maximum conduction velocity is calculated from the *Latency* of the evoked potential (muscle or nerve) at maximal or supramaximal intensity of stimulation at two different points. The distance between the two points (*Conduction Distance*) is divided by the difference between the corresponding latencies (*Conduction Time*). The calculated velocity represents the conduction velocity of the fastest fibers and is expressed as meters per second (m/sec). As commonly used, the term *Conduction Velocity* refers to the *Maximum Conduction Velocity*. By specialized techniques, the conduction velocity of other fibers can be determined as well and should be specified, e.g., minimum conduction velocity.

CONTRACTION—A voluntary or involuntary reversible muscle shortening that may or may not be accompanied by *Action Potentials* from muscle. This term is to be contrasted with the term *Contracture*, which refers to a condition of fixed muscle shortening.

CONTRACTURE—An electrically silent, involuntary state of maintained muscle contraction, as seen in phosphorylase deficiency. The term is also used to refer to immobility of a joint due to other local processes.

CORTICAL EVOKED POTENTIAL—See *Cerebral Evoked Potential.*

COUPLED DISCHARGE—See preferred term, *Late Component.*

CRAMP DISCHARGE—Repetitive firing of action potentials with the configuration of *Motor Unit Potentials* at a high frequency in a large area of muscle, associated with an involuntary, painful muscle contraction (cramp).

CYCLES PER SECOND—Unit of frequency. (Abbr. *c/sec* or *cps*). Preferred equivalent is *Hertz* (Abbr. *Hz*).

DECREMENTING RESPONSE—A progressive decline in the amplitude associated with a decrease in the area of the negative phase of the *M Wave* of successive responses to a series of supramaximal stimuli. The rate of stimulation and the number of stimuli should be specified. Contrast with *Incrementing Response.*

DELAY—Interval between onset of oscilloscope sweep and onset of a stimulus. Had been used in the past to designate the interval from the stimulus to the response. Compare with *Latency.*

DENERVATION POTENTIAL—Use of term discouraged. See *Fibrillation Potential.*

DEPOLARIZATION—A decrease in the electrical potential difference across a membrane from any cause, to any degree, relative to the normal resting potential. See *Polarization.*

DEPOLARIZATION BLOCK—Failure of an excitable cell to respond to a stimulus because of *Depolarization* of the cell membrane.

DISCHARGE—Synonymous with *Action Potential.*

DISCHARGE FREQUENCY—The rate of repetition of an *Action Potential.* When potentials occur in groups, the rate of recurrence of the group and the rate of repetition of the individual components in the groups should be specified. See *Firing Rate.*

DISCRETE ACTIVITY—The pattern of electrical activity at full voluntary contraction of the muscle is reduced to the extent that each individual *Motor Unit Potential* can be identified. The firing frequency of each of these potentials should be specified together with the force of contraction.

DISTAL LATENCY—See *Motor Latency* and *Sensory Latency.*

"DIVE BOMBER" POTENTIAL—Use of term discouraged. See preferred term, *Myotonic Discharge.*

DOUBLE DISCHARGE—Two action potentials of the same form and nearly the same amplitude, occurring consistently in the same relationship to one another at intervals of 2 to 20 msec. Contrast with *Paired Discharge.*

DOUBLET—Synonymous with *Double Discharge.*

DURATION—The time during which something exists or acts. (a) The duration of individual potential *Waveforms* is defined as the interval from the first deflection from the base line to its final return to the base line, unless otherwise specified. One common exception is the duration of the *M Wave*, which usually refers to the interval from the deflection of the first negative phase from the base line to its return to the base line. (b) The duration of a single electrical stimulus refers to the interval of the applied current or voltage. (c) The duration of recurring stimuli or action potentials refers to the interval from the beginning to the end of the series.

EARTHING ELECTRODE—Synonymous with *Ground Electrode.*

ELECTRICAL ARTIFACT—See *Artifact.*

ELECTRICAL SILENCE—The absence of measurable electrical activity due to biological or nonbiological sources. The sensitivity, or signal-to-noise level, of the recording system should be specified.

ELECTRODE—A device capable of conducting electricity. The material (metal, fabric), size, configuration (disc, ring, needle), and location (surface, intramuscular, intracranial) should be specified. Electrodes may be used to record an electrical potential difference (*Recording Electrodes*) or to apply an electrical current (*Stimulating Electrodes*). In both cases, two electrodes are always required. Depending on the relative size and location of the electrodes, however, the stimulating or recording condition may be referred to as "*Monopolar.*" See *Ground Electrode, Recording Electrode,* and *Stimulating Electrode.* Also see specific needle electrode configurations: *Monopolar, Concentric, Bipolar,* and *Multilead Needle Electrodes.*

ELECTRODIAGNOSIS—(Abbr. *EDX*). General term used to refer to the recording of responses of nerves and muscle to electrical stimulation and the recording of insertional, spontaneous, and voluntary action potentials from muscle. It was originally used to refer to *Strength-Duration Curve* determinations and other early techniques.

ELECTROMYELOGRAPHY—The recording and study of electrical activity from the spinal cord. The term is also used to refer to studies of electrical activity from the cauda equina.

ELECTROMYOGRAM—The record obtained by *Electromyography.*

ELECTROMYOGRAPH—An instrument for detecting and displaying *Action Potentials* from muscle and nerve.

ELECTROMYOGRAPHY—(Abbr. *EMG*). Strictly defined, the recording and study of insertional, spontaneous, and voluntary electrical activity of muscle. It is commonly used to refer to nerve conduction studies as well. Compare with *Clinical Electromyography* and the more general term, *Electrodiagnosis.*

ELECTRONEUROGRAPHY—The recording and study of the action potentials of peripheral nerves. See preferred term, *Nerve Conduction Studies,* and the more general term, *Electrodiagnosis.*

ELECTRONEUROMYOGRAPHY—A newly fabricated word used to refer to the combined studies of *Electromyography* and *Electroneurography.* See preferred terms, *Clinical Electromyography* and *Electrodiagnosis.*

ELECTROSPINOGRAM—The record obtained by *Electromyelography.*

END-PLATE ACTIVITY—Spontaneous electrical activity recorded with a needle electrode close to muscle end-plates. May be either of two forms:

1. **MONOPHASIC.** Low amplitude (10 to 20 μV), short duration (0.5 to 1 msec), monophasic (negative) potentials that occur in a dense, steady pattern and are restricted to a localized area of the muscle. Because of the multitude of different potentials occurring, the exact frequency, although appearing to be high, cannot be defined. These potentials are miniature end-plate potentials recorded extracellularly.. This form of end-plate activity has been referred to as *End-Plate Noise* and is associated with a sound not unlike that of a seashell, which has been called a *Sea Shell Noise* or *Roar.*
2. **BIPHASIC.** Moderate amplitude (100 to 300 μV), short duration (2 to 4 msec), biphasic (negative-positive) spike potentials that occur irregularly in short bursts with

a high frequency (50 to 100 Hz), restricted to a localized area within the muscle. These potentials are generated by muscle fibers excited by activity in nerve terminals. These potentials have been referred to as *Biphasic Spike Potentials*, *End-Plate Spikes*, and, incorrectly, "*Nerve*" *Potentials*.

END-PLATE NOISE—See *End-Plate Activity, Monophasic.*

END-PLATE POTENTIAL—Graded, nonpropagated potential recorded by microelectrodes from muscle fibers in the region of the neuromuscular junction.

END-PLATE SPIKE— See *End-Plate Activity, Biphasic.*

END-PLATE ZONE—The site of the neuromuscular junction, a localized area of the muscle fiber in which activity identified as end-plate activity may be recorded.

EVOKED ACTION POTENTIAL—Action potential elicited by a stimulus.

EVOKED COMPOUND MUSCLE ACTION POTENTIAL—The electrical activity of a muscle produced by stimulation of the nerves supplying the muscle. Base line-to-peak amplitude of the negative phase, duration of the negative phase, and *Latency* should be measured, and details of the method of stimulation should be recorded. See specific named potentials: *M Wave*, *F Wave*, *H Wave*, *R1* and *R2 Waves*, and *Blink Responses.*

EVOKED POTENTIAL—Electrical waveform elicited by and temporally related to a stimulus, most commonly an electrical stimulus delivered to a sensory receptor or nerve, or applied directly to a discrete area of the brain, spinal cord, or muscle. See *Auditory Evoked Potential*, *Brain Stem Auditory Evoked Potential*, *Spinal Evoked Potential*, *Somatosensory Evoked Potential*, *Visual Evoked Potential*, *Cerebral Evoked Potential*, *Compound Muscle Action Potential*, and *Compound Sensory Nerve Action Potential.*

EVOKED RESPONSE—Tautology. Use of term discouraged. Suggested term is *Evoked Potential.*

EXCITABILITY—Capacity to be activated by or react to a stimulus.

EXCITATORY POSTSYNAPTIC POTENTIAL—(Abbr. *EPSP*). A local, graded depolarization of a neuron in response to activation by a nerve terminal at a synapse. Contrast with *Inhibitory Postsynaptic Potential.*

EXPLORING ELECTRODE—Synonymous with *Active Electrode.* See *Recording Electrode.*

FACILITATION OF NEUROMUSCULAR TRANSMISSION—An increase in the amplitude of an end-plate potential of a muscle fiber with stimulation of the axon in a variety of physiological and pharmacological settings. Use of the term is not recommended for description of the phenomenon recorded in repetitive stimulation studies.

FASCICULATION—The random, spontaneous twitching of a group of muscle fibers which may be visible through the skin. The electrical activity associated with the spontaneous contraction is called the *Fasciculation Potential.* Compare with *Myokymia.*

FASCICULATION POTENTIAL—The electrical potential associated with *Fasciculation* which has dimensions of a motor unit potential that occurs spontaneously as a single discharge. Most commonly these potentials occur sporadically and are termed "single fasciculation potentials." Occasionally, the potentials occur as a grouped discharge and are termed "grouped fasciculation potentials." The occurrence of large numbers of either simple or grouped fasciculations may produce a writhing, vermicular movement of the skin called *Myokymia.* Use of the terms *Benign Fasciculation* and *Malignant Fasciculation* is discouraged. Instead, the configuration of the potentials, peak-to-peak amplitude, duration, number of phases, and stability of configuration, in addition to frequency of occurrence, should be specified.

FATIGUE—Reduction in the force of contraction of muscle fibers as a result of repeated use or electrical stimulation. More generally, it is a state of depressed responsiveness resulting from protracted activity and requiring appreciable recovery time.

FIBER DENSITY—(a) Anatomically, fiber density is a measure of the number of muscle or nerve fibers per unit area. (b) In single fiber EMG, the fiber density is the mean number of muscle fiber potentials under voluntary control encountered during a systematic search. See *Single Fiber Electromyography.*

FIBRILLATION—The spontaneous contractions of individual muscle fibers which are ordinarily not visible through the skin. This term has been used loosely in electromyography for the preferred term, *Fibrillation Potential.*

FIBRILLATION POTENTIAL—The electrical activity associated with fibrillating muscle fibers, reflecting the action potential of a single muscle fiber. The action potentials may occur spontaneously or after movement of the needle electrode. The potentials usually occur repetitively and regularly. Classically, the potentials are biphasic spikes of short duration (usually less than 5 msec) with an initial positive phase and a peak-to-peak amplitude of less than 1 mV. The firing rate has a wide range (1 to 50 Hz) and often decreases just before cessation of an individual discharge. A high pitched regular sound is associated with the discharge of fibrillation potentials and has been described in the old literature as "rain on a tin roof." In addition to this classic form of fibrillation potentials, *Positive Sharp Waves* may also be recorded from fibrillating muscle fibers; the difference in the configuration of the potentials is due to the position of the recording electrode.

FIRING PATTERN—Qualitative and quantitative description of the sequence of discharge of potential waveforms recorded from muscle or nerve.

FIRING RATE—Frequency of repetition of a potential. The relationship of the frequency to the occurrence of other potentials and the force of muscle contraction may be described. See *Discharge Frequency.*

FRACTIONATION OF MOTOR UNIT POTENTIALS—Use of term discouraged. This term has been used to describe polyphasic, short duration, low amplitude motor unit potentials, a configuration thought to imply failure to activate all of the muscle fibers in a motor unit.

F REFLEX—Use of term discouraged, as it is incorrect. No reflex is considered to be involved. See *F Wave.*

FREQUENCY—Number of complete cycles of a repetitive waveform in 1 sec. Measures in *Hertz* (Hz), a unit preferred to its equivalent, *Cycles per Second* (c/sec).

FREQUENCY ANALYSIS—Determination of the range of frequencies composing a potential waveform, with a measurement of the absolute or relative amplitude of each component frequency. It is similar to the mathematical technique of Fourier analysis.

F RESPONSE—Synonymous with *F Wave.* See *F Wave.*

FULL INTERFERENCE PATTERN—See *Interference Pattern.*

F WAVE—A late compound action potential evoked intermittently from a muscle by supramaximal electrical stimulus to the nerve. Compared with the maximal amplitude M wave of the same muscle, the F wave has a reduced amplitude and variable configuration and a longer and more variable latency. It can be found in many muscles of the upper and lower extremities, and the latency is longer with more distal sites of stimulation. The F wave is due to antidromic activation of motor neurons. It was named by Magladery and McDougal in 1950. Contrast with *H Wave.*

G1, G2—Synonymous with Grid 1, Grid 2. See *Recording Electrodes.*

"GIANT" MOTOR UNIT ACTION POTENTIAL—Use of term discouraged. It refers to a motor unit potential with a peak-to-peak amplitude and duration much greater than the range recorded in corresponding muscles in normal subjects of similar age. Quantitative measurements of amplitude and duration are preferable.

GROUND ELECTRODE—An electrode connected to a large conducting body (such as the earth) used as a common return for an electrical circuit and as an arbitrary zero potential reference point.

GROUPED DISCHARGE—Intermittent repetition of a group of *Action Potentials* with the same or nearly the same waveform and a relatively short interpotential interval within the group in comparison with the time interval between each group. It may occur spontaneously or with voluntary activity and may be regular or irregular in its firing pattern.

HABITUATION—Decrease in amplitude and/or duration of a response with repeated stimuli. Response may be eliminated.

HERTZ—(Abbr. Hz). Unit of frequency representing cycles per second.

HOFFMAN REFLEX—See *H Wave.*

H REFLEX—Abbreviation for Hoffman reflex. See *H Wave.*

H RESPONSE—Synonymous with *H Wave.*

H WAVE—A late compound muscle action potential having a consistent latency evoked regularly, when present, from a muscle by an electrical stimulus to the nerve. It is regularly found only in a limited group of physiological extensors, particularly the calf muscles. The reflex is most easily obtained with the cathode positioned proximal to the anode. Compared with the maximal amplitude *M Wave* of the same muscle, the H wave has a reduced amplitude, a longer latency, and a lower optimal stimulus intensity; its configuration is constant. The latency is longer with more distal sites of stimulation. A stimulus intensity sufficient to elicit a maximal amplitude M wave reduces or abolishes the H wave. The H wave is thought to be due to a spinal reflex, the Hoffman reflex, with electrical stimulation of afferent fibers in the mixed nerve to the muscle and activation of motor neurons to the muscle through a monosynaptic connection in the spinal cord. The reflex and wave are named in honor of Hoffman's description (1918). Compare with *F Wave.*

HYPERPOLARIZATION—See *Polarization.*

INCREASED INSERTIONAL ACTIVITY—See *Insertional Activity.*

INCREMENTAL RESPONSE—See synonym, *Incrementing Response.*

INCREMENTING RESPONSE—A progressive increase in amplitude associated with an increase in the area of the negative phase of the *M Wave* of successive responses to a series of supramaximal stimuli. The rate of stimulation and the number of stimuli should be specified. Contrast with *Decrementing Response.*

INDIFFERENT ELECTRODE—Synonymous with *Reference Electrode.* See *Recording Electrode.*

INHIBITORY POSTSYNAPTIC POTENTIAL—(Abbr. *IPSP*). A local graded hyperpolarization of a neuron in response to activation at a synapse by a nerve terminal. Contrast with *Excitatory Postsynaptic Potential.*

INJURY POTENTIAL—The potential difference between a normal region of the surface of a nerve or muscle and a region that has been injured; also called a demarcation potential. This potential was studied before intracellular recording was introduced. The injury potential approximates the potential across the membrane because the injured surface is almost at the potential of the inside of the cell. This term has been loosely used to describe *Insertional Activity* encountered in *Clinical Electromyography.*

INSERTIONAL ACTIVITY—Electrical activity caused by insertion or movement of a needle electrode. The amount of the activity may be described qualitatively as *Normal, Reduced, Increased,* or *Prolonged.*

INTERDISCHARGE INTERVAL—Time between consecutive discharges of the same potential. Measurements should be made between the corresponding points on each waveform.

INTERFERENCE—Unwanted electrical activity arising outside the system being studied.

INTERFERENCE PATTERN—Electrical activity recorded from a muscle with a needle electrode during maximal voluntary effort, in which identification of each of the contributing action potentials is not possible, because of the overlap or interference of one potential with another. When no individual potentials can be identified, this is known as a *Full Interference Pattern.* A *Reduced Interference Pattern* is one in which some of the individual potentials may be identified while other individual potentials cannot be identified because of overlapping. The term *Discrete Activity* is used to describe the electrical activity recorded when each of the motor unit potentials can be identified. It is important that the force of contraction associated with the interference pattern be specified.

INTERPOTENTIAL INTERVAL—Time between two different potentials. Measurement should be made between the corresponding parts on each waveform.

INTRAMUSCULAR ELECTRODE—An electrode usually used for recording and usually shaped like a needle to facilitate placement within a muscle belly.

INVOLUNTARY ACTIVITY—Action potentials that are not under voluntary control. The condition under which they occur should be described, e.g., spontaneous, or, if elicited by a stimulus, the nature of the stimulus. Compare with *Spontaneous Activity.*

ISOELECTRIC DISCHARGE—Recording obtained from a pair of equipotential electrodes.

ITERATIVE DISCHARGE—See preferred term, *Repetitive Discharge.*

JITTER—Synonymous with "single fiber electromyographic jitter." Jitter is the variability of the *Interpotential Interval* between two muscle fiber action potentials belonging to the same motor unit. It is usually expressed quantitatively as the mean value of the difference between the interpotential intervals of consecutive discharges (the mean consecutive difference, abbr. MCD). Under certain conditions, jitter is expressed as the mean value of the difference between the interpotential intervals arranged in the order of decreasing interpotential intervals (the mean sorted difference, abbr. MSD).

JOLLY TEST—A technique, described in 1895 by Jolly, of application of a Faradic current to a motor nerve while recording the muscle contraction. This test has been refined and replaced by the technique of *Repetitive Stimulation* of motor nerves and the recording of successive M waves to detect a defect of neuromuscular transmission; use of the term is discouraged for modern testing techniques.

LATE COMPONENT OF A MOTOR UNIT POTENTIAL—A potential separated from a *Motor Unit Potential* by a segment of base line recording, but firing in a time-locked relationship to the motor unit potential.

LATE RESPONSE—A general term used to describe an evoked potential having a longer latency than the *M Wave*. See *H Wave*, *F Wave*.

LATENCY—Interval between the onset of a stimulus and the onset of a response unless otherwise specified. Latency always refers to the onset unless specified, as in *Peak Latency*.

LATENCY OF ACTIVATION—The time required for an electrical stimulus to depolarize a nerve. In the past this had been estimated to be 0.1 msec.

LATENT PERIOD—See synonym, *Latency*.

MALIGNANT FASCICULATION—Use of term discouraged. See *Fasciculation Potential*.

MAXIMAL STIMULUS—See *Stimulus*.

MAXIMUM NERVE CONDUCTION VELOCITY—See *Conduction Velocity*.

MEMBRANE INSTABILITY—Tendency of a cell membrane to depolarize spontaneously or after mechanical irritation or voluntary activation.

MICRONEUROGRAPHY—The technique of recording peripheral nerve action potentials in man by means of intraneural microelectrodes.

MINIATURE END-PLATE POTENTIAL—When recorded with microelectrodes, monophasic negative discharges with amplitudes less than 100 μV and duration of 4 msec or less, occurring irregularly and recorded in an area of muscle corresponding to the myoneural junction. They are thought to be due to small quantities (quanta) of acetylcholine released spontaneously. Compare with *End-Plate Activity*.

MIXED NERVE ACTION POTENTIAL—See *Compound Nerve Action Potential*.

MONOPHASIC ACTION POTENTIAL—An action potential with one phase.

MONOPHASIC END-PLATE ACTIVITY—See *End-Plate Activity*.

MONOPOLAR NEEDLE ELECTRODE—A solid wire, usually of stainless steel, coated, except at its tip, with an insulating material. Variations in voltage between the tip of the needle (active or exploring electrode) positioned in a muscle and a conductive plate on the skin surface or a bare needle in subcutaneous tissue (reference electrode) are measured. By convention, this recording condition is referred to as a monopolar needle electrode recording; it should be emphasized, however, that potential differences are always recorded between two electrodes.

MOTOR LATENCY—Interval between the onset of a stimulus and the onset of the resultant *Compound Muscle Action Potential*. The term may be qualified as *Proximal Latency* or *Distal Latency*, depending on the relative position of the stimulus.

MOTOR NERVE ACTION POTENTIAL—See *Compound Motor Nerve Action Potential*.

MOTOR NERVE CONDUCTION VELOCITY—(Abbr. MNCV). See *Conduction Velocity.*

MOTOR POINT—The point over a muscle where a contraction of a muscle may be elicited by a minimal intensity, short duration electrical stimulus.

MOTOR RESPONSE—Either (a) the compound muscle action potential recorded over a muscle with stimulation of the nerve to the muscle or (b) the muscle twitch or contraction elicited by stimulation of the nerve to a muscle. As commonly used, the motor response refers only to the evoked potential, the *M Wave.*

MOTOR UNIT—The anatomic unit of an anterior horn cell, its axon, the neuromuscular junctions, and all of the muscle fibers innervated by the axon.

MOTOR UNIT ACTION POTENTIAL—(Abbr. MUAP). See synonym, *Motor Unit Potential.*

MOTOR UNIT POTENTIAL—(Abbr. MUP). Action potential reflecting the electrical activity of that part of a single anatomic motor unit that is within the recording range of an electrode. The action potential is characterized by its consistent appearance with and relationship to the force of a voluntary contraction of a muscle. The following parameters should be specified, quantitatively if possible, after the recording electrode is placed so as to minimize the *Rise Time* (which by convention should be less than 0.5 msec), which generally also maximizes the amplitude:

I. Configuration
   A. *Amplitude*, peak to peak (μV or mV)
   B. *Duration*, total (msec)
   C. Number of *Phases* (*Monophasic*, *Biphasic*, *Triphasic*, *Tetraphasic*, *Polyphasic*)
   D. Direction of each *Phase* (negative, positive)
   E. Number of *Turns of Serrated Potential*
   F. Variation of shape with consecutive discharges
   G. Presence of *Late Components*

II. *Recruitment* characteristics
   A. Threshold of activation (first recruited, low threshold, high threshold)
   B. *Onset Frequency* (Hz)
   C. *Recruitment Frequency* (Hz) or *Recruitment Interval* (msec) of individual potentials

Descriptive terms implying diagnostic significance are not recommended, e.g., *Myopathic*, *Neuropathic*, *Regeneration*, *Nascent*, *Giant*, *BSAP*, and *BSAPP.*

MOTOR UNIT SUBUNIT—Abandoned concept of muscle physiology. Fibers of a motor unit were considered to be arranged in groups of subunits containing an average of 10 fibers that fired synchronously. This is no longer accepted.

MOTOR UNIT TERRITORY—(a) The area in which *Motor Unit Potentials* from a single motor unit may be recorded with a *Rise Time* of less than 0.5 msec. (b) The area in a muscle over which the muscle fibers of an individual motor unit are distributed anatomically.

MOVEMENT ARTIFACT—See *Artifact.*

M RESPONSE—See synonym, *M Wave.*

MUAP—Abbreviation for motor unit action potential. See synonym, *Motor Unit Potential.*

MULTIELECTRODE—See *Multilead Electrode.*

MULTILEAD ELECTRODE—Three or more insulated wires inserted through a common metal cannula with their bared tips at an aperture in the cannula and flush with the outer circumference of the cannula. The arrangement of the bare tips relative to the axis of the cannula and the distance between each tip should be specified.

MULTIPLE DISCHARGE—Four or more motor unit action potentials of the same form and nearly the same amplitude occurring consistently in the same relationship to one another. See *Double* and *Triple Discharge.*

MULTIPLET—See *Multiple Discharge.*

MUP—Abbreviation for *Motor Unit Potential.*

MUSCLE ACTION POTENTIAL—Strictly defined, the term refers to the action potential recorded from a single muscle fiber. However, the term is commonly used to refer to a compound muscle action potential. See *Compound Muscle Action Potential.*

MUSCLE FIBER CONDUCTION VELOCITY—The speed of propagation of a single muscle fiber action potential, usually expressed as meters per second. The muscle fiber conduction velocity is usually less than most nerve conduction velocities, varies with the rate of discharge of the muscle fiber, and requires special techniques for measurement.

MUSCLE UNIT—An anatomic term referring to the group of muscle fibers innervated by a single motor neuron. See *Motor Unit.*

M WAVE—A *Compound Action Potential* evoked from a muscle by a single electrical stimulus to its motor nerve. By convention, the M wave elicited by supramaximal stimulation is used for motor nerve conduction studies. The recording electrodes should be placed so that the initial deflection of the evoked potential is negative. The *Latency*, commonly called the *Motor Latency*, is the latency (milliseconds) to the onset of the first negative phase. The amplitude (millivolts) is the base line-to-peak amplitude of the first negative phase, unless otherwise specified. The *Duration* (milliseconds) refers to the duration of the first negative phase, unless otherwise specified. Normally, the configuration of the M wave (usually biphasic) is quite stable with repeated stimuli at slow rates (1 to 5 Hz). See *Repetitive Stimulation.*

MYOKYMIA—Involuntary, continuous quivering of muscle fibers which may be visible through the skin as a vermiform movement. It is associated with spontaneous, rhythmic discharge of *Motor Unit Potentials.* See *Myokymic Discharges*, *Fasciculation*, and *Fasciculation Potential.*

MYOKYMIC DISCHARGES—Action potentials with the configuration of *Motor Unit Potentials* that occur spontaneously, recur regularly, and may be associated with clinical myokymia. Two distinct firing patterns are recognized. Commonly, the discharges are grouped with a short period (up to a few seconds) of firing at a uniform rate (2 to 20 Hz) followed by a short period (up to a few seconds) of silence, with repetition of the same sequence for a particular potential. Less commonly, the potential recurs continuously at a fairly uniform firing rate (1 to 5 Hz). Myokymic discharges are a subclass of *Grouped Discharges* and *Repetitive Discharges.*

MYOPATHIC MOTOR UNIT POTENTIAL—Use of term discouraged. It is used to refer to low amplitude, short duration, polyphasic motor unit action potentials. The term incorrectly implies specific diagnostic significance of a motor unit potential configuration. See *Motor Unit Potential.*

MYOPATHIC RECRUITMENT—Use of term discouraged. It is used to describe an increase in the number of and firing rate of motor unit potentials compared with normal for the strength of muscle contraction.

MYOTONIC DISCHARGE—Repetitive discharge of 20 to 80 Hz of biphasic (positive-negative) spike potentials less than 5 msec in duration or monophasic positive waves of 5 to 20 msec recorded after needle insertion, or less commonly after voluntary muscle contraction or muscle percussion. The amplitude and frequency of the potentials must both wax and wane to be identified as myotonic discharges. This change produces a characteristic musical sound in the audio display of the electromyograph due to the corresponding change in pitch, which has been likened to the sound of a "dive bomber." Contrast with *Waning Discharge.*

MYOTONIC POTENTIAL—See preferred term, *Myotonic Discharge.*

MYOTONIC RESPONSE—Delayed relaxation of muscle after voluntary contraction or percussion and associated with a myotonic discharge. See *Myotonic Discharge.*

NASCENT MOTOR UNIT POTENTIAL—From the Latin "nascens," to be born. Use of term is discouraged as it incorrectly implies diagnostic significance of a motor unit potential configuration. Term has been used to refer to very low amplitude, long duration, highly polyphasic motor unit potentials observed during early stages of reinnervation of muscle. See *Motor Unit Potential.*

NASCENT UNIT—Use of term discouraged. See *Nascent Motor Unit Potential.*

NEEDLE ELECTRODE—An electrode for recording or stimulating, shaped like a needle. See specific electrodes: *Bipolar Needle Electrode, Concentric Needle Electrode, Monopolar Needle Electrode, Multilead Electrode.*

NERVE ACTION POTENTIAL—Strictly defined, refers to an action potential recorded from a single nerve fiber. The term is commonly used to refer to the compound nerve action potential. See *Compound Nerve Action Potential.*

NERVE CONDUCTION STUDIES—Refers to all aspects of electrodiagnostic studies of peripheral nerves. However, the term is generally used to refer to the recording and measurement of *Compound Nerve* and *Compound Muscle Action Potentials* elicited in response to a single supramaximal electrical *Stimulus* under standardized conditions that permit establishment of normal ranges of amplitude, duration, and latency of *Evoked Potentials* and the calculation of the *Maximum Conduction Velocity* of individual nerves. See *Compound Nerve Action Potential, Compound Muscle Action Potential, Conduction Velocity,* and *Repetitive Stimulation.*

NERVE CONDUCTION VELOCITY—(Abbr. NCV). Loosely used to refer to the maximum nerve conduction velocity. See *Conduction Velocity.*

NERVE POTENTIAL—Equivalent to *Nerve Action Potential.* Also commonly, but inaccurately, used to refer to the biphasic form of *End-Plate Activity.* The latter use is incorrect because muscle fibers, not nerve fibers, are the source of these potentials.

NERVE TRUNK ACTION POTENTIAL—See preferred term, *Compound Nerve Action Potential.*

NEUROMYOTONIA—Clinical syndrome of continuous muscle fiber activity manifested as continuous muscle rippling and stiffness. It may be associated with a variety of electrical discharges.

NEUROMYOTONIC DISCHARGES—Bursts of *Motor Unit Potentials* firing at more than 150 Hz for ½ to 2 sec. The amplitude of the response typically wanes. Discharges may occur spontaneously or be initiated by needle movement.

NEUROPATHIC MOTOR UNIT POTENTIAL—Use of term discouraged. It is used to refer to abnormally high amplitude, long duration, polyphasic *Motor Unit Potentials.* The term incorrectly implies a specific diagnostic significance of a motor unit potential configuration. See *Motor Unit Potential.*

NEUROPATHIC RECRUITMENT—Use of term discouraged. It has been used to describe a recruitment pattern with a decreased number of *Motor Unit Potentials* firing at a rapid rate. See preferred terms, *Discrete Activity, Reduced Interference Pattern.*

NOISE—Strictly defined, an *Artifact* consisting of low amplitude, random potentials produced by an amplifier and unrelated to the input signal. It is most apparent when high gains are used. It is loosely used to refer to end-plate noise. Compare with *End-Plate Activity.*

ONSET FREQUENCY—The lowest stable frequency of firing for a single *Motor Unit Potential* that can be voluntarily maintained by a subject.

ONSET LATENCY—Tautology. See *Latency.*

ORDER OF ACTIVATION—The sequence of appearance of different

Motor Unit Potentials with increasing strength of voluntary contraction. See *Recruitment.*

ORTHODROMIC—Said of *Action Potentials* or stimuli eliciting action potentials propagated in the same direction as physiological conduction, e.g., motor nerve conduction away from the spinal cord and sensory nerve conduction toward the spinal cord. Contrast with *Antidromic.*

PAIRED DISCHARGE—Two action potentials of the same form and nearly the same amplitude occurring consistently in the same relationship to each other at intervals of 20 to 80 msec. Contrast with *Double Discharge.*

PAIRED RESPONSE—Loosely used to refer to either the preferred term *Paired Discharge* or the preferred term *Late Component.*

PAIRED STIMULI—Two temporally linked stimuli. The time interval between the two stimuli and the intensity of each stimulus should be specified. The first is called the *Conditioning Stimulus* and the second the *Test Stimulus.*

PARASITE POTENTIAL—See Preferred term, *Late Component of a Motor Unit Potential.*

PEAK LATENCY—Interval between the onset of a stimulus and a specified peak of the evoked potential (usually the negative peak).

PHASE—That portion of a *Wave* between the departure from and the return to the *Base Line.*

POLARIZATION—As used in neurophysiology, the presence of an electrical *Potential* difference across an excitable cell membrane. The potential across the membrane of a cell when it is not excited by input or spontaneously active is termed the *Resting Potential*; it is at a steady state with regard to the electrical potential difference across the membrane. *Depolarization* describes a decrease in polarization to any degree, relative to the normal resting potential. *Hyperpolarization* describes an increase in polarization relative to the resting potential. *Repolarization* describes an increase in polarization from the depolarized state toward, but not above, the normal or resting potential.

POLYPHASIC ACTION POTENTIAL—An *Action Potential* having five or more phases. See *Phase.* Contrast with *Serrated Action Potential.*

POSITIVE SHARP WAVE—Strictly defined, one form of electrical activity associated with fibrillating muscle fibers. It is recorded as a biphasic, positive-negative *Action Potential* initiated by needle movement and recurring in a uniform, regular pattern at a rate of 2 to 50 Hz, which may decrease just before cessation of discharge. The amplitude and duration vary considerably, but the initial positive deflection is usually less than 5 msec in duration and up to 1 mV in amplitude. The negative phase is of low amplitude, with a duration of 10 to 100 msec. A sequence of positive sharp waves is commonly referred to as a *Train of Positive Sharp Waves.* Positive sharp waves are recorded from the damaged area of fibrillating muscle fibers. Loosely defined, positive sharp waves refer to any action potential recorded with the wave form of a positive wave, without reference to the firing pattern or method of generation.

POSITIVE WAVE—Strictly defined, the positive phase of a waveform. Loosely defined, the term refers to a positive sharp wave. See *Positive Sharp Wave.*

POSTACTIVATION DEPRESSION—The reduction in the amplitude of an *Evoked Potential* in response to a single *Stimulus* which occurs after *Repetitive Stimulation* or after voluntary contraction.

POSTACTIVATION EXHAUSTION—The reduction of the amplitude associated with a decrease in the area of the negative phase of the initial *M Wave* and/or the exaggeration of the *Decrementing Response* seen 2 to 4 min after either a brief (10 to 30 sec), strong voluntary contraction or a period of nerve stimulation causing tetanic muscle contraction. Compare with *Postactivation facilitation.*

POSTACTIVATION FACILITATION—The increase in amplitude associated with an increase in the area of the negative phase of the initial *M Wave* and/or the diminution of the *Decrementing Response* seen a few seconds after either a brief (10 to 30 sec), strong voluntary contraction or a period of nerve stimulation causing tetanic muscle contraction. Compare with *Postactivation Exhaustion.*

POSTACTIVATION POTENTIAL—Synonymous with preferred term, *Postactivation Facilitation.*

POSTTETANIC POTENTIATION—Enhancement of excitability following a long period of high frequency stimulation. This phenomenon is known mainly in the mammalian spinal cord, where it lasts minutes or even hours. Use of the term is not recommended to describe the phenomenon of *Postactivation facilitation.*

POTENTIAL—Strictly, *Voltage*; loosely, synonymous with *Action Potential.* See *Polarization.*

PROLONGED INSERTIONAL ACTIVITY—See *Insertional Activity.*

PROPAGATION VELOCITY OF A MUSCLE FIBER—The speed of transmission of a muscle fiber action potential.

PROXIMAL LATENCY—See *Motor Latency* and *Sensory Latency.*

PSEUDOFACILITATION (OF NEUROMUSCULAR TRANSMISSION)—Use of term discouraged. It refers to an increase in amplitude with a corresponding reduction in duration of the negative phase of the *M Wave,* resulting in no change in the area of the negative phase of the M wave. This probably reflects a reduction in the temporal dispersion of a constant number of summated muscle fiber action potentials, and must be differentiated from *Postactivation Facilitation.* See *Postactivation Facilitation.*

PSEUDOMYOTONIC DISCHARGE—Use of term discouraged. It has been used to refer to different phenomena, including (a) *Myotonic Dis-*

charges occurring in the presence of a neurogenic disease, (b) *Complex Repetitive Discharges*, and (c) *Repetitive Discharges* that wax or wane in either frequency or amplitude but not in both. See *Waning Discharge.*

PSEUDOPOLYPHASIC ACTION POTENTIAL—Use of term discouraged. See preferred term, *Serrated Action Potential.*

R1, R2 WAVES—See *Blink Responses.*

RECORDING ELECTRODE—Device used to monitor electrical current or potential. All electrical recordings require two *Electrodes.* The electrode close to the source of the activity to be recorded is called the *Active* or *Exploring Electrode*, and the other electrode is called the *Reference Electrode.* Active electrode is synonymous with the older terminology G1 or Grid 1, and the reference electrode with G2 or Grid 2. By current convention, a potential difference that is negative at the active electrode relative to the reference electrode causes an upward deflection on the oscilloscope screen. The term "monopolar recording" is not recommended, because all recording requires two electrodes; however, it is commonly used to describe the use of an intramuscular needle exploring electrode in combination with a surface disc or subcutaneous needle reference electrode.

RECRUITMENT—The orderly activation of the same and new motor units with increasing strength of voluntary muscle contraction. See *Motor Unit Potential.*

RECRUITMENT FREQUENCY—Firing rate of a *Motor Unit Potential* when an additional motor unit potential first appears during gradually increasing strength of voluntary muscle contraction.

RECRUITMENT INTERVAL—The *Interdischarge Interval* between two consecutive discharges of a *Motor Unit Potential* when an additional motor unit potential first appears during gradually increasing strength of voluntary muscle contraction. The reciprocal of the recruitment interval is the *Recruitment Frequency.*

RECRUITMENT PATTERN—A qualitative and/or quantitative description of the sequence of appearance of *Motor Unit Potentials* with increasing strength of voluntary muscle contraction. The *Recruitment Frequency* and *Recruitment Interval* are two quantitative measures commonly used. See *Interference Pattern* for qualitative terms commonly used.

REDUCED INSERTIONAL ACTIVITY—See *Insertional Activity.*

REDUCED INTERFERENCE PATTERN—See *Interference Pattern.*

REFERENCE ELECTRODE—See *Recording Electrode.*

REFLEX—A stereotyped *Motor Response* elicited by a *Stimulus.*

REFRACTORY PERIOD—Time after an *Action Potential* during which the response to an additional stimulus is altered. The *Absolute Refractory Period* is that segment of the refractory period during which no stimulus, however strong, evokes an additional action potential. The *Relative Re-*

fractory Period is that segment of the refractory period during which a stimulus must be greater than a normal threshold stimulus to evoke a second action potential.

RELATIVE REFRACTORY PERIOD—See *Refractory Period.*

REPETITIVE DISCHARGES—General term for the recurrence of an *Action Potential* with the same or nearly the same form. The term may refer to recurring potentials recorded in muscle at rest, during voluntary contraction, or in response to a single nerve stimulus. The discharge may be named for the number of times a potential recurs in a group (e.g., *Double Discharge, Triple Discharge, Multiple Discharge, Coupled Discharge*) or other characteristics (e.g., *Complex Repetitive Discharge, Myokymic Discharge*).

REPETITIVE STIMULATION—The technique of utilizing repeated supramaximal stimulation of a nerve while quantitatively recording *M Waves* from muscles innervated by the nerve. It should be described in terms of the frequency of stimuli and number of stimuli (or duration of the total group). For descriptions of specific patterns of responses, see the terms *Incrementing Response, Decrementing Response, Postactivation Facilitation,* and *Postactivation Exhaustion.*

REPOLARIZATION—See *Polarization.*

RESIDUAL LATENCY—Refers to the calculated time difference between the measured distal latency of a motor nerve and the expected distal latency, calculated by dividing the distance between the stimulus cathode and the active recording electrode by the maximum conduction velocity measured in a more proximal segment of a nerve.

RESPONSE—Used to describe an activity elicited by a *Stimulus.*

RESTING MEMBRANE POTENTIAL—Voltage across the membrane of an excitable cell at rest. See *Polarization.*

RHEOBASE—The intensity of an electrical current of infinitely long duration necessary to produce a minimal visible twitch of a muscle when the cathode is applied to the motor point of the muscle. In practice a duration of at least 300 msec is used to determine the rheobase.

RISE TIME—By convention, the shortest interval from the nadir of a positive phase to the peak of a negative phase of a *Wave.*

SATELLITE POTENTIAL—Synonymous with preferred term, *Late Component.*

SEA SHELL NOISE (SEA SHELL ROAR)—Use of term discouraged. See *End-Plate Activity, Monophasic.*

SENSORY DELAY—See preferred terms, *Sensory Latency* and *Sensory Peak Latency.*

SENSORY LATENCY—Interval between the onset of a stimulus and the onset of the *Compound Sensory Nerve Action Potential.*This term has been loosely used to refer to the *Sensory Peak Latency.* The term may be qualified as *Proximal Sensory Latency* or *Distal Sensory Latency*, depending on the relative position of the stimulus.

SENSORY NERVE ACTION POTENTIAL—See *Compound Sensory Nerve Action Potential.*

SENSORY NERVE CONDUCTION VELOCITY—See *Conduction Velocity.*

SENSORY PEAK LATENCY—Interval between the onset of a *Stimulus* and the peak of the negative phase of the *Compound Sensory Nerve Action Potential.* Note that the term "*Latency*" refers to the interval between the onset of a stimulus and the onset of a response.

SENSORY POTENTIAL—Used to refer to the compound sensory nerve action potential. See *Compound Sensory Nerve Action Potential.*

SENSORY RESPONSE—Used to refer to a sensory evoked potential, e.g., *Compound Sensory Nerve Action Potential.*

SERRATED ACTION POTENTIAL—An action potential waveform with several changes in direction (turns) which do not cross the base line. This term is preferred to the terms *Complex Action Potential* and *Pseudopolyphasic Action Potential.* See *Turns.*

SHOCK ARTIFACT—See *Artifact.*

SILENT PERIOD—Time during which there is no electrical activity in muscle following rapid unloading of a muscle.

SINGLE FIBER ELECTROMYOGRAPHY—(Abbr. SFEMG). General term referring to the technique and conditions that permit recording of a single muscle fiber *Action Potential.* See *Single Fiber Needle Electrode.*

SINGLE FIBER NEEDLE ELECTRODE—A needle *Electrode* with a small recording surface (usually 25 μm in diameter) permitting the recording of single muscle fiber action potentials. See *Single Fiber Electromyography.*

SOMATOSENSORY EVOKED POTENTIAL—(Abbr. SSEP). Electrical *Waves* recorded from the head or trunk in response to electrical or physiological stimulation of peripheral sensory fibers. Recordings over the spine may be referred to as *Spinal Evoked Potentials.*

SPIKE—Transient *Wave* with a pointed peak and a short duration (a few milliseconds or less). See *End-Plate Spike* and *Fibrillation Potentials.*

SPINAL EVOKED POTENTIAL—Electrical *Wave* recorded over the spine in response to electrical stimulation of peripheral sensory fibers. See *Somatosensory Evoked Potential.*

SPONTANEOUS ACTIVITY—Action potentials recorded from muscle or nerve at rest after insertional activity has subsided and when there is no voluntary contraction or external stimulus. Compare with *Involuntary Activity.*

STAIRCASE PHENOMENON—The progressive increase in the force of a muscle contraction observed with repeated nerve stimulation at low rates.

STIGMATIC ELECTRODE—Synonymous with active or exploring electrode. See *Recording Electrode.*

STIMULATING ELECTRODE—Device used to apply electrical current. All electrical stimulation requires two electrodes; the negative terminal is termed the *Cathode* and the positive terminal, the *Anode.* By convention, the stimulating electrodes are called "*Bipolar*" if they are roughly equal in size and separated by less than 5 cm. The stimulating electrodes are called "*Monopolar*" if the cathode is smaller in size than the anode and is separated from the anode by more than 5 cm. Electrical stimulation for *Nerve Conduction Studies* generally requires application of the cathode to produce depolarization of the nerve trunk fibers. If the anode is inadvertently placed between the cathode and the recording electrodes, a focal block of nerve conduction (*Anodal Block*) may occur and cause a technically unsatisfactory study.

STIMULUS—Any external agent, state, or change that is capable of influencing the activity of a cell, tissue, or organism. In clinical *Nerve Conduction Studies*, an electrical stimulus is generally applied to a nerve or a muscle. The electrical stimulus may be described in absolute terms or with respect to the evoked potential of the nerve or muscle. In absolute terms, the electrical stimulus has a strength or intensity measured in voltage (volts) or current (milliamperes) and a duration (milliseconds). With respect to the evoked potential, the stimulus may be graded as subthreshold, threshold, submaximal, maximal, or supramaximal. A *Threshold Stimulus* is that electrical stimulus just sufficient to produce a detectable response. Stimuli less than the threshold stimulus are termed *Subthreshold.* The *Maximal Stimulus* is the stimulus intensity after which a further increase in the stimulus intensity causes no increase in the amplitude of the evoked potential. Stimuli of intensity below this and above threshold are *Submaximal.* Stimuli of intensity greater than the maximal stimulus are termed *Supramaximal.* Ordinarily, supramaximal stimuli are used for nerve conduction studies. By convention, an electrical stimulus of approximately 20% greater voltage than required for the maximal stimulus may be used for supramaximal stimulation. The frequency, number, and duration of a series of stimuli should be specified.

STIMULUS ARTIFACT—See *Artifact.*

STRENGTH-DURATION CURVE—Graphic presentation of the relationship between the intensity (Y axis) and various durations (X axis) of the threshold electrical stimulus for a muscle with the stimulating cathode positioned over the motor point.

SUBMAXIMAL STIMULUS—See *Stimulus.*

SUBTHRESHOLD STIMULUS—See *Stimulus.*

SUPRAMAXIMAL STIMULUS—See *Stimulus.*

SURFACE ELECTRODE—Conducting device for stimulating or recording placed on a skin surface. The material (metal, fabric), configuration (disc, ring), size, and separation should be specified. See *Electrode (Ground, Recording, Stimulating).*

S-X INTERVAL—The total duration of the *Silent Period* produced by electrical stimulation of the mixed nerve to a voluntarily contracting muscle, measured from the stimulus artifact to resumption of uninterrupted voluntary activity.

TEMPORAL DISPERSION—A waveform of longer duration than normal. Commonly used to refer to an increase in the duration of an evoked potential with more proximal sites of stimulation of a greater degree than that normally seen.

TERMINAL LATENCY—Synonymous with preferred term, *Distal Latency.* See *Motor Latency* and *Sensory Latency.*

TEST STIMULUS—The stimulus producing the event being measured. Contrast with *Conditioning Stimulus.*

TETANIC CONTRACTION—State of a muscle in sustained contraction resulting from stimulation at a frequency high enough for individual twitches to summate to a smooth tension and with associated electrical activity of muscle action potentials. It may be attained in normal muscle voluntarily or in response to repetitive nerve stimulation. Contrast with *Cramp Discharge.*

TETANUS—Loosely used to refer to *Tetanic Contraction.* The term is also used to refer to the acute infectious disease. See *Tetanic Contraction* and *Tetany.*

TETANY—A clinical syndrome manifested by muscle twitching, cramps, and sustained muscle contraction (*Tetanus*). These clinical signs are manifestations of peripheral and central nervous system nerve irritability from several causes. In these conditions, *Repetitive Discharges* (double discharge, triple discharge, multiple discharge) occur frequently with voluntary activation of motor unit potentials or may appear as spontaneous activity with systemic alkalosis or local ischemia.

TETRAPHASIC ACTION POTENTIAL—*Action Potential* with four phases.

THRESHOLD—The level at which a clear and abrupt transition occurs from one state to another. The term is generally used to refer to the voltage level at which an *Action Potential* is initiated in a single axon or a group of axons. It is also operationally defined as the intensity that produced a response in about 50% of equivalent trials.

THRESHOLD STIMULUS—See *stimulus.*

TIME CONSTANT OF ACCOMMODATION—(lambda, λ). The time

constant of the rate at which, after accommodation, the threshold of an excitable tissue reverts to its initial level. It is the reciprocal of the slope of the *Accommodation Curve.*

TRAIN OF POSITIVE SHARP WAVES—See *Positive Sharp Waves.*

TRAIN OF STIMULI—A group of stimuli. The duration of the group and the frequency of the individual components should be specified.

TRIPHASIC ACTION POTENTIAL—*Action Potential* with three phases.

TRIPLE DISCHARGE—Three action potentials of the same form and nearly the same amplitude, occurring consistently in the same relationship to one another. The interval between the second and the third action potential often exceeds that between the first two, and both are usually in the range of 2 to 20 msec.

TRIPLET—See *Triple Discharge.*

TURNS—Changes in direction of a waveform which do not necessarily pass through the base line. The minimal excursion required to constitute a turn should be specified.

UNIPOLAR NEEDLE ELECTRODE—See synonym, *Monopolar Needle Electrode.*

VISUAL EVOKED POTENTIAL—Electrical waveforms of biological origin recorded over the cerebrum and elicited by light stimuli.

VISUAL EVOKED RESPONSE—(Abbr. VER). See *Visual Evoked Potential.*

VOLTAGE—Potential difference between two points.

VOLUME CONDUCTION—Spread of current from a potential source through a conducting medium, such as the body tissues.

VOLUNTARY ACTIVITY—In electromyography, the electrical activity recorded from a muscle with consciously controlled muscle contraction. The effort made to contract the muscle, e.g., minimal, moderate, or maximal, and the strength of contraction in absolute terms or relative to a maximal voluntary contraction of a normal corresponding muscle should be specified.

WANING DISCHARGE—General term referring to a repetitive discharge that decreases in frequency or in amplitude. Compare with *Myotonic Discharge.*

WAVE—An undulating line constituting a graphic representation of a change, e.g., a changing electrical potential difference.

WAVEFORM—The shape of a *Wave.* The term is often used synonymously with wave.

WEDENSKY-LIKE NEUROMUSCULAR FAILURE—Use of term discouraged. The term has been used to describe a decrease in the strength of the sustained muscle contraction during repeated nerve stimulation at frequencies within the physiological range (less than 50 Hz). See preferred term, *Decrementing Response.*

WEDENSKY PHENOMENON—A decrease in strength of a sustained muscle contraction during sustained nerve stimulation at frequencies above the physiological range, e.g., greater than 50 Hz. This phenomenon is seen in normal muscle.

Index